Applied Statistics

Third Edition

Applied Statistics

Analysis of Variance and Regression

Third Edition

Ruth M. Mickey
Olive Jean Dunn
Virginia A. Clark

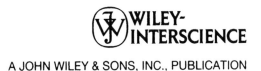

WILEY-
INTERSCIENCE

A JOHN WILEY & SONS, INC., PUBLICATION

Library of Congress Cataloging-in-Publication Data

Mickey, Ruth M., 1954–
   Applied statistics : analysis of variance and regression.—3rd ed. / Ruth M. Mickey,
Olive Jean Dunn, Virginia A. Clark.
       p. cm.—(Wiley series in probability and statistics)
   Includes bibliographical references and index.
   ISBN 0-471-37038-X (acid-free paper)
     1. Analysis of variance. 2. Regression analysis. I. Dunn, Olive Jean. II. Clark, Virginia,
1928– III. Title. IV. Series

   QA279.M45   2004
   519.5'38—dc21   20033053461

10 9 8 7 6 5 4 3 2 1

Contents

Preface

What This Book Is About

The objectives of this third edition of *Applied Statistics: Analysis of Variance and Regression* are to be a textbook for a one year or, with omissions, a one-semester course in analysis of variance and regression and also to be a useful reference. In each chapter, we give an example, discuss how to summarize the data, state the model and the assumptions, give confidence intervals and tests, describe how to tell if the assumptions are satisfied, and offer advice on what to do if they are not satisfied. To illustrate the analysis of data that do not meet all the assumptions, in some of the examples the assumptions are not fully met. The statistical methods are given in a general context and are illustrated in terms of the chapter example. With this organization, the student is exposed to the whole data analysis process, starting from a data set to the presentation and interpretation of its statistical analyses. A low level of mathematics is assumed and clear statements of the model assumptions are made.

What Changes Have Been Made in this 3rd Edition

There is now greater emphasis on data screening. This is introduced in the first chapter and continues to be addressed in subsequent chapters. Interpretation of computer program results are included so the reader will know how to perform and interpret real life analyses. We have added sections on how to explain the statistical methods used and the results of the analyses.

We have included a wider variety of homework problems at the end of each chapter. Some problems make use of small, artificial data sets, which lend themselves to focusing on the statistical methods addressed in each chapter. These emphasize straightforward applications of the statistical methods or their verification by spreadsheet or by hand. Other problems make use of larger, real data sets; these are particularly useful for illustrating violations of the assumptions and other practical problems that can arise in real world applications. Finally, we have developed a limited number of problems that involve simulations. Large data sets are available on the Wiley ftp given below.

Some of the more technical material (such as general rules for deriving the formulae given in the chapters and some illustrative examples) is now in an appendix. Students can read through the material in a chapter and stay focused on the application and interpretation of the statistical methods; for interested students who need or want to verify formulae, the appendix is a good source of information. We reference relevant books and journal articles at the end of each chapter. We have tried to include both standard references as well as some very practical articles that have appeared in *The American Statistician*.

The first four chapters of the second edition were deleted as this introductory material would likely not now be covered in a course in analysis of variance and regression. However, some key topics in those deleted chapters are incorporated into other chapters or included in the appendix. We also dropped material that seems more appropriate for a course in experimental design: factorial designs with each factor at two levels and the Latin square design. Finally, we eliminated detailed computing formulas.

Use of the Computer and the Wiley ftp Site

We recognize that there are numerous software packages that are available and have not written this book with any particular one in mind. We performed our data analyses using SAS and Minitab and occasionally S-PLUS; the graphs were generated using S-PLUS. We have tried to be aware of alternative names that the different packages use to describe the same thing and mention them in the text. The ftp site associated with this book is ftp:// ftp.wiley.com / public / sci_tech_med / applied_statistics. We will use this site to store the larger data sets used in the text, selected computer programs that we created, additional homework problems, and errata.

Acknowledgements

Many people contributed to this revision. Dr Mickey, who has used this material in her teaching, has taken a lead role in this new edition and she has been backstopped by Dr Clark. We both have benefited from the clarity of thinking and writing of Dr Dunn in earlier editions. We thank Dr Philip Ades, Dr Lorraine Berkett, Dr Richard Branda, Dr Elena Garcia, Neil Kamman, and Scott Pfister for generously giving us their data sets. We thank Welden Clark for his assistance with figures and tables and his help in putting the entire work together. We thank Steve Quigley, Executive Editor, and the editorial and production staff at Wiley—Heather Bergman, Rosalyn Farkas, and Susanne Steitz, for their patience and advice.

RUTH M. MICKEY (PROFESSOR, UNIV. OF VERMONT)

OLIVE JEAN DUNN (PROFESSOR EMERITA, UCLA)

VIRGINIA A. CLARK (PROFESSOR EMERITA, UCLA)

1
Data Screening

The process of reaching conclusions from surveys or experiments involves taking a series of steps. Initially, the investigator develops his or her major research hypothesis and a study is designed to test this hypothesis. Decisions are made on what type of data to collect, the necessary sample size, and who will actually obtain the data. After this planning phase is completed, the data collection phase of the study is carried out. If it is an extensive study, checks will be made during its course to determine if the data collection is going as planned in terms of both the speed of collection and the quality of the data. After the data collection is completed more checks are made on the data. Finally, statistical analyses are performed on the data and, on the basis of these analyses, conclusions are reached about the research hypothesis.

To help ensure the best possible analyses, the investigator needs to become well acquainted with the data and to make sure they are ready to analyze, prior to performing detailed statistical analyses and tests. The process by which this is done is frequently referred to as data screening. Screening is done with two objectives in mind: to detect errors in the data and to detect departures from the assumptions on which the analyses are based.

There are two types of data screening. The first type is performed one variable at a time on the entire data set, prior to any formal analysis. Here we will call this preliminary data screening. The second type of data screening is done in conjunction with the statistical analysis and is dependent on the specific analysis being performed. For example, in this book analysis of variance and regression analysis will be covered. Special screening techniques exist for each of these two major statistical procedures. These special techniques will be given later in conjunction with the explanation of the statistical analysis.

In this introductory chapter, we provide an overview of the first type of data screening.

In Section 1.1 we define variables and give one system for classifying different types of variables. In Section 1.2 we consider the detection of the more obvious errors in the data and address summarizing data in terms of descriptive statistics and graphical presentation. Since two assumptions — those of normally distributed data and independence of observations — are made for most of the techniques described in subsequent chapters, we consider assessment of normality and independence in Section 1.3. Finally, in Section 1.4 a brief chapter summary is given. To illustrate some of the concepts, we will make use of data determined from water samples collected from 40 lakes in Vermont (VT) and New Hampshire (NH). Surveys were conducted to determine the distribution of algae in lakes in VT and NH. These data were supplied by the Vermont Department of Environmental Conservation.

1.1 VARIABLES AND THEIR CLASSIFICATION

The word *variable* is used for a characteristic or attribute that we can measure and that varies from subject to subject, place to place, or time to time. If we measure something, we assign a number to each of its levels. Sometimes this is done directly; we simply measure something such as height using physical instruments. Alternatively, we may wish to measure the quality of life for patients with coronary heart disease; we may make up some questions that the patients answer, and use their answers as an indication of their quality of life. In this latter example, we obtain an indirect measurement that we hope relates well to quality of life. Variables are sometimes classified by whether they are measured directly or indirectly.

Investigators want to consider the types of variables they have measured, as this will have an impact of the sorts of analyses that are appropriate for the data set. There are a variety of ways people have gone about classifying their variables; we describe Stevens's classification system [17]. In that system, there are four types of variables: nominal, ordinal, interval, and ratio. We characterize these and provide examples, many of which are used in subsequent chapters in the book.

A *nominal* variable is a variable that assumes categories which have no ordering associated with them. Examples that everyone is familiar with include gender, race, and religion. Patients with cardiac disease might be classified according to diagnostic category: angioplasty, bypass surgery, chronic angina, or myocardial infarction. Sites along streams might be classified according to the potential for contamination from adjacent agricultural use: cow pastures, cornfields, or no adjacent agriculture. Corn seeds might be classified according to the type of genetic modification that has been made to them.

An *ordinal* variable is a variable that assumes categories which have an ordering. A physical therapist might classify patients with mild, moderate, or severe carpal tunnel syndrome. Most scales developed to measure something that can't be directly measured, such as quality of life or depression, are considered ordinal.

An *interval* variable not only has the characteristic that it has ordering associated with it, but in addition, a specified difference between any two points has the same interpretation, regardless of where the two points are. We don't encounter many variables which are strictly interval, but one example is year. A study may have been conducted during 1999, 2000, and 2001. The difference between 2001 and 2000 is one year, as is the difference between 2000 and 1999. The difference between 2001 and 1999 is two years. (In contrast with ordinal variables, we can't say that the difference between moderate and mild carpal tunnel syndrome is the same as the difference between severe and moderate carpal tunnel syndrome.) We could have used another calendar, and the differences in time would have been the same. But what is year 0 in the Common Era does not correspond to year 0 in other systems; a ratio of years is not a meaningful quantity.

A *ratio* variable has the characteristics that it is ordered, differences can be interpreted, and furthermore, the ratio of two values can be interpreted. Put another way, there is a meaningful origin or zero. Examples are concentration of cadmium or folic acid, distance from a location on a river or stream to a sampling site, the height of an apple tree, or the diameter of an apple.

Stevens's classification system is not without its limitations [20]. For example, if the measurements are counts (for example, the number of species of algae in a sample of water), the variable doesn't really fit into any of his types. Such variables are often handled as interval variables.

While data screening is relevant to all types of variables, we direct most attention here to ratio or interval variables. For our purposes, nominal variables and ordinal variables with few categories are frequently referred to as categorical variables, while interval and ratio variables are referred to as continuous variables.

1.2 DESCRIBING THE DATA

1.2.1 Errors in the Data

One of the first things to do with a data set is to look at the variables one at a time. This can be done manually if the data set is small or through the use of computer software if it is large. An objective of the first look at the data is to detect obvious errors. One very simple type of error is missing values. Missing values can occur in two ways. First, the data may simply not have been collected. Second, the information may have been collected but deleted later because they appear to be incorrect (see the following discussion on outliers). For example, missing values may be a problem in surveys if respondents refuse to answer a question, or in laboratory data if some procedures are prone to problems. Missing values are sometimes an indication of problems in data collection and may be an indication that a particular variable has not been accurately measured. If there are very few missing values, then this is usually not considered a major problem. If considerable data are missing, then special techniques should be considered, which are not covered in this book [11, 13].

A more common way to look for errors is to search for outliers, that is, observations that are far removed in some sense from the rest of the data. Outliers can occur in several ways. One way is through sampling problems, whereby the sample obtained contains individuals or objects that do not come from the population we would like to sample (the *target* population). For example, if we wish to sample women of age 40 or older, but a woman of age 35 incorrectly gets included, her age could be considered an outlier. Another way is through errors in taking a measurement, recording it, or entering it into the computer. For example, a height may be measured in centimeters instead of inches, a woman who is really 45 may have her age incorrectly entered as 35, or a decimal point may be put in the wrong place. A third way an outlier can occur is through extreme biological, psychological, or environmental variation resulting in unusual values. For example, due to unusual conditions, some lakes will contain unusually large numbers of algae; we shall see an illustration of this in the example below.

Gross outliers can be detected visually by simply scanning the data. If the data set is so large that careful scanning is impractical, gross outliers can be spotted from printouts of maximum and minimum values of the data. Often a data analyst compares these printouts with known or reasonable ranges of the data (e.g., a weight of 13 lb for an adult male is unreasonable) to detect outliers caused by a misplaced decimal point, typing error, and so on. For categorical data, outliers are commonly detected by obtaining the frequencies for each outcome and checking whether or not all the outcomes are the ones expected. For example, if one of the variables being measured is gender, which was coded as male=1, female=2, and unknown=9, then if there were cases where a 3 was entered as an outcome, these would be considered outliers.

When a gross outlier is detected, we must decide what to do with the observation. In part, the decision depends on the source of the outlier. For example, if we believe data were collected from an object or individual that is not in our target population, we may wish to delete the entire case. Or, if we believe that the outlier is due to an error in measurement, recording, or data entry, it is sometimes possible to replace the value with a corrected value or to retake the observation. If no reason for the unusual value can be found, the problem is more difficult. Investigators vary in their opinions; there are some investigators of the "if in doubt, throw it out" school of thought and some who believe that it is unethical to throw observations away. It seems foolish to use, in a statistical analysis, observations that are clearly errors, yet discarding observations without a convincing explanation can reduce the confidence felt in the results of the analysis. We suggest that gross outliers be eliminated in the statistical analysis (made into missing values). If there are very few such values and their removal is at all questionable, then they should be reported along with the statistical analysis; this allows the readers of the report to judge for themselves.

Not all outliers are errors; they may represent genuine observations. This will be the case for the third source of outliers mentioned above: extreme biological, psychological, or environmental variation resulting in unusual values. Here, the presence of outliers appropriately indicates that the sample is from a nonnormal distribution, for example, one with a long upper tail. Thus, rather than identifying an error, the outlier suggests that some distributional assumptions (here, that a sample was drawn from a normally distributed population) may be violated.

Note that the detection and removal of outliers is no guarantee that all incorrect observations have been identified and removed. If a measurement error occurs that lowers the height of a tall person, it could result in a height in the normal range and would not then be identified as an error in preliminary data screening. It may be detected later when data screening is repeated for a particular analysis. For computation of descriptive statistics such as means or standard deviations, such outliers usually do not have a major effect unless they are numerous.

Example. The algae data set supplied by the VT Department of Environmental Conservation included 40 lakes, so the total sample size was $n = 40$. The names of lakes as well as two variables, species richness and total biovolume, are presented in Table 1.1. Observations were made on a number of other variables; some of them are used in the problem set at the end of this chapter. Species richness is defined as the total number of algal species present in a sample of lake water. Total biovolume of algae is defined as the total volume of algal cells in 1 ml of lake water, in units of of $\mu m^3/ml$. Species richness is regarded as an interval variable, while total biovolume is a ratio variable.

In this particular data set, no data were missing; there were 40 determinations of species richnesses and total biovolume. Species richness ranged from 9 to 31; neither the smallest nor the largest stands out as unusual. Thus, there do not appear to be any outliers for species richness in this data set.

However, for the other variable, biovolume, there are two values that are unusually high, when compared with the biovolumes of the other lakes — 2,018,630 for Lake Wolcott and 3,935,994 for Lake Carmi. Investigators from the VT Department of Environmental Conservation felt that these values were genuine and did reflect lakes with large amounts of algae, and so it was not appropriate to discard them. Thus, the two biovolumes were outliers, but there was no indication that they were errors in the data. The effect of these two biovolumes will be illustrated in Sections 1.2.2 and 1.2.3.

If errors had been found, it would have been necessary to decide how to address them. However, as no errors were found, we are ready to look further at the data.

First, we'll describe some summary statistics, which will be used to help understand graphical summaries. With both the numerical and graphical summaries in hand, further data screening will be done.

1.2.2 Descriptive Statistics

Once errors in the data have been identified and decisions have been made about what to do with them, it is helpful to continue looking at the variables one at a time and to further examine summary statistics. Summarization is useful in itself — the statistics convey a lot of information that is easily communicated to others. In addition, they also are useful for further data screening — they allow the investigator to determine if the data seem reasonable and will help the data analyst learn about the distributions of the variables. Of particular interest is how symmetric the distribution is.

There are many summary statistics available; here we focus on ones that are of particular interest for data screening. As described above, the sample size for each variable is still important, as it indicates how many observations have been declared missing. Similarly, the minimum and maximum values are useful to verify that all observations are within a plausible range.

A variety of descriptive statistics are calculated using the n observations when they have been ordered from smallest to largest. We will first define percentiles, quantiles, and quartiles, as these will be used throughout this chapter. Percentiles divide the total observations into 100 equal parts. The pth percentile corresponds to a value for which $p\%$ of the observations lie at or below it and $(100-p)\%$ of the observations lie at or above it. Quantiles divide the observations into n equal parts, and the quantile is the fraction of the observations that are at or below it. The only difference between quantiles and percentiles is that quantiles refer to fractions and percentiles to percentages of the observations. Quantiles are used more than percentiles when the number of observations is small. When a set of ordered observations is divided up into four equal-size sets, the cutpoints are referred to as quartiles; there are three quartiles: Q_1, Q_2, and Q_3. Q_1 corresponds to the 25th percentile or 0.25 quantile, Q_2 corresponds to the 50th percentile or 0.50 quantile, and Q_3 corresponds to the 75th percentile or 0.75 quantile. These can be used to summarize ordinal, interval, and ratio data.

The median, or 50th percentile, conveys information about what a typical value is. It is informative to compare it with the mean (denoted $\bar{Y}$), as the comparison of these two statistics will provide information about how symmetric the distribution of the variable is. When the mean is close to the median, the distribution is likely symmetric. When the mean and median are

Table 1.1 Lake, Total Biovolume and Species Richness for 40 Lakes in Vermont and New Hampshire

Lake	Total Biovolume	Species Richness
Bald Hill	568,072	25
Beaver	232,816	19
Branch	123,542	16
Butternut	108,894	29
Carmi	3,935,994	13
Caspian	61,223	11
Cole	155,687	17
Crystal	79,282	18
Curtis	221,882	17
Dudley	133,772	18
Dunmore	307,262	18
Eden	147,930	26
Ewell	230,236	9
Fairfield	486,378	11
French	462,969	19
Gilman	195,615	20
Great Hosmer	258,359	19
Hatch	328,656	25
High	128,932	11
Hinkum	64,946	17
Holland	66,829	18
Intervale	129,889	19
Little (Elmore)	487,253	24
Long (Greens)	668,498	23
Long (Shef)	136,884	17
Maidstone	254,018	18
Marshfield	305,301	27
McConnell	283,305	26
Nathan	190,739	31
Russell	11,408	16
Sessions	189,202	21
Shadow (Glov)	138,649	15
Smith	157,883	22
Spring (Shrews)	256,201	10
St. Catherine	606,308	16
Stratton	247,099	15
Wallingford	318,376	17
Wheeler (Brun)	327,977	16
Willard	92,436	16
Wolcott	2,018,630	21

quite dissimilar, there may be some outliers or the distribution of the variable is not symmetric. Because the mean is more sensitive to extreme values than the median, a value of the mean appreciably greater than the median would suggest that there are some large outliers or an excessive number of observations in the right or upper tail, and the distribution may be skewed to the right. Similarly, a mean less than the median would indicate that there are some outlying small values for the variable or an excessive number of observations in the left or lower tail, and the distribution may be skewed to the left.

Two other percentiles that are of particular interest are the 25th percentile, or first quartile (Q_1), and the 75th percentile, or third quartile (Q_3). When compared with the median, they provide some information about the symmetry of a distribution. For a symmetric distribution, the difference between the median and Q_1 should be approximately the same as the difference between Q_3 and the median; if Q_3 − median > median − Q_1, the distribution is skewed to the right. The advantage to looking at the differences between the median and the quartiles over looking at the differences between the median and the maximum or the minimum is that there is less certainty about the extreme values than about the quartiles. However, comparing the median with the extremes is worthwhile, as in some cases the lack of symmetry can be found in the tails but not in the middle of the distribution.

The difference between the third and first quartile is the *interquartile range*, IQR = $Q_3 - Q_1$. The advantage of the IQR as a measure of variability is that it is not affected by outliers as much as the variance or standard deviation is. Frequently, observations that are 2 to 3 times the IQR above the third quartile or below the first quartile are considered outliers. Statistical programs which generate descriptive statistics routinely provide these estimates.

The *skewness* also can be examined. Skewness is a measure of how non-symmetric a distribution is. Symmetric distributions, such as a normal distribution or a t distribution, have a skewness of 0. A distribution that is skewed to the right has a skewness > 0, and a distribution that is skewed to the left has a skewness < 0. Skewness is an appropriate summary statistic for either interval or ratio data.

Before estimating skewness, let us introduce some notation. Suppose a sample of size n is drawn from a population. Let Y denote a variable, $Y_1, \ldots, Y_n$ the n observations, and $\bar{Y}$ the sample mean.

Skewness can be estimated as

$$\frac{\frac{1}{n} \sum_{i=1}^{n} (Y_i - \bar{Y})^3}{[\frac{1}{n} \sum_{i=1}^{n} (Y_i - \bar{Y})^2]^{3/2}}. \tag{1.1}$$

Note that the numerator (and thus the skewness) will be close to zero when the observations are symmetric about the sample mean $\bar{Y}$. In this case, $Y_i - \bar{Y}$, and therefore its cube, will be positive or negative depending on whether the observation is above or below the sample mean, but $\sum_{i=1}^{n} (Y_i - \bar{Y})^3$ should be near zero, since equal numbers of observations would be expected above and below the mean. If the upper tail is more spread out than the lower tail, so that the magnitudes of the $Y_i - \bar{Y}$ are large compared with those of the lower tail, the numerator will be positive, and the skewness will be greater than zero. Since the denominator is a sum of squared terms, it is always positive.

The above formula for skewness may or may not correspond exactly to what is seen in other books or to what a particular software package uses. There are a variety of expressions for skewness, and some have suggested modifying this basic formula to get estimators which are less biased than the one presented here. The important point lies in why skewness is greater than, equal to, or less than 0, which can be seen from the expression presented in Equation 1.1.

Example. For the algae data, summary statistics are given in Table 1.2. For species richness, the sample size ($n = 40$), minimum (9), and maximum (31) were discussed previously. The median is 18, which is the mean of the 20th and 21st ordered observations; the number of species was 18 for both. $Q_1 = 16$ and is calculated as the mean of the 10th and 11th ordered observations (the species richness for both is 16); likewise, $Q_3 = 21.5$ is the mean of the 30th and 31st ordered observations (species richnesses of 21 and 22). (Note that Q_3 assumes a value that cannot actually be observed.) There is an indication of some slight skewness to the right: the mean (18.7) exceeds the median (18); $Q_3 -$ median $= 21.5 - 18 = 3.5$, which is greater than median $- Q_1 = 18 - 16 = 2$; the skewness is 0.4. The IQR is $21.5 - 16 = 5.5$. There are no observations which exceed $Q_3 + 2(\text{IQR}) = 21.5 + 2(5.5) = 32.5$; using this criterion, there are no indications of outliers.

A different situation is apparent from examining the summary statistics for total biovolume. The mean is 377,983.3, which is over one and a half times higher than the median, 226,059. Q_1 is equal to 131,830.5, and Q_3 equals 323,176.5. Thus, the difference between Q_3 and the median is $323,176.5 - 226,059$ or 97,117.5; the difference between the median and Q_1 is $226,059 - 131,830.6$, or 94,228.4. The similarity in these two differences suggests that total biovolume is symmetric in the middle half of the distribution, between the first and third quartiles. A large positive skewness of 4.6 was determined. In combination, these indicators suggest that the distribution of total biovolumes is skewed to the right, and that the lack of symmetry is apparent mainly in the lower and upper tails of the distribution. Note that the two high values, obtained from Lakes Carmi and Wolcott, have a large effect on the skewness: when they are deleted from the data set, the skewness drops from 4.6 to 1.1. That, however, is still a sizable value.

1.2.3   Graphical Summarization

The simplest techniques for looking for outliers or learning about the shapes of data distributions are graphical. These may include histograms, stem and

Table 1.2 Summary Statistics for Species Richness and Total Biovolume

Statistic	Species Richness	Total Biovolume
n	40	40
Minimum	9	11,408
Q_1	16	131,830.5
Median	18	226,059
Maximum	31	3,935,994
Q_3	21.5	323,176.5
Mean	18.7	377,983.3
Skewness	0.4	4.6
Interquartile range	5.5	191,346

leaf plots, and box and whisker plots, among others. These are primarily used as exploratory techniques with continuous data. (Bar charts are useful for categorical data, and are not discussed here.) They provide an opportunity to take a quick look at the data. We generally rely on computer packages to construct these graphs for us. General methods to construct histograms, stem and leaf plots, and box and whisker plots can be found elsewhere (e.g., [2, 10, 19]). Here, we will briefly discuss the general information that can be obtained from each kind of graph. This will be followed by some illustrations of the graphs (Figures 1.1 and 1.2) and more discussion about their interpretation, using the algae data.

The graph that is easiest to communicate to others is the histogram. What a histogram looks like will depend on the number or width of the bins (also known as class intervals), that is, how many dividing points there are and where the dividing points are made for the continuous data. A variety of rules have been suggested for bin width [8, 10, 14]. Many software packages will create histograms, and some give the user the option of specifying the bin widths. The histogram is useful for detecting asymmetric distributions and outliers.

The stem and leaf plot provides a bit more information than the histogram, in that it will allow detection of observations which seem unusually common or uncommon. This could suggest that there were unexpected limitations to the measurement device or some other source of measurement error in the data. For example, if observations that only end in 5 or 0, or only even-numbered observations, are observed, this will alert the analyst to digit preference in the data collection phase. Many software packages produce stem and leaf plots, although they use different criteria for selecting stems, so the plots created by different packages may not be the same. As with the histogram, if the user doesn't have control over the setting of stems, the plot may not be useful to examine. Another advantage of the stem and leaf plot is that it can be done relatively quickly by hand.

The box and whisker plot contains more specific information than either the histogram or the stem and leaf plot, although it doesn't provide any indication of digit preference. From the plot, five numbers can be roughly determined: the smallest observation, the first quartile (Q_1), the median, the third quartile (Q_3), and the largest observation; these were described in Section 1.2.2. Outlying observations and the symmetry of the distribution of data can be quickly assessed. One point to keep in mind is that different software packages have different ways of presenting a boxplot, so that it is important to know how a package creates its boxplots in order to interpret them correctly. The procedures that are used by different packages are summarized in [9].

Example. First, let's compare the histograms, stem and leaf plots, and box and whisker plots for species richness (Figure 1.1). These plots were all created using the package S-PLUS. Each one indicates that the distribution of species richness is nearly symmetric, although some skewness to the right is apparent. The Y axis for the histogram (Figure 1.1a) is the number of lakes with a species richness within the bin. This particular histogram was produced with bin widths of 5. The first one goes from 5 to 10 and the last one goes from 30 to 35. Note that the cutpoints are possible values, so we need to know how the package allocated species richness to a particular bin. The default for this particular package is that the upper cutpoint of each bin is included in the bin; the lower cutpoint is not. So the second bin includes values of richness greater than 10 but less than or equal to 15; note that there are five of them.

The stem and leaf plot did not do a lot of summarization of the data as the stem included each value of species richness (Table 1.3). But we can see immediately that there was one 9 (indicated by a single 0 associated with the value of 9), the minimum value, and one 31 (indicated by the single 0 associated with this value), the maximum value. The distribution looks fairly symmetric, with most values between 16 and 19.

The box and whisker plot for species richness (Figure 1.1b) highlights the median value of 18 by the dot within the box. The left and right sides of the box indicate the first and third quartiles, 16 and 21.5, respectively. We can quickly see the range of values within which the middle half of the observations lie and note that the median is slightly off to the left; this would indicate some skewness of the distribution within its middle half. In S-PLUS, the vertical bars indicating the ends of the whiskers are drawn at the observations not beyond $Q_1 - 1.5\,IQR$ or $Q_3 + 1.5\,IQR$. Since the IQR for this variable is 5.5 (Table 1.2) they are drawn at the observations not below $16 - 1.5(5.5) = 7.75$ and not above $21.5 + 1.5(5.5) = 29.75$. The nearest observations are 9 and 29 (Lakes Ewell and Butternut), which is where the bars are drawn. The observed value of 31 (Lake Nathan) is not far enough away from the bar to be of concern as an outlier (see circle with vertical line).

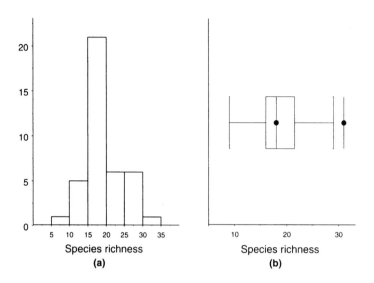

Fig. 1.1 (a) Histogram and (b) box and whisker plot for species richness.

Now, let's take a look at the histogram for total biovolume. We can see that most of the biovolumes are between 0 and 500,000, but mostly the histogram (Figure 1.2a) highlights the two very high values. The way the plot is constructed, there is little information available about total biovolumes below 500,000.

The stem and leaf plot (Table 1.4) shows that the distribution of the total biovolume is skewed to the right:

Note that the data for biovolume are summarized somewhat differently from species richness. The stem ranges between 0 and 6. Since the decimal point is five places to the right of the vertical line, the first stem includes numbers below 100,000, the second stem includes numbers from 100,000 to below 200,000, and so forth. The leaves for the first stem correspond to 10,000, 60,000, and so forth. While these numbers are only approximations to the actual observations, we can tell by examining the shape of the plot that this variable is skewed to the right. In the software package we used, the largest two values were excluded as outliers from the plot itself and noted separately; the package considered a value to be an outlier if it was above $Q_3 + 2\,\text{IQR}$ or below $Q_1 - 2\,\text{IQR}$.

The box and whisker plot for total biovolume (Figure 1.2b) shows that the middle half of the distribution is within a relatively small range, and is symmetric about the median. From the plot, it appears that the IQR is close to 200,000; using the computed values, it is 191,346, which is the difference

Table 1.3   Stem and Leaf Plot for Species Richness.

Stem	Leaf
9	0
10	0
11	000
12	
13	0
14	
15	00
16	00000
17	00000
18	00000
19	0000
20	0
21	00
22	0
23	0
24	0
25	00
26	00
27	0
28	
29	0
30	
31	0

Decimal is at the center line.

between the third quartile (323,176.5) and first quartile (131,830.5). We have 1.5 IQR = 287,019, so the ends of the whiskers should correspond to the observations not beyond $131,830.5 - 2,870,189 = -155,188.5$ or $323,176.5 + 287,019 = 610,195.5$. Examination of the data in Table 1.1 verifies that the vertical bars denoting the ends of the whiskers are drawn at 11,408 and 606,308, corresponding to Lakes Russell and St. Catherine. The most dramatic part of this box and whisker plot is the two outliers, which appear to be at least four times the IQR beyond Q_3; the skewness of the data is also evident. Note also that the median, indicated by the large dot in the box, is at the midpoint between Q_1 and Q_3, suggesting that the middle 50% of the distribution is symmetric; excessively large values have the effect of moving the upper bar to the right.

Table 1.4   Stem and Leaf Plot for Biovolume.

Stem	Leaf
0	166789
1	123334456699
2	023355668
3	11233
4	699
5	7
6	17

Decimal is five places to the right of the center line.

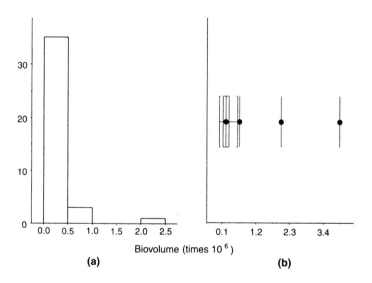

Fig. 1.2   (a) Histogram and (b) box and whisker plot for biovolume.

1.3   DEPARTURES FROM ASSUMPTIONS

The methods discussed in this book are based on a variety of assumptions. We focus on two here: data in each sample were obtained from a normally distributed population, and all observations are independent. We discuss how to assess departures of the data from the assumptions and some suggested procedures for dealing with them.

1.3.1   The Normal Distribution

First, let us briefly review the normal distribution. If we say that a variable such as blood pressure of college women has a normal distribution, we mean that an infinite population of blood pressures has as its distribution a curve that is symmetric and bell-shaped; it can be represented by a particular formula. The curve extends an infinite distance in both directions but comes very close to the horizontal axis. Thus, if the population of systolic blood pressures followed a normal distribution, an extremely small proportion of blood pressures would be above any large number such as 400. This obviously would not occur, and of course it is out of the question for even a small proportion of the population to have blood pressures below zero. Thus it is clearly impossible for an infinite population of systolic blood pressures to be exactly normally distributed. For practical purposes, however, blood pressures for young women might be considered to be normally distributed. That is, areas under the normal curve might closely approximate the proportions of the population with the corresponding blood pressures.

A normal distribution has two parameters that describe it completely — the population mean μ and the population variance σ^2 (or its square root, the standard deviation, σ). That is, if we know that blood pressures are (approximately) normally distributed, that the mean blood pressure for the population is 120 mm Hg, and that the standard deviation of the population of blood pressures is 11 mm Hg, we can plot the distribution curve for blood pressures. The mean tells us where the central point of the distribution lies. The standard deviation tells us how spread out the distribution is. Approximately 68% of the blood pressures lie within one standard deviation of the mean, or between 109 and 131 mm Hg, and approximately 95% of them lie within 2σ of μ, or between 98 and 142. Because the normal distribution is symmetric, its skewness is zero. Figure 1.3 shows a distribution of blood pressures for normal individuals with mean systolic blood pressure $\mu = 120$ mm Hg and $\sigma = 11$ mm Hg.

1.3.2   The Normality Assumption

Distributions of observations such as heights and weights often tend to be slightly skewed to the right rather than being normally distributed. For example, since we find some extremely heavy persons and no one who weighs less than zero, the distribution of weights tends to have a long right-hand tail. In most problems concerning the mean of such a distribution, this slight skewness causes no difficulty and we can proceed as if we had normality. Extreme skewness can be handled by making a transformation on the data that lowers larger values more than it lowers smaller values (see Section 1.3.3). Statements are then made in terms of the transformed data. Assessments of the

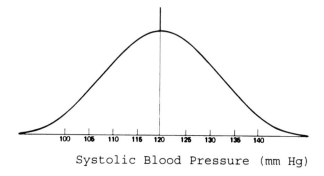

Systolic Blood Pressure (mm Hg)

Fig. 1.3 Normal distribution where $\mu = 120$ and $\sigma = 11$.

appropriateness of the normality assumptions can be made using graphical procedures, summary statistics, or formal hypothesis tests.

Example. For the algae data set, we have considered two variables, species richness and total biovolume. There may be concern about the species richness being normally distributed, because, strictly speaking, it is not a continuous variable but a discrete one; possible values are the whole numbers. Furthermore, the median lies closer to Q_1 than Q_3. While total biovolume is continuous (it can assume values ≥ 0), we have seen from the data summarizations that it is clearly skewed.

1. Graphical Approaches
   A way to assess whether a sample could have come from a normally distributed population is to construct a *normal probability* or *normal quantile plot*; this tends to be more informative for this purpose than the graphs described for general data description.
   These plots have the property that points fall on a straight line if data are normally distributed. As with other graphs, we rely on statistical software to produce them; how different software actually constructs a plot, and its degree of resolution, vary, so different interpretations of the plot can arise from use of different software. A brief explanation of how a normal quantile graph may be constructed is given here. The observations are ordered, and each ordered observation is plotted against the value it would be expected to assume if the data came from the standard normal distribution (i.e., came from a normal distribution with $\mu = 0$ and $\sigma = 1$), sometimes referred to as *normal quantiles*. Suppose we were to draw a sample of size n from a standard normal population. The value that the smallest observation assumed would have a distribution associated with it, the value that the second observation assumed would have a distribution associated with it, ..., and the largest observation

would have a distribution associated with it. Because it is complicated to determine expected values of these order statistics, a variety of ways have been proposed for estimating them. One commonly used procedure is to compute, for the ith ordered observation, the probability $p_i = (i - 0.5)/n$. Then, we would determine the value of z_i such that $P(Z < z_i) = p_i$. If the observed data were normally distributed, the plot of the ith ordered observation versus z_i, the normal quantiles, should be linear.

We have $n = 40$ observations. For the smallest observation, $p_1 = (1 - 0.5)/40 = 0.0125$, and, using the table of the standard normal distribution in Appendix B, we determine that $P(Z < -2.24) = 0.0125$. That is, if we had a sample of size 40 from a standard normal distribution, we would expect the value that the smallest observation assumed would be close to -2.24; this is the smallest quantile. On the plot, the smallest observation, 9, is plotted versus -2.24. Similarly, for the largest observation, $p_{40} = (40 - 0.5)/40 = 0.9875$ and $P(Z > 2.24) = 0.9875$, so the largest observation, 31, is plotted versus 2.24, the largest quantile. This is repeated for all 40 observations.

This plot has the property that points fall on a straight line if data are normally distributed; the point $z = 0$ should correspond to the mean and median. If the points do not fall on a straight line, the plot is informative in that its the shape can suggest the nature of the departure from normality. The plot can identify departures from normality due to outliers, tails of a distribution that are either too large or too small, or skewness, among other reasons. Examination of a normal quantile plot can suggest a transformation of a variable to a new one which will approximately follow a normal distribution. (This will be discussed in more detail in Section 1.3.3.)

Here, the observations are plotted on the vertical axis and the normal quantiles are plotted on the horizontal axis. Some software packages present their normal quantile plots in this way, while others present the reverse — normal quantiles on the vertical axis and observations on the horizontal axis. Some packages also draw straight lines through the plot to aid in its interpretation.

Example. Normal quantile plots for the algae data are shown in Figures 1.4 and 1.5. Note that for the species richness data (Figure 1.4), for the smallest observation of 9, the point that is plotted is $(9, -2.24)$ and for the largest value of 31, the point that is plotted is $(31, 2.24)$. Examination of the plot reveals evidence of departures from normality. There are multiple circles denoting observations; the five observations of 16 is one such example. This reflects the fact that values of species richness can only assume whole values; no 16.5 could be observed. The observations are counts rather than continuous measurements. There are gaps in the plot which reflect this (for example, the gap between 16 and 17).

The package that was used to construct this probability plot drew a line through Q_1 and Q_3. By drawing a vertical line at the point $z = 0$, we can see that the median (18) is clearly below what it should be if the data were indeed normally distributed between Q_1 and Q_3. Because of this departure, we should be wary of reading too much into the line through the first and third quartiles. If the line is eliminated, the points do appear more or less on a straight line. While there is departure from normality, the departure doesn't seem extreme.

For total biovolume, the shape of the normal quantile plot is convex (Figure 1.5). (A convex curve has the appearance of an upright bowl.) This is consistent with a distribution that is skewed to the right. A straight line through the set of points shows a tendency for the points corresponding to the smaller observations and those corresponding to the larger observations to be above the line. The lower points above the line suggest that the observations in the lower tail are closer to the middle of the distribution than what would be observed if the data were normally distributed. Similarly, the higher points above the line indicate that the observations in the upper tail are farther away from the middle of the distribution than what would be observed if the data were normally distributed. This is what is expected with a distribution that is skewed to the right. (In contrast, a concave plot suggests a distribution that is skewed to the left.) The two outliers are also readily apparent. Note that if the axes were reversed, so that normal quantiles were on the vertical axis and observations were on the horizontal axis, the shape of the plot would be concave, having the appearance of an upside down bowl. (A convex plot suggests a distribution that is skewed to the left with this plotting scheme.)

Even though the total biovolume is symmetric between the first and third quartiles (suggesting that the line drawn through Q_1 and Q_3 is appropriate), note that when z is < -1.5, the line drops below 0. Since the total biovolume cannot be negative, this provides further indication of lack of normality of the plot.

Besides straight lines and concave or convex curves, sometimes an S-shaped curve is observed. In these situations, a straight line can be drawn through the middle points of the plot, but lower observations may fall below the line and higher observations fall above it. This would be consistent with a distribution that has heavier tails than a normal distribution. Similarly, the lower observations may fall above the line and the higher observations may fall below it. This situation would correspond to one in which the tails are lighter than those of the normal distribution.

To summarize, the following should aid in interpreting a normal quantile plot:

(1) Points that fall approximately on a straight line indicate a normal distribution.

(2) Points at either end that are far away from the majority of points in the middle indicate outliers.

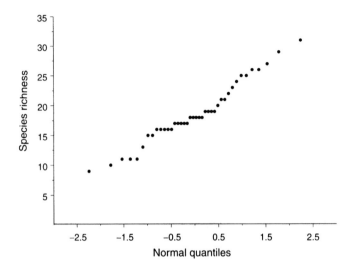

Fig. 1.4 Normal quantile plot for species richness.

(3) If the normal quantiles are on the horizontal axis, a concave curve indicates a distribution that is skewed to the right; a convex curve indicates a distribution that is skewed to the left.

(4) If the normal quantiles are on the vertical axis, a convex curve indicates a distribution that is skewed to the right; a concave curve indicates a distribution that is skewed to the left.

(5) An S-shaped curve indicates a distribution with tails that are heavier or lighter than a normal distribution.

(6) Gaps on the curve may indicate counts rather than continuous data.

For further discussion, Chambers et al., [2] provide a good overview of normal quantile plots.

2. Tests for Normality

The Shapiro-Wilk W test is often used to test for normality [12, 15]. The null hypothesis for this test is that the observations form a random sample from a normally distributed population. W can range between 0 and 1, and is an indicator of the linearity of the points on a normal quantile plot. The maximum value that W can assume is 1, which occurs when all points on the normal quantile plot fall on a straight line. The null hypothesis is rejected for smaller values of W. If the hypothesis is rejected, the test doesn't provide any information about what, if anything, to do about the lack of normality. Examination of normal quantile plots would be the next step. This test could be regarded as a screening device: if the hypothesis is not rejected, assume normality, and if it is rejected, get more information from the normal quantile plots. Several software packages will compute the value of W and its associated p value.

Example. For the species richness data, the calculated value of the W statistic is 0.97 and $p = 0.54$. Thus, we do not reject the hypothesis that the species richness data come from a normal distribution. The test indicates that the slight skewness and the discontinuity of the variable itself were not significant enough departures from normality to be of concern. In contrast, for the total biovolume, $W = 0.44$ and $p < 0.0001$. Thus, we reject the hypothesis that the biovolume data come from a normal distribution. Note the smaller values of W and p for the total biovolume than for the species richness; lack of normality is a much bigger problem for total biovolume.

1.3.3 Transformations

If data are skewed, it may be necessary to consider transforming them so that the transformed data are approximately normally distributed. An inves-

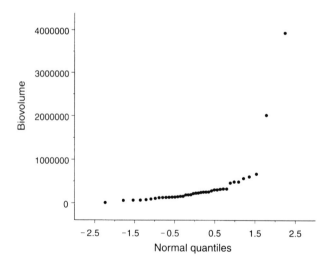

Fig. 1.5 Normal quantile plot for biovolume.

tigator may realize the advisability of a transformation from (1) theoretical considerations, (2) literature dealing with data of a similar type, or (3) examination of the current data set (through graphical means, summary statistics, and hypothesis tests, as discussed in Section 1.3.1).

Use of statistical software greatly facilitates trying various transformations. Finding the best transformation is often an iterative process involving considerable trial and error. Variables can be transformed and plots, summary statistics, and hypothesis tests obtained for the transformed values. Visual inspection of plots frequently indicates whether an acceptable transformation has been found.

Which transformations are potentially useful candidates to try depends on whether the original data are skewed to the right or skewed to the left. We will first consider transformations for data which are skewed to the right, the far more common situation. While there are many possible transformations, we will focus on two which are most commonly used: log and square root. A *log* transformation of a variable Y has the form $\log(Y + A)$, where A is some constant. The log transformation has the effect of compressing larger values of Y to a greater extent than smaller values. If the data are skewed to the right, the larger observations will be closer together on a log scale and the resulting distribution will be closer to being symmetric.

Often, the constant A is chosen to be zero. There are at least two reasons, however, why one would want to consider adding a constant to each of the observations in a data set before taking a log. First, all observations must be greater than zero in order to take a log, so that A can be chosen such that each $Y + A$ is greater than zero. So, for example, if some of the original observations are 0, one will want to add a positive number, say $A = 1$, to each of the observations; otherwise, the 0 observations would become missing data. Second, simply taking a log won't necessarily remove all the asymmetry. Note that A will have a larger effect on smaller values of Y.

Sometimes A is selected by trying several values and transforming the data with each value. The final value of A is selected by examining normal quantile plots or, alternatively, by making tests with the W statistic on the transformed data.

Sometimes, the observations are also multiplied by a constant, so that the transformation $\log(CY + A)$ is made. Certainly a value of C below zero would be indicated in the rare situation when the observations are negative. Another reason for selecting C different from one is to create a particular scale associated with it. For example, the transformed variable may be of particular interest if the researcher wants the scale to have a particular range associated with it.

It is possible to take the log to many different bases, the most common being $\log_{10}$ and $\log_e$; less commonly $\log_2$ is used. In most situations, it doesn't really matter which base is used, since the values obtained with one log transformation are proportional to the values of another; for example, the $\log_e$ of a number is 2.3 times the $\log_{10}$ of the same number. In most applications, $\log_{10}$ is used.

Another commonly used transformation when data are skewed to the right is the *square root* transformation. The square root transformation of a variable Y has the form $\sqrt{Y + A}$. This transformation does not compress the larger values of Y as much as a log transform would, so it will not be as effective in removing more extreme skewness, if it is present. As a rule, the square root transformation is used if the data have a Poisson distribution [5, 6]; count data [6] or data on rare events often follow the Poisson distribution [5]. The constant A should be chosen so that all transformed observations are nonnegative, and, as with the log, by changing the value of A, different degrees of skewness can be controlled; A is frequently chosen to be 0.

In contrast, data which are skewed to the left can be made more symmetric by using a transformation which spreads out the larger values. For example, when all observations are greater than one, squaring them will have the effect of increasing the larger observations to a greater extent than the smaller observations. This transformation will be of the form $Y' = (Y + A)^2$. Or, if a more extreme transformation is needed, one of the form $Y' = 10^{CY+A}$ or e^{CY+A} could be considered.

When data are proportions or percentages, the *arcsine square root*, or angular, transformation, is considered. The arcsine square root transformation of a variable $P = Y/n$, where P is a proportion and n is a sample size, is $\arcsin\sqrt{P}$, or $\arcsin\sqrt{Y/n}$. The proportions of different kinds of algae are examples of variables for which this transformation may be appropriate. The arcsine is also called the inverse sine and denoted $\sin^{-1}$. Recall that the sine of a 0 degree angle is 0, and the sine of a 90 degree angle is 1. The arcsine is the value of the angle which corresponds to a sine. Thus, 0 is the arcsine of 0 degrees, and 1 is the arcsine of 90 degrees. Since $\sqrt{P}$ can range between 0 and 1, the arcsine $\sqrt{P}$ can assume values between 0 and 90 degrees. Between 0 and 1 (the range of values that a proportion can assume) there is a one-to-one correspondence between the proportion and the angle. Frequently in statistics (in statistical software in particular), an angle is expressed in radians rather than degrees (1 degree $= \pi/180$ radians). So we can say that since P can assume values between 0 and 1, $\arcsin\sqrt{P}$ can assume values between 0 and $90 \cdot \pi/180 = \pi/2 = 1.57$ radians. This transformation spreads out the small and large proportions. A variety of modifications to this transformation have been proposed.

Numerous other methods have been proposed for finding appropriate transformations. For example, Tukey [19] gives a method for choosing a transformation from the shape of the curve obtained from plotting the transformed observations versus the nontransformed ones. He also gives a diagram summarizing possible transformations.

One point to keep in mind if a variable is transformed and used in subsequent statistical analyses is that the conclusions must be expressed in terms of the transformed variable and not the original one. Making the transformation can give the advantage that the assumptions of the analyses are satisfied, but it can also produce the disadvantage that their interpretation is much more difficult to understand and communicate. Some investigators will perform the analysis with and without the transformation, and use the transformation only if it makes an appreciable difference. Others will use the transformed variables for their statistical inferences, and then present their main findings in terms of statistics which have been back-transformed to the usual scale.

Sometimes it is not possible to find a transformation which will induce normality. For example, if there are two very distinct modes (observations that occur more frequently than their neighbors), then it may not be possible to determine such a transformation. Or if the mode is at zero and there are no negative values, the methods given previously will not work. In these and other situations, it may be necessary to consider transformations which don't attempt to transform a variable to one with a normal distribution. One is the *rank* transformation, in which observations are replaced with their ranking. Generally some form of rank transformation is used when nonparametric or distribution-free methods are applied [4]. (We will consider these alternatives to the traditional analysis of variance and regression methods when appropriate.)

In other cases, due to small sample sizes, one can be quite uncertain about the form of the distribution. Different analysts will follow different procedures in these cases. Some will perform the desired statistical analysis anyway and warn the reader that the assumptions are not met. Others will describe their outcome in a descriptive fashion and not perform formal tests of hypotheses. Still others will use procedures that require less assumptions.

Often investigators are uncertain whether a transformation is needed. Will it really change the results? Some have suggested guidelines. For example, Hoaglin et al. [10, page 125] suggest that when the largest observation divided by the smallest observation is less than two, a transformation may not have much effect on the shape of the distribution. This rule only applies for ratio data.

Example. Assessments of the biovolume of algal cells made earlier revealed that the data did not come from a normally distributed population. All of the graphs and the positive skewness indicated that the distribution was skewed to the right. The ratio of the maximum to the minimum for this variable is 3,935,994 / 11,407.7 = 345, suggesting that transformation could be worthwhile. Both the presence of the extreme values and the lack of symmetry of the distribution would pose problems for analyses described later on in this book. Thus, if one wanted to apply the techniques described later on, it would be necessary to transform the variable. A reasonable candidate transformation is the log transformation. A log transformation would have the effect of lessening the extreme high values relative to the other observations, while making the smaller observations farther apart from each other. A histogram and boxplot for the log transformed biovolume are presented in Figure 1.6, and its stem and leaf plot is shown in Table 1.5. In this plot, the stems are two digits and the leaf is one digit. Since the decimal point is one place to the left of the line, the first log biovolume is read as 4.79. The smallest value (4.06) and the largest two values (6.31 and 6.59) were excluded from the plot. Comparing these plots with those found in Figure 1.2, we see that the distribution of the log transformed biovolume is much more symmetric.

The normal quantile plot in Figure 1.7 can be compared with the plot for the nontransformed variable in Figure 1.5. With the log biovolume, the shape of the curve is much closer to a straight line.

The log transformed variable more closely follows a normal distribution. The histogram and stem and leaf plot are more symmetric, the box and whisker plot indicates that the transformation was effective in bringing down the largest values, and the points nearly fall on a straight line on the normal quantile plot. The skewness is 0.2. The Shapiro-Wilk test statistic is $W = 0.95$ ($p = 0.09$), so that we conclude that log total volume of algal cells may be normally distributed.

In this example, we were trying to find a transformation that would produce a variable that was approximately normally distributed. An alternative transformation, $5\log_2[0.001(\text{algal biovolume} +1)]$ was used to create the Sweet trophic state index (TSI) [18], a scale for measuring nutrient content that was adapted from [1]. Larger values indicate that there is too much biota growing

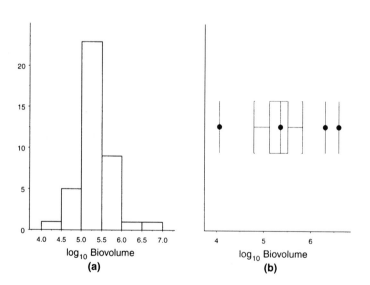

Fig. 1.6 (a) Histogram and (b) box and whisker plot for log total biovolume.

Table 1.5   Stem and Leaf Plot for Log$_{10}$ Biovolume.

Stem	Leaf
47	9
48	12
49	07
50	49
51	1134479
52	0889
53	5679
54	011589
55	022
56	799
57	58
58	3

Decimal is one place to the left of the center line.

in the water. As the biota dies off, there is insufficient oxygen to decompose the material. There is a pile-up of organic matter which does not decompose and which causes odor and scum. This index was established to correspond to a theoretical range from 0 (when there are no algae in a lake) to 100. The addition of the constant $A = 1$ was made to ensure that the index could be computed when no algae were detected. In the 40 VT and NH lakes, the Sweet TSI ranged from 18.2 to 59.7, suggesting that there was not an excessive problem with algae in the lakes.

To make a rank transformation of the 40 total biovolume values, we would assign a value of 1 to the smallest biovolume, (associated with Lake Russell) and 40 to the largest biovolume (associated with Lake Carmi). To categorize species richness variable into four categories, we might select the categories 0 – 9, 10 – 19, 20 – 29, and 30 – 39. Species richness would still be an ordinal variable, but would have fewer categories.

1.3.4   Independence

A simple random sample is a subset of the population chosen in such a way that any subset of equal size is equally likely to be chosen. When a random sample is chosen from a very small population without replacement, it seems clear that two individuals in the sample are not statistically independent of each other. Knowledge of the first individual chosen gives us information concerning the second individual (e.g., it cannot be the first individual). For

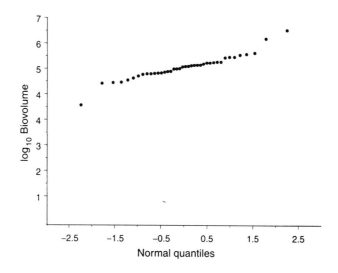

Fig. 1.7   Normal quantile plot for $\log_{10}$ biovolume.

an infinite population, however, any two observations in a random sample are statistically independent of each other.

Lack of independence among observations within a sample occasionally arises because measurements have not been taken in a random order and a dependence exists from observation to observation. Such dependence can be caused by factors such as equipment drifting out of calibration, physical effects of the location of experimental animal cages, natural time trends, or the learning curve on the part of the investigator performing the experiment. The simplest way to detect gross lack of independence is to plot the observations over time or space. A trend over time or space would suggest lack of independence; a lack of trend would suggest independence.

Oftentimes, dependence among observations is not expected. To detect it, the analyst should be well acquainted with the design and data collection procedures of the research study.

Example. In a separate investigation, the VT Department of Environmental Conservation determined the Sweet TSI every week from June through August for some of these lakes over a period of years. To illustrate the tendency of the total biovolume of algae in Lake Carmi to increase over time, we plot the 13 observations by week in Figure 1.8; this leads us to suspect that the observations are not independent. In particular, there is a tendency for the

Sweet TSI to slowly increase over time, suggesting that there is an increase in algae over the summer.

The *serial correlation* is sometimes calculated as a summary statistic to describe the strength of a linear trend over time. Most software packages compute a serial correlation. We will present the formula here, to illustrate its interpretation. (The more general concept of correlation will be discussed in greater detail in Chapter 11.) The serial correlation is calculated as the correlation between an observation at one time point and the observation at the next time point. Let Y_i denote the observation at the ith time point, and Y_{i+1} denote the observation at the $(i+1)$th time point. If there are n time points, then there are $n-1$ pairs of consecutive time points: 1 and 2, 2 and 3, ..., $n-1$ and n. Let $\bar{Y}_1$ denote the mean of the Y's for time points 1 through $n-1$, and $\bar{Y}_2$ denote the mean of the Y's for time points 2 through n. Then the expression for the serial correlation is

$$ r = \frac{\sum_{i=1}^{n-1}(Y_i - \bar{Y}_1)(Y_{i+1} - \bar{Y}_2)}{\sqrt{\sum_{i=1}^{n-1}(Y_i - \bar{Y}_1)^2 \cdot \sum_{i=2}^{n}(Y_i - \bar{Y}_2)^2}}. \tag{1.2} $$

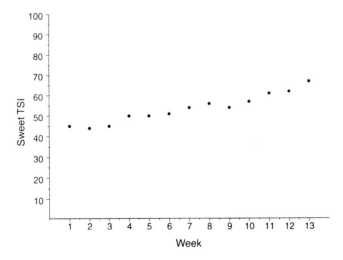

Fig. 1.8 Plot of Sweet TSI, by week, for Lake Carmi.

Note that it is the numerator that determines the sign of the serial correlation; the denominator is always > 0. The serial correlation ranges between -1 and 1. When there is a trend for the observations to increase over time, the statistic will assume positive values and will assume a value of 1 if all pairs of time points fall on a straight line. Similarly, when there is a decreasing time trend, the statistic will assume negative values and will assume a value of -1 if all pairs of time points fall on a straight line. A serial correlation close to 0 indicates no linear time trend.

Table 1.6   Values of Sweet TSI by Week for Lake Carmi

Week	Sweet TSI for Week	Week + 1	Sweet TSI for Week + 1
1	45	2	44
2	44	3	45
3	45	4	50
4	50	5	50
5	50	6	51
6	51	7	54
7	54	8	56
8	56	9	54
9	54	10	57
10	57	11	61
11	61	12	62
12	62	13	67
$\bar{Y}_1$	52.4	$\bar{Y}_2$	54.3

Example. Using Equation 1.2 and the data in Table 1.6, the serial correlation of the Sweet TSI during a given summer for Lake Carmi, VT can be computed. For the first six pairs of time points, both observations are below their sample means $\bar{Y}_1$ and $\bar{Y}_2$, and for the last six pairs, both observations are above the sample means. Thus, all terms in the numerator of the expression for serial correlation are positive. The serial correlation is $r = 0.95$, consistent with the strong increasing trend over time of the Sweet TSI index.

1.4 SUMMARY

In this chapter, we have discussed ways of initially screening and then summarizing data, using both numerical and graphical procedures. We assume that we have taken a random sample from a single population and focus on one variable at a time. We looked at two example variables in detail; one needed to be transformed to achieve a distribution that more closely follows a normal distribution, and one probably didn't. As this example illustrates, often there is ambiguity about whether to transform variables and, if so, which transformation should be selected. In subsequent chapters, we consider the design and analysis of studies which deal with multiple populations or multiple variables simultaneously. The information given in this chapter will form the basis for more specialized methods of data screening that will be presented along with methods of data analysis and presentation of results in subsequent chapters. In Chapter 2, we start with a commonly used method for analyzing data from two or more populations.

Problems

1.1   Other measurements taken from the 40 VT and NH lakes, in addition to species richness and biovolume, are used for this problem and the next one. The algae data and documentation are available on the Wiley web site, `ftp://ftp.wiley.com/sci_tech_med/applied_statistics`.

   a)   Since species richness is count data, try taking the square root transformation. Recompute the descriptive statistics and replot the graphs. Do you think anything is gained by transforming the data? Comment on the normality of species richness and square root of species richness.

   b)   Eliminate the largest two values of total biovolume, recompute the descriptive statistics, and replot the graphs. Compare the results you obtained when you did and did not delete these two observations. Comment on the normality of total biovolume when the two observations are and are not deleted.

1.2   Answer the following questions for the following variables in the algae file: total density, % biovolume of green algae, brown algae, blue algae and % by density of green algae, brown algae, and blue algae.

   a)   Do the data appear to have come from normally distributed populations? Why or why not?

   b)   If the data do not appear to have come from a normally distributed population, can you find a transformation which will induce normality? (Note: This is a good problem for stimulating class discussion.)

1.3   For another year, the values of the Sweet TSI were determined weekly, June – September, for Lake Carmi, VT.

Week	TSI
1	46
2	45
3	51
4	50
5	44
6	51
7	60
8	58
9	63
10	60
11	63
12	62
13	57
14	62

a)   Plot the data by week. Based on the graph, do the data suggest lack of independence? If so, describe the time trend.

b)   Calculate the serial correlation. What does the value of the serial correlation indicate about the time trend?

1.4   Data obtained from a sample of patients who participated in a program of cardiac rehabilitation, and related documentation, are available on the Wiley ftp site given in the Preface or in the first problem. Use graphs and numerical summaries to describe the distributions of the following variables: age (in years), weight (in pounds), and height, waist, and hip measurements (in inches). Which variables seem approximately normally distributed and which ones appear skewed?

1.5   Repeat Problem 1.4 for the following two subsets of the data.
a)   Restrict the data to the males (coded as sex = 1).
b)   Restrict the data to the females (coded as sex = 2).
c)   Compare the distributions of the five variables for females and males.

1.6   Using a statistical software package of your choice, randomly generate 50 observations from a normal distribution with $\mu = 5$ and $\sigma = 1$. Compute the following summary statistics: mean, median, first quartile (Q_1), third quartile (Q_3), interquartile range (IQR), skewness. Obtain the following graphs: histogram, stem and leaf plot, boxplot. Assess normality using normal quantile plots and the W test. Use this information to summarize characteristics of the normal distribution.

1.7 Transform the data in Problem 1.6 using the transformation $Y' = 10^Y$. (The distribution that you generate is called the log normal distribution.) Repeat the computer runs you did in the previous problem, and summarize the characteristics of the log normal distribution.

1.8 Randomly generate 50 observations from a uniform (rectangular) distribution with lower limit of 0 and upper limit of 1. Repeat Problem 1.6. Do you think a suitable transformation to a normal distribution could be found for this data? Why or why not?

REFERENCES

1. Carlson, R.E. [1977]. A Trophic State Index for Lakes, *Limnology and Oceanograph*, 22, 361–369.

2. Chambers, J.M., Cleveland, W.S., Kleiner, B., and Tukey, P.A. [1983]. *Graphical Methods for Data Analysis*, Belmont, CA: Wadsworth Incorporated, 9–42, 191–238.

3. Cleveland, W.S. [1993]. *Visualizing Data*, Summit, NJ: Hobarth Press, 29–33.

4. Conover, W.J. [1999]. *Practical Nonparametric Statistics*, New York: John Wiley & Sons, 269–272.

5. Dixon, W.J. and Massey, F.J. [1983]. *Introduction to Statistical Analysis*, 4th ed., New York: McGraw-Hill Book Company.

6. Fisher, L.D. and van Belle, G. [1993]. *Biostatistics: A Methodology for the Health Sciences*, New York: John Wiley & Sons, 211–217.

7. Fox, J. and Long, J.S. [1990]. *Modern Methods of Data Analysis*, Newbury Park, CA: Sage Publications, Inc., 80–88.

8. Freedman, D. and Diaconis, P. [1981]. On the Histogram as a Density Estimator: L_2 Theory, *Zeitschrift für Wahrscheinlichkeitstheorie und Verwandte Gebiete*, 57, 453–476.

9. Frigge, M., Hoaglin, D.C., and Iglewicz, B. [1989]. Some Implications of the Boxplot, *The American Statistician*, 43, 50–54.

10. Hoaglin, D.C., Mosteller, F., and Tukey, J.W. [1983]. *Understanding Robust and Exploratory Data Analysis*, New York: John Wiley & Sons, 7–31, 58–127.

11. Little, R.J.A. and Rubin, D.B. [2000]. *Statistical Analysis with Missing Data*, New York: John Wiley & Sons.

12. Roylston, J.P. [1982]. An Extension of Shapiro and Wilk's *W* Test for Normality for Large Samples. *Applied Statistics*, 31, 115–124.

13. Rubin, D.B. [1986]. *Multiple Imputation in Surveys*, New York: John Wiley & Sons, 1–23.

14. Scott, D.W. [1979]. On Optimal and Data-Based Histograms, *Biometrika*, 66, 605–610.

15. Shapiro, S.S. and Wilk, M.B. [1965]. An Analysis of Variance Test for Normality (Complete Samples), *Biometrika*, 52, 591–612.

16. Shapiro, S.S., Wilk, M.B. and Chen, H.J. [1968]. A Comparative Study of Various Tests for Normality, *Journal of the American Statistical Association*, 63, 1343–1372.

17. Stevens, S.S. [1951]. Mathematics, Measurement and Psychophysics, in Stevens, S.S., editor, *Handbook of Experimental Psychology*, New York: John Wiley & Sons, 1–49.

18. Sweet, J. [1986]. A Survey and Ecological Analysis of Oregon and Idaho Phytoplankton. Final Report submitted to Environmental Protection Agency. Portland, OR: Aquatic Analysts.

19. Tukey, J.W. [1977]. *Exploratory Data Analysis*, Reading, MA: Addison-Wesley, 57–93.

20. Velleman, P.F. and Wilkinson, L. [1993]. Nominal, Ordinal, Interval, and Ratio Typologies Are Misleading, *The American Statistician*, 47, 65–72.

2

One-Way Analysis of Variance Design

In the previous chapter, we assumed we had a sample from a single population and considered ways to perform data screening and to describe the data using both numerical and graphical approaches. In many situations, more than one population is of interest and the investigator wishes to compare their means. Samples are drawn from each of them, and one of the first questions to be asked is: on the basis of the sample data, are the means of the populations equal? Another way to ask this question is: does the population from which an individual is drawn affect its mean? Here the focus is on making an inference or drawing a conclusion about the populations on the basis of the samples. When there are only two populations involved, the two-sample t test for the equality of population means or a confidence interval for the difference of the population means can be used to answer these questions. In this chapter, we are concerned principally with how to go about answering this question when there are multiple populations. The technique that is used to perform the test for equality of population means is one-way analysis of variance (ANOVA).

In Section 2.1, we describe what is called one-way ANOVA with fixed effects. This section goes into greater detail than is provided in other sections of the book; we are laying the foundation for other applications of ANOVA which appear in this and subsequent chapters. Section 2.2 considers one-way ANOVA with random effects. Then in Section 2.3 we step back and consider what to think about when designing an experiment or observational study in which one-way ANOVA is an appropriate statistical analysis technique. We consider how to check if the data fit the one-way ANOVA model in Section 2.4, and what to do if they don't in Section 2.5. How to present and interpret results of one-way ANOVA is discussed in Section 2.6. Finally, the chapter is summarized in Section 2.7.

2.1   ONE-WAY ANALYSIS OF VARIANCE WITH FIXED EFFECTS

2.1.1   Example

To illustrate one-way ANOVA we will first consider a small example. An investigator wishes to study lung function in relation to smoking behavior. People are classified into four categories: nonsmokers (category 1), former smokers who stopped smoking more than two years ago, called early smokers (category 2), former smokers who stopped smoking within the past two years, called recent smokers (category 3), and current smokers (category 4). Samples of size 6 are drawn from each of these four populations of people, and the lung function of each person is measured. The volume of air that can be forcibly expired in the first second of exhalation, referred to as FEV1, is the measure of lung function which is determined for each individual. These measurements, in liters, are given in Table 2.1.

What the investigator would be interested in is whether or not the mean FEV1 is the same across the four categories of smokers, or equivalently, whether smoking status affects mean FEV1. Note than in an actual study, many more measurements would be made than on smoking behavior and FEV1. Typically, other variables, such as age, gender, weight, height, and other measures of lung function, would be measured.

As in the previous chapter, we will use Y to denote a variable for which we have a set of measurements. Here, Y is an outcome or dependent variable and is FEV1. We use Y_1 to denote FEV1 among nonsmokers, and Y_2, Y_3, Y_4 to denote FEV1 for early smokers, recent smokers, and smokers, respectively. Smoking status is a *classification variable*, or *factor*; it has four levels, corresponding to the four categories of smokers.

Each observation will be identified as a Y with two subscripts; the first subscript will specify the category level or group, and the second will identify the observation. Y_{ij} denotes the jth observation from the ith smoking group. So, for example, Y_{11}, the value of FEV1 for the first nonsmoker, is 4.41. In this example, the sample size is the same for each category of smokers. This sample size is denoted by n; here, n is equal to 6. The data are graphed, by smoking category, in Figures 2.1 and 2.2. Figure 2.1 provides a scatter plot of the data, and Figure 2.2 plots the mean plus or minus one standard deviation for each smoking category. Both show the greatest lung function among nonsmokers; the FEV1 values decrease as time since last smoking increases (i.e., among people who had smoked, early smokers have higher FEV1's than recent smokers; current smokers have the lowest FEV1). No obvious outliers can be detected from these graphs.

Table 2.1 Forced Expiratory Volume, in Liters, During First Second by Four Smoking Categories

Observation	1	2	3	4	5	6	$\bar{Y}_{i.}$	s_i^2
Category:								
1 Nonsmokers	4.41	4.96	3.50	3.66	4.68	4.11	4.22	0.33
2 Early smokers	3.69	3.90	3.82	4.08	3.76	4.38	3.94	0.06
3 Recent smokers	3.54	4.40	3.28	2.28	3.34	3.92	3.46	0.51
4 Smokers	2.98	2.95	2.15	3.41	3.97	3.86	3.22	0.46
Mean							3.71	0.34

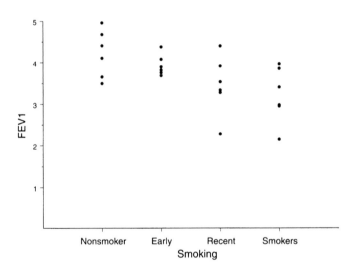

Fig. 2.1   Plot of the lung function data, by smoking category.

For the mean of the ith sample, we use $\bar{Y}_{i.}$; the dot in the second place indicates that we have averaged over the second subscript. For the mean of all observations in the sample, we use $\bar{Y}_{..}$; the dots indicate we have averaged over both subscripts. The variance of the ith sample is denoted by s_i^2, and its square root, the standard deviation, by s_i. Thus, the mean FEV1 of the six nonsmokers is $\bar{Y}_{1.} = 4.22$ liters, the variance is $s_1^2 = 0.33$ liters, and the standard deviation is $s_1 = 0.57$ liters.

While Figures 2.1 and 2.2 and the summary statistics presented in Table 2.1 are informative for summarizing the samples for the four smoking categories, we cannot use these statistics to conclude that the mean lung functions are equal or unequal in the populations from which the samples are taken. To do this, we will perform a hypothesis test called the ANOVA F test.

2.1.2 The One-Way Analysis of Variance Model with Fixed Effects

In this section, the assumptions needed to test the equality of means will be given first, followed by the model. In order to test for equality of population means, we need to make some assumptions. For the lung function example, we have three assumptions about the samples and their underlying populations:

(1) The four samples, each consisting of six measurements, are independent random samples from four populations of FEV1 measurements. That is, there is a population of FEV1 measurements for nonsmokers, one for early smokers, one for recent smokers, and one for smokers.

(2) Each of the four populations of FEV1 measurements is normally distributed.

(3) The variances of these four populations of FEV1 measurements are equal.

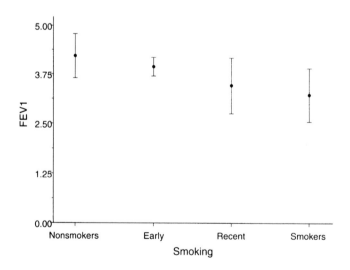

Fig. 2.2 Plot of sample mean plus or minus one standard deviation, by smoking category.

As indicated in Chapter 1, a normal distribution is uniquely identified by its mean and variance. The four population means may be designated μ_1, μ_2, μ_3, and μ_4. We arbitrarily divide each of these four means into two parts. The first part is the mean of the four population means, which we call the overall mean, and the second part is the difference between the mean of each population and the overall mean. In symbols, the means are written as $\mu_1 = \mu + \alpha_1, \ldots, \mu_4 = \mu + \alpha_4$, where μ denotes the overall mean and α_i is the difference $\mu_i - \mu$. The overall mean μ has been chosen in such a way that $\sum_{i=1}^{4} \alpha_i = 0$, where 4 is the number of smoking categories. No additional assumption is being made here; any four means can be expressed in this way.

If in our example the four population means were $\mu_1 = 4.2$, $\mu_2 = 3.5$, $\mu_3 = 3.4$, and $\mu_4 = 3.3$, we should have $\mu = (4.2 + 3.5 + 3.4 + 3.3)/4 = 3.6$. The population means could then be written

$$
\begin{aligned}
\mu_1 = \mu + \alpha_1 &= 3.6 + (+0.6), \\
\mu_2 = \mu + \alpha_2 &= 3.6 + (-0.1), \\
\mu_3 = \mu + \alpha_3 &= 3.6 + (-0.2), \\
\mu_4 = \mu + \alpha_4 &= 3.6 + (-0.3).
\end{aligned}
$$

The difference $\alpha_i = \mu_i - \mu$ is often called the effect of the ith category. We think of a population mean as the sum of two parts: an overall mean μ (which, as an average of the four population means, may be of little interest to us) and the part that we attribute to the particular smoking category. Thus, in this example, the population of nonsmokers has a mean FEV1 0.6 liters above the average of the four mean FEV1's, while the population of current smokers has a mean FEV1 0.3 liters below the average. The α_i should not be confused with the level of significance α, the probability of rejecting a true null hypothesis.

Not everyone who is in the same smoking category has the same value of FEV1; there is variation among lung functions within a category. The variability is assumed to be the same in the four populations of smokers; the common variance is denoted by σ^2. If in our example, the populations of nonsmokers, early smokers, recent smokers, and smokers each had population variance of 0.3 liter^2, then σ^2 would be equal to 0.3.

We can summarize the assumptions in terms of a model, called the *fixed effects one-way ANOVA model*. A model is a mathematical expression; it allows us to formally state something about the underlying populations and how the samples were obtained from them.

For the lung function example, the model can be specified as

$$
Y_{ij} \sim \text{IND}(\mu + \alpha_i, \sigma^2), \qquad \sum_{i=1}^{4} \alpha_i = 0, \quad i = 1, \ldots, 4, \quad j = 1, \ldots, 6. \quad (2.1)
$$

This statement is read as "The Y_{ij} are independent and normally distributed (IND) with means $\mu + \alpha_i$, and constant variance σ^2; there are samples of size 6 from each of the four populations." The model implies the assumptions that were given at the start of this subsection: all observations are independent; the four populations are normally distributed; the variances of the four populations are equal.

Each Y_{ij} is made up of $\mu + \alpha_i$, the mean for the population of people of the ith category, plus whatever is left over, the ε_{ij}. In our data, for example, $Y_{23} = 3.82$; therefore, if the population mean expiratory volume for people who stopped smoking more than two years ago is 3.50, then $\varepsilon_{23} = 3.82-3.50 = +0.32$. In our data there are 24 deviations ε_{ij}; they form a random sample of size 24, all from a normal population with zero mean and variance σ^2. Thus, an alternative, equivalent way of specifying the model is

$$Y_{ij} = \mu + \alpha_i + \varepsilon_{ij}, \tag{2.2}$$

$$\sum_{i=1}^{4} \alpha_i = 0, \quad \varepsilon_{ij} \sim \text{IND}(0, \sigma^2), \quad i = 1,\ldots,4, \quad j = 1,\ldots,6.$$

This model is referred to as a *one-way ANOVA model with fixed effects*. It is specified as "one-way" because the populations differ with respect to levels of a single factor, here smoking status. It is called "fixed effects" to indicate that conclusions will be drawn only about the populations that were sampled, here the four populations of smokers. (This point is indicated by $\sum_{i=1}^{4} \alpha_i = 0$.)

Using this notation, we can summarize the model just described more generally:

$$Y_{ij} \sim \text{IND}(\mu + \alpha_i, \sigma^2), \quad \sum_{i=1}^{a} \alpha_i = 0, \quad i = 1,\ldots,a, \quad j = 1,\ldots,n \tag{2.3}$$

where a is the number of levels the factor assumes, n is the number of observations at each level, and IND is read as "independently normally distributed". Note that in this model expression, the sample sizes from each population, n, are equal. (We are considering equal sample sizes here because this is the simplest case; we will generalize our model to allow for unequal sample sizes in Section 2.1.8.) In the fixed effects model, we are studying only these particular a populations. An equivalent way of writing down the model given in Equation 2.3 which is often convenient is

$$Y_{ij} = \mu + \alpha_i + \varepsilon_{ij}, \tag{2.4}$$

where

$$\sum_{i=1}^{a} \alpha_i = 0, \qquad \varepsilon_{ij} \sim \text{IND}(0, \sigma^2), \quad i = 1, \ldots, a, \quad j = 1, \ldots, n.$$

Here ε_{ij} indicates how much the ijth variable deviates from the ith population mean.

The assumptions implied by the model can be restated in general terms:

(1) The a samples, each consisting of n measurements, are independent random samples from a populations.

(2) Each of the a populations is normally distributed.

(3) The variances of the a population are equal.

There are advantages to specifying a model. First, the expression "one-way analysis of variance model with fixed effects" is commonly used, so that it is easy to communicate to others the specifics of which statistical analyses are used. Second, many software packages require that the user specify the underlying model in order to perform the ANOVA to test for equality of means. In later chapters, more complex models will be specified when more complex designs are considered.

2.1.3 Null Hypothesis: Test for Equality of Population Means

The objective is to test for equality of population means. There are a variety of ways that the null hypothesis, H_0, can be specified. We can state it in words: the mean of the first population equals the mean of the second population, the third population, ..., and the ath population. Alternatively, we can make use of the model to state what the hypothesis should be. Examples include

$$H_0 : \mu_1 = \cdots = \mu_a$$

and

$$H_0 : \alpha_i = 0, \quad i = 1, \ldots, a.$$

To help reinforce the null hypothesis, it is helpful to express it in terms of the problem at hand. So, for example, in the lung function example, we might state that the null hypothesis is that the mean FEV1 is equal among nonsmokers, early smokers, recent smokers, and smokers.

2.1.4 Estimation of Model Terms

We can estimate the values of μ, α_i, σ^2, and ε_{ij} from our data. These are related to some of the summary statistics which investigators would initially calculate for their data.

For example, the first calculations performed by the investigator with the data in Table 2.1 are the sample means $\bar{Y}_{i.}$, the sample variances s_i^2, and the sample standard deviations s_i. Note that we are still assuming equal sample sizes here.

The mean of the ith sample is calculated as

$$\bar{Y}_{i.} = \frac{Y_{i1} + \cdots + Y_{in}}{n}; \tag{2.5}$$

this is an estimate of $\mu_i = \mu + \alpha_i$. Similarly, $\bar{Y}_{..}$ can be expressed as

$$\bar{Y}_{..} = \frac{(Y_{11} + \cdots + Y_{1n}) + \cdots + (Y_{a1} + \cdots + Y_{an})}{an} \tag{2.6}$$

and is an estimate of μ.

With $\bar{Y}_{i.}$ as an estimate of $\mu + \alpha_i$ and $\bar{Y}_{..}$ as an estimate of μ, we have $\bar{Y}_{i.} - \bar{Y}_{..}$ as our estimate of α_i.

To estimate the population variance σ^2, we make use of the category-specific sample variances. Each one by itself is an estimate of σ^2. However, these can be combined, or pooled, into a single estimate, s^2. Recall that

$$s_i^2 = \frac{\sum_{j=1}^{n}(Y_{ij} - \bar{Y}_{i.})^2}{n-1}. \tag{2.7}$$

When sample sizes are equal, s^2 is the mean of the s_i^2; we don't believe one of the s_i^2 provides a better estimate of σ^2 than any of the others, so each one is given equal weight:

$$s^2 = \frac{s_1^2 + \cdots + s_a^2}{a}. \tag{2.8}$$

For a given data set, the ε_{ij} can be estimated as $Y_{ij} - \bar{Y}_{i.}$. These are frequently referred to as *residuals*, and represent deviations of an individual observation from its category mean.

Example. Using the formulas given in Equations 2.5 and 2.6, we could verify that $\bar{Y}_{..}$ is 3.71 liters and the mean FEV1 for non-smokers is $\bar{Y}_{1.} = 4.22$ liters (see Table 2.1). The effect of not smoking is estimated as the difference between the mean of the nonsmokers and the overall mean, i.e. $4.22 - 3.71 = 0.51$ liters.

The sample variances are $s_1^2 = 0.33$, $s_2^2 = 0.06$, $s_3^2 = 0.51$, and $s_4^2 = 0.46$; s^2, the pooled estimate of σ^2, is the mean of the four sample variances, or 0.34 (see Table 2.1).

The residual for the first individual in the data set is estimated as the difference of $Y_{11} - \bar{Y}_{1.}$ or $4.41 - 4.22 = 0.19$ liters. That is, the first individual has an FEV1 measurement that is 0.19 liters above the mean FEV1 of nonsmokers.

In summary, the model parameters and their point estimates are as follows:

Parameter	Estimate	Interpretation of Estimate
μ	$\bar{Y}_{..}$	Overall mean
α_i	$\bar{Y}_{i.} - \bar{Y}_{..}$	Effect of ith category
$\mu + \alpha_i$	$\bar{Y}_{i.}$	Mean of ith category
σ^2	s^2	Common variance

Note: Estimators of the population parameters are defined in such as way that they are *unbiased*; that is, their expected value is equal to the parameter being estimated. Interested students should see Appendix A for properties of expected values and expected values of estimators relevant to this chapter.

2.1.5 Breakdown of the Basic Sum of Squares

When the terms in the model $Y_{ij} = \mu + \alpha_i + \varepsilon_{ij}$ are replaced by their estimates from the data, we have

$$Y_{ij} = \bar{Y}_{..} + (\bar{Y}_{i.} - \bar{Y}_{..}) + (Y_{ij} - \bar{Y}_{i.}), \qquad (2.9)$$

an algebraic identity. (To be an identity, the equation must hold for any values of Y_{ij}. Note that if we cancel out the two $\bar{Y}_{i.}$ and $\bar{Y}_{..}$ we have the same thing on the right-hand side of the equation as on the left.)
    Instead, however, we usually write

$$Y_{ij} - \bar{Y}_{..} = (\bar{Y}_{i.} - \bar{Y}_{..}) + (Y_{ij} - \bar{Y}_{i.}), \qquad (2.10)$$

subtracting $\bar{Y}_{..}$ from both sides of the identity in Equation 2.9. Written in this way, the total deviation of an individual observation from the overall mean is broken down into two parts: the deviation of the category mean from the overall mean, and the deviation of the individual observation from its category mean.
    Squaring both sides of the equation and making use of the identity $(a+b)^2 = a^2 + b^2 + 2ab$ on the right-hand side, and then summing over all an observations in the data set, gives the following:

$$\sum_{i=1}^{a}\sum_{j=1}^{n}(Y_{ij} - \bar{Y}_{..})^2 = \sum_{i=1}^{a}\sum_{j=1}^{n}(\bar{Y}_{i.} - \bar{Y}_{..})^2 + \sum_{i=1}^{a}\sum_{j=1}^{n}(Y_{ij} - \bar{Y}_{i.})^2$$

$$+2\sum_{i=1}^{a}\sum_{j=1}^{n}(\bar{Y}_{i.} - \bar{Y}_{..})(Y_{ij} - \bar{Y}_{i.}).$$

Since $\sum_{j=1}^{n}(Y_{ij} - \bar{Y}_{i.}) = 0$, the cross product term equals 0 and the resulting equation is

$$\sum_{i=1}^{a}\sum_{j=1}^{n}(Y_{ij} - \bar{Y}_{..})^{2} = \sum_{i=1}^{a}\sum_{j=1}^{n}(\bar{Y}_{i.} - \bar{Y}_{..})^{2} + \sum_{i=1}^{a}\sum_{j=1}^{n}(Y_{ij} - \bar{Y}_{i.})^{2} \qquad (2.11)$$

Thus, the sum of squared deviations from the overall mean, the *total* sum of squares, has been broken into two parts. The first sum of squares, $\sum_{i=1}^{a}\sum_{j=1}^{n}(\bar{Y}_{i.} - \bar{Y}_{..})^{2}$, is the sum of squared deviations of individual means from the overall mean. This quantifies the amount of variation that is due to the classification variable or factor. It may be referred to by various names, such as "factor" or "between groups"; we shall call it *factor*. The second sum of squares, $\sum_{i=1}^{a}\sum_{j=1}^{n}(Y_{ij} - \bar{Y}_{i.})^{2}$, represents the variation of the individual observations about their own sample means and quantifies the amount of variation that is attributable to sources other than the factor. It may be referred to as "residual", "error", or "within groups"; we shall call it the *residual*. The total, factor, and residual sums of squares are denoted SS_{t}, SS_{a}, SS_{r}, respectively, below. Thus, Equation 2.11 can be reexpressed as $SS_{t} = SS_{a} + SS_{r}$.

In the expression $\sum_{i=1}^{a}\sum_{j=1}^{n}(\bar{Y}_{i.} - \bar{Y}_{..})^{2}$ there is no subscript j within the summation sign; thus over j we add the same expression n times. Therefore, $\sum_{i=1}^{a}\sum_{j=1}^{n}(\bar{Y}_{i.} - \bar{Y}_{..})^{2}$ can be written $n\sum_{i=1}^{a}(\bar{Y}_{i.} - \bar{Y}_{..})^{2}$.

Example. Let us consider the lung function example to illustrate this breaking apart of the total sum of squares. Following the pattern outlined above, we could express, for example, Y_{23} as $3.82 = 3.71 + (3.94 - 3.71) + (3.82 - 3.94) = 3.71 + 0.23 - 0.12$ using the sample estimates obtained in Table 2.1. Subtracting the overall mean 3.71 from both sides of the equation gives $0.11 = 0.23 - 0.12$. In other words, we look at the deviation of this particular measurement from the overall mean $(3.82 - 3.71 = 0.11)$ and break that deviation into two terms. The first term represents the deviation of the average FEV1 value for the early smokers from the average FEV1 for all smoking categories $(3.94 - 3.71 = 0.23)$; the second term represents the difference between the measurement for this particular individual and the average FEV1 for early smokers $(3.82 - 3.94 = -0.12)$. Squaring the deviation $0.12 = 0.23 - 0.11$, we obtain

$$(0.11)^{2} = (0.23)^{2} + (-0.12)^{2} + 2(0.23)(-0.12),$$

or

$$0.0121 = 0.0529 + 0.0144 - 0.0552.$$

When these calculations are performed, the cross product terms (i.e., $2ab$) add to zero when summed over the entire set of 24 observations. In this example, the sum of squared deviations of observations from the overall mean, the total sum of squares, is $SS_t = 10.48$, which is divided into two parts: (1) the sum of squared deviations of the individual means from the overall mean, the *smoking* variation, $SS_a = 3.69$, and (2) the sum of squared deviations of the observations from the individual means, the *residual* variation, $SS_r = 6.79$.

2.1.6   Analysis of Variance Table

The division of the basic sum of squared deviations is usually summarized in an ANOVA table. The table displays in a particular order the sums of squares and certain other quantities involved in the computations. Table 2.2 shows the general form of the analysis of variance table for the fixed effects one-way design with equal n.

In the first column of the table, we write the *source of variation*, that is, which sum of squares is listed in each row of the table. As shown in Section 2.1.5, the total variation in the observations is divided into two parts: factor and residual variation. The second column of the table contains the sums of squares, denoted by SS_a, SS_r, and SS_t in Section 2.1.5.

The third column contains the number of *degrees of freedom* (df) for each sum of squares. That is the number by which we divide the sum of squares in order to obtain the mean squares in column 4. For one way ANOVA, the number of degrees of freedom associated with the total sum of squares is equal to the total number of observations minus 1, or $an - 1$. The number of degrees of freedom associated with variation due to the factor equals the number of levels of the factor minus one, or $a - 1$. The number of degrees of freedom associated with the residual is $a(n - 1)$. This can be explained in various ways. There are $n - 1$ degrees of freedom associated with each category-specific sample variance s_i^2, and when these are pooled over the a categories, the result is $a(n - 1)$. Alternatively, the *total* number of degrees of freedom is of course $an - 1$, so that the residual number can be obtained

Table 2.2   One-Way Analysis of Variance Table: Fixed Effects with Equal Numbers

Source of Variation (1)	Sum of Squares (2)	df (3)	Mean Square (4)	Expected Mean Square (5)	Computed F (6)
Factor	SS_a	$a - 1$	MS_a	$\sigma^2 + n\phi(\alpha)$	MS_a^2/s^2
Residual	SS_r	$a(n - 1)$	s^2	σ^2	
Total	SS_t	$an - 1$			

by subtraction: $(an - 1) - (a - 1) = an - a = a(n - 1)$. Note that the number of degrees of freedom associated with the factor and the residual always add up to that for the total sum of squares. (In most computer programs, the df column precedes the sum of squares column; we have reversed these two columns in this book, as the material seemed easier to explain in this order.)

The mean square associated with the factor variation is MS_a. This is $SS_a/(a-1)$, and it is an estimate of $\sigma^2 + n \sum_{i=1}^{a} \alpha_i^2/(a-1)$. [For convenience, we will use the notation $\phi(\alpha)$ for $\sum_{i=1}^{a} \alpha_i^2/(a-1)$.] For the residual mean square, we use the symbol s^2; this estimates the parameter σ^2. Note that s^2 is $SS_r/a(n-1)$, or equivalently, the pooled estimate of the variance, as defined in Section 2.1.4.

The values in the mean square column are used as estimates of the population parameters in column (5). These are referred to as the expected mean squares (EMS). Each entry in the EMS column is the parameter (or sum of parameters) that can be estimated by the corresponding statistic in the mean square column. By choosing the degrees of freedom as specified, the mean squares have the property of being *unbiased*. This means that if we were to repeatedly take samples of size n from each of the a populations and calculate the means of the mean squares, the values would correspond to the values given in column (5). The EMS column is an important one, since it provides one justification for how to perform the F test in analysis of variance. Note that if we divide $\sigma^2 + n\phi(\alpha)$ by σ^2 and the ratio is greater than 1, this indicates $\phi(\alpha)$ is greater than 0 or the α_i are not all 0. (See Appendix A for derivation of the EMS column parameters.)

The test statistic for testing equality of population means is given in column (6). The F statistic is calculated as MS_a/s^2. The use of the statistic in the hypothesis test, and the justification for that use is given in Section 2.1.7.

Example. Table 2.3 is an ANOVA table for the lung function example. In this case, the factor is smoking, so the two sources of variation are smoking and residual. The sums of squares were calculated earlier, using the formulas given in Table 2.2: 3.69 for smoking and 6.79 for residual, which sum to the total sum of squares, 10.48. Because there are four populations in this problem, the degrees of freedom for smoking are $a - 1 = 4 - 1 = 3$. The residual degrees of freedom are 20. There are 5 degrees of freedom associated with each category specific sample variance s_i^2, and when these are pooled over the four categories, the result is 4 times 5, or 20. Alternatively, the total degrees of freedom are $24 - 1 = 23$, so that the residual degrees of freedom can be obtained by subtraction $24 - 4 = 20$.

When the sums of squares are divided by the number of degrees of freedom, the resulting mean squares are $3.69/3 = 1.23$ for smoking and $6.79/20 = 0.34$ for the residual. The calculated $F = 1.23/0.34 = 3.62$.

Table 2.3   Analysis of Variance Table for FEV1

Source of Variation (1)	SS (2)	df (3)	MS (4)	EMS (5)	Computed F (6)	p Value (7)
Smoking	3.69	3	1.23	$\sigma^2 + 6\phi(\alpha)$	3.62	0.030
Residual	6.79	20	0.34	σ^2		
Total	10.48	23				

2.1.7 The F Test

We will now explain how and why we make use of these mean squares to test for equality of population means. The usual estimate of the variance σ^2 is simply s^2, obtained from the residual sum of squares divided by the number of degrees of freedom, $a(n-1)$. It can be shown that s^2 is an unbiased estimator of σ^2 *whether or not* the means of the populations are equal.

Let us consider what happens to the ratio MS_a/s^2 when the population means differ widely from one another. We would expect that the a sample means $\bar{Y}_{i.}$ will probably vary considerably around the overall mean $\bar{Y}_{..}$; thus $\mathrm{MS}_a = n\sum_{i=1}^{a}(\bar{Y}_{i.} - \bar{Y}_{..})^2/(a-1)$ tends to be large. On the other hand, $s^2 = \sum_{i=1}^{a}\sum_{j=1}^{n}(Y_{ij} - \bar{Y}_{i.})^2/a(n-1)$ has no tendency to be large because of large differences among the population means. In repeated sampling, it still estimates σ^2. The ratio of MS_a to s^2 will become larger than one.

In repeated sampling when the population means are *unequal*, MS_a estimates something larger than σ^2 . It can be shown mathematically that the expected value for the factor mean square equals $\sigma^2 + n\sum_{i=1}^{a}\alpha_i^2/(a-1)$, or, as given in column (5) of Table 2.2, $\sigma^2 + n\phi(\alpha)$, as shown in Appendix A. For convenience, and only for convenience, the quantity $\sum_{i=1}^{a}\alpha_i^2/(a-1)$ has been denoted by $\phi(\alpha)$. In the fixed effects model, we are concerned with only a α's, based on a populations chosen in some purposeful fashion; we are not interested in any other populations.

When the population means are *equal*, it can be shown that the factor sum of squares $\mathrm{SS}_a = n\sum_{i=1}^{a}(\bar{Y}_{i.} - \bar{Y}_{..})^2$, when divided by the proper number of degrees of freedom $(a-1)$, also provides an unbiased estimate of the variance σ^2. That is, all the α_i are zero, and $\sum_{i=1}^{a}\alpha_i^2/(a-1)$ is also zero. Then the expected value of the factor mean square is σ^2 . In this case the ratio of the expected factor mean square to the expected residual mean square is one. For a given data set, the ratio of their estimates, the factor mean square to the residual mean square, should be close to 1.

Thus, we can justify rejection of the null hypothesis of equality of population means for *large* values of $F = \mathrm{MS}_a/s^2$ through use of the expected mean squares. A value of $F < 1$ occurs when the residual variance s^2 is large relative to MS_a. This can occasionally occur by chance, or it can be an indication of lack of independence, as discussed in Section 2.4.3.

Next, we need to consider the distribution of the test statistic F when the null hypothesis is true. First, the two statistics MS_a and s^2 can be shown to be statistically independent of each other. In other words, the value of s^2, whether particularly large or small, tells us nothing about whether the value of MS_a is particularly large or small.

When H_0 is true, the quantity $(a-1)MS_a/\sigma^2$ has a χ^2 distribution with $a-1$ degrees of freedom; for under H_0, MS_a is simply a variance calculated from a sample of size a to estimate σ^2. The quantity $a(n-1)s^2/\sigma^2$ has a χ^2 distribution with $a(n-1)$ degrees of freedom. Because the two χ^2 variables are independent, after dividing each by its number of degrees of freedom, their ratio has an F distribution with $\nu_1 = a-1$ and $\nu_2 = a(n-1)$ degrees of freedom. The ratio is

$$F = \frac{MS_a/\sigma^2}{s^2/\sigma^2} = \frac{MS_a}{s^2}. \tag{2.12}$$

The unknown σ^2 has canceled out of the ratio, and F can be written down directly from the ANOVA table. The justification of the χ^2 and F distributions requires the three assumptions that were made when the one-way ANOVA model with fixed effects was written down: the a populations are normally distributed, with the same variance σ^2, and all observations are independent.

When there are just two treatments or categories, we can perform either a two-sided two-sample t test or the F test as given in this chapter. These two tests are equivalent in that for any particular level of significance they result in the same decision. In fact, the calculated F statistic is equal to the square of the calculated t statistic.

Example. For the lung function example, we can now specify the distribution of the test statistic F when H_0 is true: when the mean lung function values of the four populations defined by smoking status are equal, the test statistic follows an F distribution with $\nu_1 = 3$ and $\nu_2 = 20$ degrees of freedom. The distribution of the test statistic is shown in Figure 2.3.

The calculated F statistic is

$$F = 1.23/0.34 = 3.62 \tag{2.13}$$

and is written under Computed F in the sixth column of Table 2.3. Is this value large enough that the null hypothesis is rejected?

One way to make this decision is to compare the level of significance with the p value. Suppose we wish to test the hypothesis at a level of significance $\alpha = 0.05$. This means that the probability of rejecting the hypothesis when the means really are equal, sometimes referred to as making an α or Type I error, is 0.05. The α level is determined prior to performing the test.

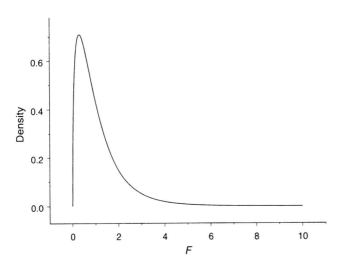

Fig. 2.3 Distribution of the test statistic when the means of all four smoking groups are equal.

In contrast, the p value is associated with a calculated F statistic. It provides information about how unusual the calculated F statistic is if the population means are the same. In the lung function example, the p value is $p = 0.03$. The probability of getting an F value larger than the calculated value of 3.62 when the population means really are equal is 0.03. When the p value is less than α, the null hypothesis of equal population means is rejected.

The 95th percentile of an F distribution with 3 and 20 degrees of freedom is 3.10. (A table of the F distribution is given in Appendix B. The values in the table are given according to ν_1 and ν_2.) Thus, for any calculated F above 3.10, the corresponding p value is less than 0.05. Similarly, for calculated F values below 3.10, the null hypothesis would not be rejected and the p value would exceed 0.05. If this were the case, we would conclude that the means might be equal, or that there was no evidence to say that the means are unequal. The p value can be obtained from a table of F values and is routinely produced, along with the ANOVA table, by software packages when ANOVA is performed. Note that the conclusion that is made involves only whether or not all of the means are equal; it doesn't say anything about which means are unequal.

What is the distribution of the test statistic when H_0 is not true? When the null hypothesis is not true, $(a - 1)\mathrm{MS}_a/\sigma^2$ has a *noncentral* χ^2 distribution. The non-central χ^2 distribution depends on two parameters: the

Table 2.4   One-Way Analysis of Variance Table: Fixed Effects with Unequal Numbers

Source of Variation (1)	Sum of Squares (2)	df (3)	Mean Square (4)	Expected Mean Square (5)	Computed F (6)
Factor	SS_a	$a-1$	MS_a	$\sigma^2 + \dfrac{\sum_{i=1}^a n_i(\alpha_i - \bar{\alpha})^2}{a-1}$	MS_a^2/s^2
Residual	SS_r	$N-a$	s^2	σ^2	
Total	SS_t	$N-1$			

on having greater sample size in one group than in another. Insight into the importance of examining the reason for the lack of equal sample sizes can be gained by viewing it as a problem of missing values. See Section 2.4.5 for discussion of this problem.

2.2   ONE-WAY ANALYSIS OF VARIANCE WITH RANDOM EFFECTS

Sometimes, the populations that are sampled are not the only ones of interest. The populations that are selected constitute a random sample of those that could have been studied. To say this another way, there are many possible levels of the classification variable that could have been selected; the levels that were selected were chosen at random. The objective is to draw inferences about *all* possible populations (all possible levels of the classification variable) that could have been selected. When the researcher wishes to make inferences to the populations from which these samples were selected, then the *random effects* model should be used. This model is sometimes also called the "components of variance model" or "Model Two".

2.2.1   Data Example

Suppose there is a new method of determining vitamin C content, which requires the skills of a laboratory technician. One question of interest is whether one technician makes the same determinations as another, or whether there is any variation in determinations among technicians. To study this question, $a = 4$ laboratory technicians each use the same new method to make $n = 10$ determinations of vitamin C content. We are not interested per se in the four laboratory technicians who participate in the investigation; we wish to study the new method as applied to laboratory technicians in general. If we consider that the four technicians form a random sample from a large population of laboratory technicians, then a random effects model is appropriate.

Recall that when interest was only in the sampled a populations, the hypothesis that we were particularly interested in concerned the means of these populations (e.g., $H_0 : \mu_1 = \cdots = \mu_a$ or $H_0 : \alpha_1 = \cdots = \alpha_a = 0$) and we were interested in estimating the mean of the ith population or the *effect* of population i. In contrast, when our populations are a random subset of possible populations, our hypotheses and what we want to estimate are different.

2.2.2 The One-Way Analysis of Variance Model with Random Effects

In the context of the above example, we make the following assumptions:

(1) There is a random sample of size $a = 4$ laboratory technicians, from a large population of laboratory technicians.

(2) For each laboratory technician, there is a normally distributed population of vitamin C contents.

(3) For each laboratory technician, the normally distributed population of vitamin C contents has the same variance.

(4) Vitamin C determinations made by one technician are independent of determinations made by other technicians, that is, they provide no information about vitamin C determinations from another technician.

(5) Vitamin C determinations made by a particular technician may not be independent.

We want to consider the possibility that there is an effect of technician on vitamin C determination. The means of the four technicians are not of interest, since they are simply a sample of possible technicians. Instead we want to find out if there is a significant variation in the determinations among technicians. We are not interested in α_i, but instead want to know their variance σ_a^2.

We can express these assumptions more precisely in terms of a random effects one-way ANOVA model:

$$Y_{ij} = \mu + \alpha_i + \varepsilon_{ij}, \qquad i = 1, \ldots, a, \quad j = 1, \ldots, n, \qquad (2.14)$$

$$\alpha_i \sim \mathrm{IND}(0, \sigma_a^2), \qquad \varepsilon_{ij} \sim \mathrm{IND}(0, \sigma^2).$$

Here μ denotes the overall mean for the infinite number of populations that could have been selected, and α_i denotes the effect of the ith population; these effects are independent and normally distributed with mean 0 and variance σ_a^2. The ε_{ij} are similarly independent and normally distributed with mean 0 and variance σ^2. The variances of random effects, such as σ_a^2 and σ^2, are known as *variance components*. For simplicity, we are restricting our discussion to the special case of equal sample size n from each of the populations sampled.

One consequence of this model is that the variance of each observation Y_{ij} is equal to the sum of the variance components, $\sigma_a^2 + \sigma^2$. The dependence between observations from the same sample can be measured in terms of the covariance σ_a^2 or in terms of their correlation, $\rho = \sigma_a^2/(\sigma_a^2+\sigma^2)$. (See Appendix A for derivations.) This correlation is often referred to as the *intraclass correlation* and provides a measure of how correlated (similar) the observations are within a particular population. Note that the intraclass correlation can range from 0 to 1. It assumes a value of 0 when $\sigma_a^2 = 0$; in this situation, observations sampled from one population are no more alike than observations sampled from all populations combined. It assumes a value of 1 when $\sigma^2 = 0$; in this extreme situation, there is no variation in observations drawn from the ith population, $i = 1, \ldots, a$.

2.2.3 Null Hypothesis: Test for Zero Variance of Population Means

For the random effects one-way ANOVA, the null hypothesis can be expressed as

$$H_0 : \sigma_a^2 = 0.$$

The null hypothesis specifies that there is no variation in outcome among all possible populations or levels of the factor. When there is an effect of the factor, $\sigma_a^2 > 0$.

For the vitamin C example, the null hypothesis is that technician has no effect on vitamin C determination. If this hypothesis were rejected, we would conclude that vitamin C determinations are influenced by who is making the determination, or that there was an effect of technician.

2.2.4 Estimation of Model Terms

With the random effects model, we are particularly interested in estimating the two parameters which are variance components: σ_a^2 and σ^2. These are frequently referred to as variance components. σ^2 is estimated as before, as the residual mean square, s^2. The estimate of $\sigma^2 + n\sigma_a^2$ is MS_a. Subtracting s^2 from MS_a and dividing by n, we estimate σ_a^2 by

$$s_a^2 = \frac{MS_a - s^2}{n}.$$

Note that using this method of estimation, it is possible that the estimate of the variance component σ_a^2 will be negative. This occurs when $\text{MS}_a < s^2$. Should this occur, σ_a^2 is generally reestimated as 0.

The intraclass correlation ρ may also be estimated by replacing the population parameters with their sample estimates, so

$$r = \frac{s_a^2}{s_a^2 + s^2}.$$

TABLE D.13. Dilemma data

Source: Hocking and Pendleton (1983)

CASE	X1	X2	X3	Y
1	12.980	0.317	9.998	57.702
2	14.295	2.028	6.776	59.296
3	15.531	5.305	2.947	56.166
4	15.133	4.738	4.201	55.767
5	15.342	7.038	2.053	51.722
6	17.149	5.982	-0.055	60.446
7	15.462	2.737	4.657	60.715
8	12.801	10.663	3.048	37.447
9	17.039	5.132	0.257	60.974
10	13.172	2.039	8.738	55.270
11	17.081	1.551	1.950	67.010
12	14.340	4.077	5.545	54.027
13	12.923	2.643	9.331	53.199
14	14.231	10.401	1.041	41.896
15	15.222	1.220	6.149	63.264
16	15.740	10.612	-1.691	45.798
17	14.958	4.815	4.111	58.699
18	18.225	3.224	-0.053	68.111
19	16.391	9.698	-1.714	48.890
20	16.452	3.912	2.145	62.213
21	13.535	7.625	3.851	45.625
22	14.199	4.474	5.112	53.923
23	15.837	5.753	2.087	55.799
24	14.123	0.578	-0.543	59.117
25	13.322	8.598	4.011	43.145
26	15.949	8.290	-0.248	50.706
27	16.565	8.546	8.974	55.112

same way as for the fixed effects model:
 OVA table and the F test are identical
 , the total variation is broken apart into
 he sums of squares, numbers of degrees
 lculated in the same way as before. The
 ual is the same as for the fixed effects
 es in the interpretation of the expected
 $_{1}^{2}$; here σ_a^2 represents the variance of the
 st just the a that were selected for study.
 square factor is σ^2; the expected mean
 less of whether $\sigma_a^2 = 0$. Thus, as with
 the expected factor mean square to the
 . For a given data set, the ratio of their
 $r_a^2 > 0$, the factor mean square estimates
 l hypothesis is rejected for large values

he F statistic follows an F distribution
 edom. When the null hypothesis is not
 tion which is a function of the F distri-
 $(\sigma^2 + n\sigma_a^2)/\sigma^2$ times the F distribution
 legrees of freedom. Since the constant
 lues of the calculated test statistic will
 l from the F distribution; the null hy-
 the test statistic. Greater detail can be

equal sample sizes here. Consideration
 of applying the one-way ANOVA model with random effects and unequal
sample sizes is available elsewhere [9].

2.3 DESIGNING AN OBSERVATIONAL STUDY OR EXPERIMENT

In designing a one-way ANOVA, several steps must be considered. The first
step is deciding on the objectives of the study. Some investigators find it useful
to write out ahead of time the statements they wish to make after the final
analysis is done. For example, in a study of lung function, an investigator
may want to determine the magnitude of the effect of smoking on healthy
forty-year-old males.

The lung function study is an observational study, since the investigators
cannot control who smokes. They simply observe the effects of smoking later.
In observational studies such as surveys, units are not randomized to treatments.

Alternatively, an investigator may be interested in effects of diet on a body's response to chemotherapy drugs. In one study, the effect of folate on levels of a metabolite in the liver of rats exposed to the chemotherapy drug cytotoxin was investigated (see Problem 2.1 for details). Rats were randomly assigned to diets that varied according to folate in the diet: standard rat chow, or chow that had been modified to contain low, medium, or high levels of folate. The objective of this study was to find out whether folate has an effect on mean metabolite levels, and if so, whether there is a trend of increasing mean metabolite level associated with increasing level of folate in the diet.

In an experiment, individual sampling units (such as persons, animals, or objects) are randomized to a treatment group. The factor is the treatment, and the levels of the factor correspond to the experimental groups. If there are a treatments of interest, then each unit is randomized to one of the a groups. The diet study described in the previous paragraph is an experiment, since the experimenter controls the treatments and the rats are randomly assigned to treatment groups. In the context of experimental studies, treatment is the factor or classification variable.

2.3.1 Randomization for Experimental Studies

Randomization to treatment groups can be done in several ways. One of the simplest is to use a random number table. In a random number table, numbers from 0 to 9 are arranged in a random order. If, for instance, there were three treatment groups, then sampling units could be assigned to treatment by taking successive random numbers between 1 and 9 assigning the unit to the first treatment if the chosen random number was a 1, 2, or 3; to the second treatment if it was 4, 5, or 6; and to the third treatment if it was 7, 8, or 9. Methods comparable to this are commonly used. For example, many software packages will do the same thing by producing numbers at random from a uniform random number generator. One difficulty with this method is that it does not ensure that each treatment group will have the same sample size. In order to accomplish that, some restriction on how the units are assigned is needed.

The second method can be most easily understood by using chips. Suppose again that three groups are desired and that the total sample size is 60. We take 60 chips and write 1 on 20 of them, 2 on 20 of them, and 3 on the remaining 20. Then we mix them up completely and randomly assign the chips to the sampling units. All sampling units given a chip labeled with a 1 are assigned to group 1, and so on. To get away from the physical use of chips, tables have been made of random permutations (orderings) [12]. Say a table of sets of numbers from 1 to 100 is given. Each number only appears once. The 100 distinct numbers in each set are in a random order. Again, suppose we want to have three treatment groups and want 20 in each. Each sampling unit is assigned a distinct number between 1 and 60. The sampling units with numbers that correspond to the first 20 numbers between 1 and 60 in the random permutation are assigned to the first treatment, the sampling units with numbers corresponding to the the next 20 numbers between 1 and 60 are assigned to the second treatment, and the remaining 20 sampling units are assigned to the third treatment. The results will be a random assignment of the units to the treatment groups with an equal number of units in each group.

In designing either an observational study or an experimental treatment study, if significant differences exist between the a groups, the investigators would like to be able say what caused them. If the units in the various groups differ in ways that affect the outcome variable being tested, then it is not possible to determine the cause of the differences from a one-way analysis of variance. The use of randomization in experiments is done in the hope that the treatment groups will be similar in all other ways than the treatment itself. In general this works, but in rare instances it is still possible that a particular treatment group sample will be different from the other treatment group samples prior to treatment. This is more apt to affect the results in cases where the individual units vary considerably from one another, for instance among people, than it is among laboratory animal or chemical compounds.

But clearly, the experiment is the better choice of the two. For example, earlier studies demonstrating the effectiveness of hormone replacement therapy in reducing risk factors for cardiovascular disease were *observational* in nature. That is, women who were taking the hormones were compared with women who were not taking them, but they were not randomized to treatment. In these studies, samples were drawn from populations of women who were and were not taking the therapy. Various authors have raised concerns that these populations were different with respect to other variables, such as lifestyle choices, access to medical care, and medical compliance [1, 6, 13, 19]. These authors, and others, urged caution in the interpretation of findings from the observational studies because it couldn't be determined from them whether differences in risk factors for cardiovascular disease were due to hormone replacement therapy or to other factors; *experimental* studies, with women randomized to different treatment groups, were needed.

Recent studies have been or are currently being conducted which randomize women to either receive or not receive hormone replacement therapy [18, 28, 20]. Any differences due to other factors (such as access to medical care and lifestyle choices) should be averaged out in the randomization. The Women's Health Initiative found that women randomized to taking hormone replacement therapy actually were at greater risk of experiencing coronary events than those who were randomized to a placebo [29]. The investigators concluded that the risks exceeded the benefits. (However, the issue has not been resolved to everyone's satisfaction [25].)

2.3.2   Sample Size and Power

Another important step concerns determining the size of the sample to be drawn from each of the populations. Ideally, this will help ensure that there is adequate power to detect a hypothesized difference in population means. *Power* is the probability of rejecting the null hypothesis of equality of means when in fact the means are unequal. High power is important because if the population means are unequal, one wants to be able to detect that.

There are a variety of ways to decide on what sample size is needed. One is on the basis of the power of the F test to detect a hypothesized difference in means (for the fixed effects model). Attention is given to the fixed effects model here. We go through an example for someone who has access to software that produces probabilities for a specified noncentral F distribution. Alternatively, the same results can also be obtained by using software packages specifically designed for computing sample size and power, such as nQuery [11] or more general packages such as SAS (starting with version 9). Tables that give the power for one-way ANOVA are also available [10]. More detailed treatment of sample size and power calculations for one-way ANOVA can be found elsewhere [7, 14, 27].

To perform sample size calculations, the following information must be specified: the level of significance, α (usually assumed to be 0.05), the desired power (usually assumed to be 0.80 or greater), the populations means μ_i, and variance σ^2.

The sample size calculations are only as good as the assumptions that go into them. It should be noted that minor differences in values assumed can have appreciable effects on sample size. For some practical guidelines, see [15, 24].

For the fixed effects model, the distribution of the calculated test statistic follows an F distribution with $\nu_1 = a - 1$ and $\nu_2 = N - a$ when the null hypothesis is true and follows a noncentral F distribution when it is not true, as described in Section 2.1.7. The noncentral F distribution depends on three parameters: ν_1, ν_2, and the noncentrality parameter λ, which is a function of the population means and the variance σ^2. The power of the F test corresponds to the area under the specified noncentral F distribution that is to the right of the $100(1 - \alpha)$th percentile of the corresponding F distribution (see Figure 2.4).

Example. Suppose plans are being made to conduct the lung function study and that the investigator believes that the means of the four populations are 4.2, 3.5, 3.4, and 3.3 (so the overall mean is 3.6) and that the variances of the four populations are 0.3. What sample size would be required in order for the power of the study to be 0.8 when a one-sided test at level of significance of 0.05 is specified?

The noncentrality parameter λ is estimated as $n[(4.2-3.6)^2+(3.5-3.6)^2+(3.4-3.6)^2+(3.3-3.6)^2]/0.3 = 1.87n$, as in Section 2.1.7. The power could be obtained using software which gives areas under the curve of a noncentral F distribution, something that is readily available in many statistical packages. Suppose we select $n = 6$. Then the power would be the probability that the F statistic falls in the critical region, $F > F_{0.95,3,20} = 3.1$ when the comparison distribution is the noncentral F with $\nu_1 = 3$, $\nu_2 = 20$, and $\lambda = 6(1.88) = 10$. Thus, the power is 0.67. When $n = 7$, so that the critical region is $F > F_{0.95,3,24} = 3.01$, we have $\lambda = 11.67$, and the power is 0.76. When $n = 8$, so that the critical region is $F > F_{0.95,3,28} = 2.95$, we have $\lambda = 13.33$, and the power is 0.83. Thus, given the assumptions about the means and variances, we need to sample at least 8 persons from each population in order to make sure that the power to detect the specified difference is at least 0.8.

Some general statements can be made about sample size. If the differences among the population means are large relative to the population residual mean squared error then a small sample size can be used. Likewise if the level of the significance chosen to perform the test is large. For example, if we choose an $\alpha = 0.01$ instead of $\alpha = 0.05$, we shall need to take a larger sample size to keep the power of the test the same.

Another aspect of the design of experiments is the decision on the number of treatment groups to use. Sometimes when investigators first find out that it is possible to test any number of treatment groups using ANOVA, they choose a large number of groups. Because of cost considerations, this may result in fewer observations in each group and the inability to reject the null hypothesis of equal means. Here it is useful to review the stated objectives of the study and use the smallest number of groups that allows those objectives to be met.

2.4 CHECKING IF THE DATA FIT THE ONE-WAY ANOVA MODEL

Recall the three assumptions of the fixed effects model that were made so that the distribution of the F statistic would follow an F distribution when the null hypothesis is true and the noncentral F distribution when the null hypothesis is not true: the observations under study from each population are normally distributed, the variances of the observations are equal, and all observations are independent. For the random effects model, the assumptions were: the observations under study from each population are normally distributed, the variances of the observations are equal, and all observations from one population are independent of all observations from another population. We will consider here how to check whether the data fit the ANOVA model. As discussed in Chapter 1, the observations should be checked for gross outliers before beginning the following procedures.

2.4.1   Normality

One method used as a visual check for normality consists in plotting the sample means of each treatment combination on the horizontal axis and the sample standard deviations (or sample variances) on the vertical axis. The mean and standard deviation (or variance) of a sample drawn from a normally distributed population are independent. Thus, when means and variances obtained from different samples are plotted, no relation between the two statistics should be apparent if the observations in the a populations are normally distributed. This is not the case for all distributions; we shall see in Section 2.5.1 that these plots can be suggestive of transformations to try so that the data provide a better fit to the underlying ANOVA model.

One benefit of using this procedure is that it allows us to take advantage of the fact that our observations have been separated into a groups. Its limitations are that with small sample sizes or with a small number of populations being compared, it can be difficult to decide whether or not there is some relation between the statistics.

In Chapter 1, we discussed evaluating normality in the context of a sample from a single population, through histograms, boxplots, or normal quantile plots. These procedures can be applied here separately for the samples drawn from the a populations. The only problem with doing this is that these procedures do not work well when the sample sizes are small in the treatment groups, as may be the case in one-way ANOVA.

For the fixed effects model, to increase the number of observations used in assessing normality, the investigator sometimes examines all of the residuals from the entire study, rather than working with the observations in each group. By residuals, we mean the difference between an observation and the estimate for the mean of the population from which it was drawn. As indicated above, the residual for Y_{ij} is calculated as $Y_{ij} - \bar{Y}_{i\cdot}$. Instead of examining histograms or boxplots, most investigators find it simpler to examine normal quantile plots of their residuals. The residuals will have a mean of zero and a standard deviation of s.

In Chapter 1, we also considered hypothesis tests, such as the Shapiro-Wilk test. This can also be applied for each sample separately. The drawback of applying tests such as these, using residuals, is that the residuals do not form a single random sample, since they are not all statistically independent of one another. Strictly speaking, then, the entire set of residuals does not satisfy the requirements for this test; in using residuals for the Shapiro-Wilk test, we have some uncertainty concerning the significance level.

For the lung function example, the normal quantile plot of the residuals is linear (Figure 2.5) and the value of the Shapiro-Wilk test statistic is 0.96 ($p = 0.51$); these suggest that the residuals are normally distributed, and that the FEV1 measurements come from populations that are normally distributed.

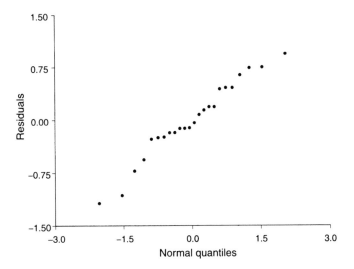

Fig. 2.5   Normal quantile plot of residuals for lung function example.

2.4.2   Equality of Population Variances

There are a variety of tests for equality of populations variances. The null hypothesis is $H_0 : \sigma_1^2 = \cdots = \sigma_a^2$ and the alternative hypothesis is that the population variances are not all equal. We will consider one such test here, Levene's test [16]. This test has the advantage that it is not dependent on the assumption that samples are drawn from normally distributed populations. It is frequently the case that unequal variances occur simultaneously with lack of normality. Thus, if data are decidedly skewed, tests that depend on the assumption of normality are not appropriate.

To perform Levene's test, the absolute value of each residual is computed for each factor level and a one-way ANOVA is performed. The F statistic is calculated and interpreted in exactly the same way as it was in the test for equality of means. Large values of the F statistic suggest that the population variances are unequal. When distributions of the observations are skewed, use of the absolute value of the deviation of an observation Y_{ij} from the median of the Y_{ij}'s is preferable, as the distribution of Levene's test statistic more closely follows an F distribution [5]. Some software packages will give users a choice of how to compute the test statistic.

For the lung function data, the calculated value of Levene's test statistic is 1.29 $(p = 0.30)$. This suggests that the variances of the FEV1 measurements may be equal.

2.4.3 Independence

In verifying the assumption of independence, there are two types we may wish to check — independence of observations within a single sample, and independence of observations between samples. Note that lack of independence within a sample is allowed in the random effects model, but not in the fixed effects model.

As with checking for independence within a sample (discussed in Chapter 1), it is difficult to decide whether observations are independent by looking at the data without investigating the actual study design. Investigation of independence serves as a check of one's knowledge of design.

One potential tip-off that there is lack of independence is a small F value. This occurs when MS_a is small in comparison with s^2. Suppose that an investigator made the first measurement (in the sense of time) in all the a samples, then went ahead and made the second measurement in all the a samples, and so on to the nth observation in each sample. If the equipment was drifting out of calibration so later measurements were larger than earlier ones and there was little or no difference among the treatment groups, the residual mean square MS_r could be larger than the factor variance. Of course, a small F can also occur by chance.

Lack of independence between the a groups can arise by design. Suppose measurements are made on a single group of patients at three time periods; one prior to an operation, one just before they leave the hospital, and one two months later. From the appearance of the data, this would look like a one-way ANOVA with three treatment groups. But the first observation in each of the three groups is made on the same person, so the observations are not independent. A different design (see Chapter 6, 8, or 9) is needed to analyze this sort of data.

Ideally, in a one-way ANOVA, all observations are made in random order, regardless of the particular treatment. Because this entails considerable effort, observations on one treatment combination are often made close together in time. Similarly, animals in a particular experiment are often caged close together. If equipment is drifting out of calibration, or if there is a time or space clustering effect, the observations and their residuals are likely to lack independence. As in the case of a single sample, if an ordering of observations is available, plots of the order versus the outcome measurement are useful in checking to see if the residuals are independent. Also, the serial correlation (i.e. the correlation between each observation and the observation adjacent to it in time or space) can be computed (see Section 1.3.4). If the observations are independent, the serial correlation is expected to be close to 0. When the observations are not dependent, the serial correlation is typically greater than 0, but, like all correlations, cannot exceed 1. Stronger dependence among observations is reflected in a higher serial correlation.

2.4.4   Robustness

We have considered how to assess departure from the assumptions. It is also important to consider whether it matters. An investigator should always consider the relative seriousness of departures from the assumptions. Considerable discussion of this matter has been published [21], but the following statements may serve as a rough guide.

Lack of independence can be the most serious, since it is usually impossible to correct and it invalidates the levels of significance. Nonnormality of the data is less serious than lack of independence; for nonnormality may be reduced by a transformation. Furthermore, small departures from normality usually do not have serious effects on the tests for equality of means. Inequality of variances is seldom serious if there are equal or nearly equal sample sizes in each group; it is also amenable to transformation. The effect of outliers depends on their size and number. Hence, outliers may be of only minor consequence, or they may completely change the results.

2.4.5   Missing Data

Missing data can sometimes cause violations of the assumptions of the one-way ANOVA model. A problem arises when samples do not represent the populations that were intended to be sampled. It may be that the population being sampled does not have mean $\mu + \alpha_i$ or variance σ^2.

To summarize, missing values are usually classified into one of three types [17]. When missing values are *missing completely at random* (MCAR), we assume that the observations that are missing are like the observations that are present. The fact that they are missing is a random event. For example, the observations could be randomly assigned to the treatment groups (factors), but by chance alone the numbers of observations in the treatment groups could be unequal. Or alternatively, a technician might just have happened to knock over a test tube so one of the results was not available. We can still assume that we have a random sample in the various treatment groups, since we can assume that being missed is independent of treatment group and the Y observation value.

The second type is called *missing at random* (MAR). Here, the values in each treatment group can be assumed to be missing at random in that treatment group but the chance of being missing varies by treatment group. In other words, one treatment group may have a greater chance of having missing values, but the values that are present are a random sample from the population of values for that group.

When the data are MAR or MCAR, the results for the one-way ANOVA can still be interpreted.

In the third type, the missing values differ in some fashion from those that are not missing. For example, suppose the instrument used to take the measurements only could measure up to a certain value. Then, all measurements larger than this value are missing. Alternatively, suppose the dose given for one treatment group was so high that it was toxic to the laboratory animals that received it and almost all of the animals died before the outcome Y was measured. Thus, the animals that survived may not be a random sample from the population of animals (the survivors are superhealthy). Means and variances that are computed from such a sample would be considered biased in the sense that they do not provide good estimates of the true population values. When this occurs, great caution should be used in interpreting the results.

2.5   WHAT TO DO IF THE DATA DO NOT FIT THE MODEL

If the data do not fit the model, several approaches may be taken: transforming the data so that the transformed data fit the model; performing a distribution-free test, in which the assumption of normality is not required; performing an alternative ANOVA test for which the assumption of equal variances is not required; or performing multiple two-sample t tests.

2.5.1   Making Transformations

As we mentioned in the previous section, for the normal distribution, the mean and variance (or standard deviation) of a sample are statistically independent. A transformation is sought that equalizes the variance regardless of the size of the mean. The first step in this procedure is to plot the sample means versus the sample variances and also versus the sample standard deviations of the separate treatment groups. Several schematic plots of this type appear in Figure 2.6.

Figure 2.6a shows a case of samples that are likely to be from normal populations, since the means and variances appear to be independent. In Figure 2.6b there seems to be a linear relation between the sample variances and the sample means; in Figure 2.6c the linear relation is between the standard deviation and the mean.

For the data graphed in Figure 2.6a, we decide that no transformation is necessary. For Figure 2.6b, the linear relation between the sample variance and sample mean suggests that the measurements follow a Poisson distribution. In this case, the following square root transformation is useful:

$$Y_i' = \sqrt{Y_i + A}.$$

As discussed in Chapter 1, this transformation is the appropriate one if the original data follow a Poisson distribution; count data or occurrence of rare events often do so [2, 3].

For Figure 2.6c, the linear relation between the sample standard deviation and sample mean suggest that the measurements follow a log normal distribution. A log transformation of the following general form may be useful:

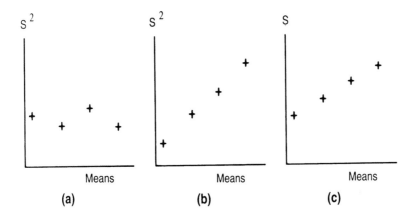

Fig. 2.6   Comparison of means with variances and standard deviations.

$$Y_i' = \log_{10}(Y_i + A).$$

Alternatively, normal quantile plots of the residuals can be examined. If the plot is not linear, then a transformation should be considered. As in Chapter 1, the shape of the normal quantile plot may suggest possible transformations.

2.5.2   Using Nonparametric Methods

Nonparametric, or distribution-free, methods do not require assumptions about the distribution of the observations. Thus, distribution-free alternatives to one-way ANOVA are not based on the assumption of normality. There are a variety of nonparametric alternatives, the most common being the Kruskal-Wallis test. The following is a very brief overview of this test. Greater detail can be found elsewhere [8]. Just as one-way ANOVA is an extension of the two sample t test, the Kruskal-Wallis test is an extension of the Wilcoxon rank sum test.

Assumptions associated with this test are that the observations in each group follow identical distributions, except for possible differences in medians (or means), and that all observations are independent.

The advantages of using this test are that it is not dependent on the assumption of normality and it is appropriate for ordinal data. The disadvantage is that, if the observations really are normally distributed, the power to detect differences in means will be slightly lower.

To compute the Kruskal-Wallis test, one ranks all of the observations from smallest (with a rank of 1) to largest (with a rank of $N = n_1 + \cdots + n_a$), regardless of the treatment group in which an observation falls. One performs one-way ANOVA on the ranked data. The test statistic is calculated as the ratio of the factor sum of squares to the mean square total (where the mean square total is total sum of squares / total df).

When the sample size is sufficiently large, the Kruskal-Wallis test statistic follows a χ^2_{a-1} distribution when the means of the a populations are equal. For small sample sizes, the exact distributions of the test statistics can be found in tables.

For the lung function example, the calculated value of the Kruskal-Wallis statistic is $W = 7.51$; the p value is 0.06. Note that the hypothesis of equality of means was rejected in the ANOVA but was not here.

In most situations, the conclusions from the nonparametric test are equivalent to those obtained from the one-way ANOVA. Practically, it isn't necessary to actually rank the observations and calculate the test statistic. Most software packages can easily compute this and other nonparametric statistics.

2.5.3 Using Alternative ANOVAs

A variety of modifications to the standard one-way ANOVA have been proposed, which are not dependent on the assumption of equality of variances. Examples are the Welch test [26] and the Brown-Forsythe test [4]. The expressions for the test statistic and the number of residual degrees of freedom are modified from the traditional ANOVA test, but both test statistics approximately follow an F distribution. These tests are not routinely available in statistical packages, although some do have them. Often, investigators will use these tests when they have unequal variances to check that they obtain similar results to the usual ANOVA test. If the results of the two tests are similar, the results of the standard ANOVA are presented.

2.6 PRESENTATION AND INTERPRETATION OF RESULTS

An important part of any statistical analyses is communicating to others what was done. Justification of the sample size or power is useful; it will let readers know that design had been considered prior to the onset of the study and is particularly useful if nonsignificant results are found.

There are a variety of ways investigators may choose to present the results of their data and ANOVAs. It's always a good idea to present some summary statistics and graphs; these should reflect the type of response variable (ordinal, interval, or ratio). They will help orient the reader as well as provide summary statistics for future sample size or power calculations.

If the response is an interval or ratio variable, means and standard deviations (or standard errors) are appropriate numerical summarizations. Bar charts with error bars can often provide a more vivid presentation of the same material. The error bars can be determined in a variety of ways. For example, standard deviations or standard errors can be chosen or the mean squared error or the sample variance for each group can be used in the calculations. The chosen style should reflect the information that is to be communicated. For example, error bars based on group-specific sample standard deviations are more appropriate if the standard deviations across the groups are unequal; otherwise the use of the square root of the mean squared error is probably a better choice. If sample sizes are equal across the groups, error bars based on the standard error are good; if sample sizes are unequal across groups, standard deviations are more appropriate.

In contrast, for ordinal data, and/or if a nonparametric ANOVA is used, presentations of medians, interquartile ranges, and boxplots provide greater consistency with the analyses.

In many cases, the assumptions are violated and it can be difficult to decide what to do. As we indicated earlier, the ANOVA test tends to be robust with respect to lack of normality and inequality of variances. Even so, it is important that the checks be made. One consequence of this robustness is that in many situations, the conclusions are the same regardless of which technique is used.

Transformations can often be found that reduce lack of normality or inequality of variances. If transformations have been made, conclusions must be made in terms of the transformed data. Frequently, an investigator must decide among using nontransformed data, using common statistical methods or presenting various alternatives. When the results are nearly independent of what method was used to present them, it's advantageous to focus on simplicity of methods and analyses, while reporting that more complex methods were investigated and found to be consistent. When the results depend on the methods, it is advantageous to use the results based on the transformed data, as the assumptions for the tests are then satisfied.

At a minimum, investigators should report their summary statistics and p values. Sometimes, the F statistic or the entire ANOVA table is presented. As we indicated earlier, if no significant differences in population means are found, the analysis does not proceed further. If significant differences are found, further work is done to identify the differences, as discussed in the following chapter.

2.7 SUMMARY

In this chapter, one of the most widely used ANOVA models has been introduced. One-way ANOVA allows the investigator to simultaneously analyze two or more (a) groups which differ with respect to a single classification variable or factor. We introduced the idea of an underlying model or equation that describes the data and the assumptions that are made. We discussed estimation of the population parameters. We described breaking the total variation in the observations into two parts: variation due to the factor, and residual variation. We motivated the F test for making inferences about the population means. When the fixed effects model is used, the results apply to tests concerning the means of the a populations. When the random effects model is used, the results apply not just to the a groups that were selected for study, but to groups that could have been selected. In most cases, the model being tested is the fixed effects model.

Methods of checking the assumptions were given, and it was pointed out that lack of independence is apt to be the most troublesome failure. For the fixed effects model, the test for equal means is quite robust to violations of the normality and equal variance assumptions.

Chapter 3 continues with further analyses for the fixed effects model. For example, if the hypothesis of equal population means is rejected, methods for determining how the means differ are explained. Tests for trends in the mean are presented. Confidence limits are also given.

Problems

2.1   Four chemicals were used to combat plant lice on sugar beets, each chemical being applied to one plot. Twenty-five leaves were picked from each plot, and the number of plant lice on each leaf was recorded. The data obtained were as follows:

Chemical	1	2	3	4	5	6	7	8	9	10	11	12	13
I	12	13	26	13	17	24	14	10	6	4	2	10	8
II	10	21	34	15	5	22	12	25	18	12	2	2	10
III	23	14	14	20	27	25	17	18	29	14	31	5	13
IV	32	26	24	16	32	18	33	16	34	18	29	14	31

Chemical	14	15	16	17	18	19	20	21	22	23	24	25
I	6	7	13	18	10	18	3	4	18	13	10	21
II	22	17	20	19	20	12	11	16	5	11	17	16
III	18	23	16	13	23	4	16	17	9	28	23	19
IV	30	18	25	20	21	27	31	25	33	24	16	24

Assume that $Y_{ij} = \mu + \alpha_i + \varepsilon_{ijk}$, where $\sum_{i=1}^{4} \alpha_i = 0$ and $\varepsilon_{ijk} \sim \text{IND}(0, \sigma^2)$.

a)   Determine point estimates of the following population parameters: (i) the overall mean number of plant lice per leaf for the four chemicals, i.e. μ; (ii) $\mu + \alpha_1$, the mean for the first chemical; (iii) $\mu + \alpha_2$, the mean for the second chemical; (iv) $\mu + \alpha_3$, the mean for the third chemical; (v) $\mu + \alpha_4$, the mean for the fourth chemical; (vi) σ^2.

b)   Obtain the ANOVA table, and test at $\alpha = 0.05$ whether differences exist in the population mean number of lice among the four chemicals.

c)   Verify that the mean squared residual obtained from the ANOVA table is equal to the mean of the sample variances calculated for each of the four samples.

d)   Construct a normal quantile plot for each of the four distributions of numbers of plant lice. Does the assumption of normal distributions seem satisfied?

2.2   IQ scores were recorded for 20 girls classified into two equal groups according to the economic status of their parents. There were 10 girls in each group, and the scores were as follows:

High Status	Low Status
124	113
114	97
115	108
106	95
84	105
96	69
106	113
126	98
124	118
116	70

a)   Would a fixed or random effects model be appropriate for these data? State the model.

b)   Make an F test of $H_0 : \mu_1 = \mu_2$.

c)   Perform a (two-sided) two-sample t test of $H_0 : \mu_1 = \mu_2$.

d)   Verify the following relation between the two calculated test statistics: $F = t^2$. What other correspondences do you see between the two tests? Consider degrees of freedom, p values, and so on.

2.3   Twenty-four rats were sent to a research oncologist. He randomly assigned six of them to each of four rat chows (1 = standard, 2 = low folate, 3 = medium folate, and 4 = high folate). One outcome of interest was the concentration of a metabolite in the liver, measured in micromoles per milligram of tissue. The data are available on the Wiley ftp site.

a)   State the underlying model.

b)   Write out instructions for a technician to follow to randomize 25 rats to four treatments. Assume the technician is not familiar with randomization.

c)   Summarize the data in graphical and tabular form. What can you say about your summaries?

d)   Make a plot of sample variances versus sample means and a plot of sample standard deviations versus sample means. Do these plots suggest whether or not the data should be transformed using a log or a square root transformation?

   e)   Construct a normal quantile plot for the residuals. Does it appear that they are normally distributed?

   f)   Test for equality of variances. What is your conclusion?

   g)   Test the hypothesis of equal mean metabolite across the four groups at $\alpha = 0.05$. What is your conclusion?

   h)   Perform the Kruskal-Wallis test. Compare the conclusion from this test with the one-way analysis of variance test. Which of the two would you prefer to present? Why?

2.4   The experiment described in Problem 2.3 was repeated, with each group of rats also receiving 50 micromoles per kilogram of body weight of the chemotherapy drug cytoxin. As before, the investigator randomly assigned six rats to each of the four treatments. One of the rats in the high folate group died and data were not available from it. Repeat Problem 2.3, excluding part (b). Note the very low F value and high p value obtained with this dose of chemotherapy. What more information would you want to know about the experiment to help in interpreting the findings?

2.5   For the cardiac rehabilitation data set (introduced in Problem 1.4), perform the following analyses. Data are available on the Wiley ftp site.

   a)   Test for equality of mean age for different diagnostic categories.

   b)   Test for effects of gender on self-reported physical functioning.

   c)   Test for effects of age group (< 60 versus ≥ 60)

   d)   Write up the results of the three analyses.

2.6   At company A, fertilizer formulated for use in vegetable gardens is made in batches. The quality control analyst wants to test if there is a significant difference in the percentage of total nitrogen from batch to batch. A random sample of four batches is chosen and six bags of fertilizer are randomly selected from each batch. The results are as follows:

	Batch		
1	2	3	4
10.46	11.02	9.52	10.56
10.06	10.24	9.99	9.73
11.35	9.50	10.86	11.23
9.65	10.44	10.21	10.01
9.53	11.39	9.90	10.42
10.23	9.74	11.03	9.07

   a)   What model will you use to perform the ANOVA?

b)   Perform the ANOVA and state your results in the context of the model you assumed.

c)   Use Levene's test to determine if the variances for the four batches are equal.

2.7   Investigators are concerned about the reliability of a new device to measure systolic blood pressure: will repeated measures obtain the same or similar results? A random sample of six normal subjects is taken, and each subject has their systolic blood pressure measured four times using the device. Suitable rest periods between measurements are taken, so there is no reason to assume there is a time effect. The results are as follows:

		Patient			
1	2	3	4	5	6
121	140	112	127	130	127
120	134	117	124	131	122
123	137	116	125	128	130
128	133	116	129	134	126

A colleague mentions that the reliability can be estimated by computing the intraclass correlation. Perform a random effects model ANOVA and compute the intraclass correlation. Does the device appear to be reliable?

REFERENCES

1. Barrett-Connor, E. [1991].   Postmenopausal Estrogen and Prevention Bias, *Annals of Internal Medicine,* 115, 455–456.

2. Box, G.E.P. and Cox, D.R. [1964]. Analysis of Transformations, *Journal of the Royal Statistical Society, Series B.* 26, 211–252.

3. Box, G.E.P., Hunter, W.G., and Hunter, J.S. [1978]. *Statistics for Experimenters,* New York: Wiley, 144–145.

4. Brown, M.B. and Forsythe, A.B. [1974]. The Small Sample Behavior of Some Statistics Which Test the Equality of Several Means, *Technometrics,* 16, 129–132.

5. Brown, M.B. and Forsythe, A.B. [1974]. Robust Tests for the Equality of Variances, *Journal of the American Statistical Association,* 69, 364–367.

6. Chae, C.U., Ridker, P.M., and Manson, J.E. [1997].   Postmenopausal Hormone Replacement Therapy and Cardiovascular Disease, *Thrombosis and Haemostasis,* 78, 770–780.

7. Cohen, J. [1988]. *Statistical Power Analysis for the Behavioral Sciences,* Hillsdale, NJ: Lawrence Elbaum Associates.

8. Conover, W.J. [1999]. *Practical Nonparametric Statistics,* New York: John Wiley & Sons, 288–297.

9. Dean, A. and Voss, D. [1999]. *Design and Analysis of Experiments,* New York: Springer-Verlag, 596–603, 610–614, 616–618.

10. Dixon, W.J. and Massey, F.M. [1983]. *Introduction to Statistical Analysis,* New York: McGraw-Hill.

11. Elashoff, J. D. [2002]. *nQuery Advisor Version 5.0 User's Guide,* Saugus, MA: Statistical Solutions.

12. Fleiss, J.L. [1986]. *The Design and Analysis of Clinical Experiments,* New York: John Wiley & Sons, 47–51.

13. Grodstein, F. [1996]. Can Selection Bias Explain the Cardiovascular Benefits of Estrogen Replacement Therapy? *American Journal of Epidemiology,* 143, 979–982.

14. Kraemer, H.C. and Thiemann, S. [1987]. *How Many Subjects?* Newbury Park, CA: Sage Publications, Inc., 38–52.

15. Lenth, R.V. [2001]. Some Practical Guidelines for Effective Sample Size Determination, *The American Statistician,* 55, 187–193.

16. Levene, H. [1960]. Robust Tests for Equality of Variances, in Olkin, I., editor, *Contributions to Probability and Statistics,* Palo Alto, CA: Stanford University Press, 278–292.

17. Little, R.J.A. and Rubin, D.B. [1987]. *Statistical Analysis with Missing Data,* New York: John Wiley & Sons, 3–96.

18. Manson, J.E., Hsia, J., Johnson, K.C., Rossouw, J.E., Assaf, A.R., Lasser, N.L., Trevisan, M., Black, H.R., Heckbert, S.R., Detrano, R., Strickland, O.L., Wong, N.D., Crouse, J.R., Stein, E., and Cushman, M. for the Women's Health Initiative Investigators. [2003]. Estrogen Plus Progestin and the Risk of Coronary Heart Disease. *New England Journal of Medicine,* 349, 523–534.

19. Matthews, K.A., Kuller, L.H., Wing, R.R., Meilahn, E.N., and Plantinga, P. [1996]. Prior to Use of Estrogen Replacement Therapy, Are Users Healthier than Nonusers? *American Journal of Epidemiology,* 143, 971–978.

20. Matthews, K.A., Shumaker, S.A., Bowen, D.J., Langer, R.D., Hunt, J.R., Kaplan, R.M., Klesges, R.C., and Ritenbaugh, C. [1997]. Women's Health

Initiative. Why Now? What Is It? What's New? *American Psychologist*, 52, 101–116.

21. Miller, R.J. [1986]. *Beyond ANOVA: Basics of Applied Statistics*, New York: John Wiley & Sons, 67–111.

22. Schenker, N. and Gentleman, J.F. [2001]. On Judging the Significance of Differences by Examining the Overlap between Confidence Intervals, *The American Statistician*, 55, 182–186.

23. Selvin, S. [1998]. *Modern Applied Biostatistical Methods Using S-PLUS*, New York: Oxford University Press, 361–384.

24. Taylor, D.J. and Muller, K.E. [1995]. Computing Confidence Bounds for Power and Sample Size of the General Linear Univariate Model, *The American Statistician*, 49, 43–47.

25. Thacker, H.L. [2002]. The Case for Hormone Replacement: New Studies That Should Inform the Debate, *Cleveland Clinic Journal of Medicine*, 69, 670–671.

26. Welch, B. L. [1951]. On the Comparison of Several Mean Values: An Alternative Approach, *Biometrika*, 38, 330–336.

27. Winer, B. J. [1971]. *Statistical Principles in Experimental Design*, New York: McGraw-Hill Co., 167–170, 220–228.

28. The Writing Group for the PEPI Trial [1995]. Effects of Estrogen or Estrogen/Progestin Regimens on Heart Disease Risk Factors in Postmenopausal Women, *JAMA*, 273, 199–208.

29. Writing Group for the Women's Health Initiative Investigators [2002]. Risks and Benefits of Estrogen Plus Progestin in Healthy Postmenopausal Women. Principal Results From the Women's Health Initiative Randomized Controlled Trial. *JAMA*, 288, 321–333.

3

Estimation and Simultaneous Inference

In Chapter 2, we presented an overall test of whether differences exist among several population means, but it should be emphasized that preparation of the ANOVA table and performance of the F test by no means complete the analysis. In the context of the previous chapter, the investigator's purpose was not just to decide whether the mean FEV1s of the four populations are equal, but rather to estimate various differences among the means. For example, the investigators may be interested in estimating the means of the four different populations ($\mu + \alpha_i = \mu_i$). Or they may wish to estimate the difference in lung volume between each population of smokers and the population of nonsmokers ($\mu_2 - \mu_1$, $\mu_3 - \mu_1$, $\mu_4 - \mu_1$). Or they may wish to estimate the difference between any two populations, $\mu_3 - \mu_4$, for example.

The objective is to determine which means are different, or how the level of the factor affects mean response. In order to do this, we need to consider not only how to estimate population means (as in Chapter 2), but also how to estimate the variability of the estimates. Furthermore, we need to consider how to estimate linear combinations of the population means, such as $\mu_1 - \mu_2$, and how to estimate their variability. These estimates are of interest in themselves, but they are also used for making inferences, or drawing conclusions, about the a different populations. The inference may be in terms of confidence intervals (emphasized here) or of hypothesis testing. The term *simultaneous statistical inference* is sometimes applied to the procedures of making multiple inferences from a single investigation. For example, besides investigating whether μ_1 and μ_2 are equal, we may also want to investigate the equality of μ_1 and μ_3 or of μ_2 and μ_3.

Sometimes, researchers are concerned about statistical problems that can arise when many simultaneous inferences are made from one investigation. When they wish to make adjustments, the methods for constructing the confidence intervals or performing the tests are referred to as *multiple comparison procedures*.

In Section 3.1 we define the point, variance, and interval estimates for population means considered one at a time. In Section 3.2, we introduce estimation of linear combinations of means, called *contrasts*, and discuss estimation of variances and standard errors of the sample contrasts. This is followed by a consideration of simultaneous statistical inference in Section 3.3. Here, we examine the straightforward methods of simultaneous statistical inference, provide reasons why there may be problems with this approach, and finally consider three difference multiple comparison procedures: the Bonferroni, the Tukey, and the Scheffé. In Section 3.4, inference for variance components estimated when effects are random rather than fixed is introduced. Some things to keep in mind when selecting a multiple comparison method and when presenting and summarizing results are given in Section 3.5. The chapter is summarized in Section 3.6. We will continue illustrating these ideas with the lung function example introduced in Chapter 2.

3.1   ESTIMATION FOR SINGLE POPULATION MEANS

3.1.1   Parameter Estimation

In Chapter 2, we considered the estimation of parameters of the one-way ANOVA model. So, for example, we discussed the estimation of the population means, μ_1, μ_2, μ_3, and μ_4. The corresponding point estimates were $\bar{Y}_{1.}$, $\bar{Y}_{2.}$, $\bar{Y}_{3.}$, $\bar{Y}_{4.}$. We now wish to determine their variability.

Variances of the estimates can be obtained by noting that the $\bar{Y}_{i.}$'s are linear combinations of the individual Y_{ij}'s, so for example

$$\bar{Y}_{i.} = \frac{Y_{i1} + Y_{i2} + \cdots + Y_{in_i}}{n_i}. \tag{3.1}$$

The variance of $\bar{Y}_{i.}$ can be obtained by applying the rules for taking the variance of a linear combination (see Appendix A). Since all of the observations are assumed to be independent and have the same variance σ^2,

$$\text{Var}(\bar{Y}_{i.}) = \frac{\sigma^2}{n_i}. \tag{3.2}$$

The *standard error* of $\bar{Y}_{i.}$ is the standard deviation of $\bar{Y}_{i.}$, or $\sigma/\sqrt{n_i}$. The larger the sample size, the smaller the standard error of the sample mean.

How should σ be estimated? We really have two choices. One is to use the sample standard deviation of the ith sample, s_i. Alternatively, if we assume our one-way ANOVA model is appropriate, so that the a populations have the same variance, then the pooled estimate of the standard deviation, s (i.e., the square root of the mean square residual obtained from the ANOVA table) is preferable; this estimate is computed from more observations (i.e., more degrees of freedom), and it is a more precise estimate.

In many journal articles, particularly those reporting results of laboratory experiments, graphs of means with error bars, called *error bar charts* are presented. The sample mean is plotted on the Y axis, and the factor levels are identified on the X axis. Bars at plus and minus one estimated standard error away from the mean are drawn. Most commonly, for the sample mean $\bar{Y}_{i.}$, the standard error is estimated as $s_i/\sqrt{n_i}$; however, as discussed above, it is preferable to estimate it as $s/\sqrt{n_i}$. The standard error reflects the variability of the sample mean. Some prefer to use upper and lower confidence limits for the population mean. If the purpose of the error bar chart is to communicate something about the sample mean and its variability, then use of standard errors or confidence intervals is appropriate. Some investigators (mistakenly) prefer to report standard errors rather than standard deviations because the standard errors (of the $\bar{Y}_{i.}$) are smaller than the standard deviations of Y and thus the results somehow appear more accurate. (In Chapter 2, we presented an error bar chart in which bars at plus and minus one estimated standard deviation were drawn. That graph was used to communicate something about the variability of the lung function measurements, not the variability of the sample means.)

Example. For the lung function example introduced in Chapter 2, the sample means and standard errors estimated as $s_i/\sqrt{n}$ and as $s/\sqrt{n}$ are presented in Table 3.1. The sample means are referred to as point estimates of the population means; they were presented earlier in Table 2.1. The standard error of each sample mean, $\sigma/\sqrt{n}$ is estimated in two ways. For one way, the estimated standard deviation of the $n = 6$ lung function measures (s_i) was used to estimate σ. For the second way, the estimated standard deviation of the FEV1's was based on all $N = 24$ observations and computed as the square root of the pooled sample variance. The s_i^2 and s^2 were given in Table 2.1. For example, he mean squared error MS_r, or s^2, is equal to 0.34.

3.1.2 Confidence Intervals

Going back to the one-way ANOVA model in Chapter 2, recall that we assumed that the individual observations from the ith population were normally distributed with mean μ_i and variance σ^2. We can use this information to say something about the distribution of $\bar{Y}_{i.}$. In particular,

$$\bar{Y}_{i.} \sim \text{IND}\left(\mu_i, \frac{\sigma^2}{n_i}\right). \tag{3.3}$$

Table 3.1 Sample Means and Estimated Standard Errors for FEV1 by the Four Smoking Categories

Category	Parameter	Point Estimate, $\bar{Y}_{i.}$	Estimate of $\sigma/\sqrt{n}$ $s_i/\sqrt{n}$	$s/\sqrt{n}$
Nonsmokers	μ_1	4.22	0.23	0.24
Early smokers	μ_2	3.94	0.10	0.24
Recent smokers	μ_3	3.46	0.29	0.24
Current smokers	μ_4	3.22	0.28	0.24

That is, each sample mean is normally distributed with mean μ_i and variance σ^2/n_i.

We also stated in the previous chapter that when our one-way ANOVA model is assumed, s^2 is an estimate of σ^2 and $(N-a)s^2/\sigma^2$ has a χ^2 distribution with $\nu = N - a$ degrees of freedom. Furthermore, each $\bar{Y}_{i.}$ and s^2 are statistically independent. These statements allow us to formulate a $1 - \alpha$ level confidence interval for each μ_i:

$$\bar{Y}_{i.} \pm t_{[1-\alpha/2;\nu]}\sqrt{\frac{s^2}{n_i}}. \qquad (3.4)$$

As is usually the case, we compute a $100(1-\alpha)\%$ confidence interval by taking a point estimate plus or minus the product of two terms. One is the $1 - \alpha/2$ percentile of a t distribution with degrees of freedom corresponding to the degrees of freedom used in the estimation of σ^2 (here $\nu = N - a$), and the other is the estimated standard error of the point estimate.

We may be inclined to examine the confidence intervals for individual means and see if they overlap as a method of testing for equality of population means. If they do not overlap, then the conclusion would be that the means are not equal; if they do, we would conclude that the means may be equal. However, this is not recommended [3, 13]. Compared with conventional methods (described below), the procedure has *lower power*, that is, if the population means are unequal, it is more difficult to detect it. Furthermore, it is *more conservative*: the level of significance α is smaller than what the investigators believe they have specified (usually 0.05), or, the level of confidence, $1 - \alpha$, is greater than specified. This method performs most poorly when standard errors are equal — the situation that arises when an ANOVA model is assumed and equal sample sizes are used for all populations.

Thus, estimating confidence intervals for individual population means is appropriate if the objective is to determine interval estimates for the means. These intervals should not be used for testing equality of means.

Example. Suppose we wish to construct 95% confidence intervals for μ_1, μ_2, μ_3, and μ_4. The critical value of t is the 97.5 percentile of a t distribution with $\nu = 20$ degrees of freedom, or 2.086. The estimated standard error, as shown in Table 3.1, is 0.24. The length of each confidence interval is the same: $2(2.086 \times 0.24)$, or 0.50. The interval for the ith population mean is centered about the ith sample mean. The 95% confidence intervals can be viewed graphically, as in Figure 3.1, or summarized as follows:

$$
\begin{aligned}
3.72 &\leq \mu_1 \leq 4.72, \\
3.44 &\leq \mu_2 \leq 4.44, \\
2.96 &\leq \mu_3 \leq 3.96, \\
2.72 &\leq \mu_4 \leq 3.72.
\end{aligned}
\tag{3.5}
$$

We are 95% confident that the mean FEV1 is between 3.72 and 4.72 for the nonsmokers. The interval gives us a plausible range within which the true population mean μ_1 is found. A computed interval either covers or does not cover μ_1. It is not correct to say that the probability is 0.95 that μ_1 falls within this interval. Rather, if we were to repeatedly draw samples of size $n = 6$ from the four populations, 95% of the intervals would cover μ_1. Similar statements can be made for the three other populations.

In this particular example, the confidence intervals all overlapped, but we would not want to conclude that the mean FEV1 of the four populations are equal.

An alternative strategy for estimating relationships among means from different populations involves estimating linear combinations of the means; this is the subject of the Sections 3.2 and 3.3.

3.2 ESTIMATION FOR LINEAR COMBINATIONS OF POPULATION MEANS

A *linear combination* of a population means is of the general form

$$
c_1\mu_1 + c_2\mu_2 + \cdots + c_a\mu_a,
\tag{3.6}
$$

where the c's are constants and the μ's represent unknown population means which must be estimated.

A *contrast* of a population means is a linear combination

$$c_1\mu_1 + c_2\mu_2 + \cdots + c_a\mu_a \tag{3.7}$$

where $\sum_{i=1}^{a} c_i = 0$. Contrasts are of interest because they relate to inferences which an investigator wishes to make. Commonly used approaches for making the inferences involve estimating a contrast and its corresponding estimated standard error. These can then be used for confidence interval estimation or for hypothesis testing, as described in Section 3.3.

3.2.1 Differences of Two Population Means

One of the simplest contrasts is that for the difference of two population means. Paired differences are particularly of interest when the factor that distinguishes them is qualitative. Examples include exposure categories (such as smoking histories or drugs), or diagnostic categories (for medical applications), or different cultivars or insecticides (in agriculture).

Suppose investigators wish to compare the means μ_1 and μ_2. They can specify the difference of the means as $\mu_1 - \mu_2$ or as $\mu_2 - \mu_1$. Suppose there are $a = 4$ populations altogether, so that the contrast is $1 \cdot \mu_1 + (-1) \cdot \mu_2 + 0 \cdot \mu_3 + 0 \cdot \mu_4 = \mu_1 - \mu_2$. The coefficients associated with each of the four population means are $c_1 = 1$, $c_2 = -1$, $c_3 = 0$ and $c_4 = 0$. (Note that the sum of the four coefficients is $1 - 1 + 0 + 0 = 0$.)

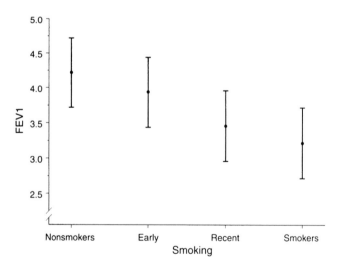

Fig. 3.1 95% confidence intervals for FEV1 by smoking category.

Table 3.2 Contrast Coefficients for All Possible Pairings of $a = 4$ Population Means

Paired Difference	c_1	c_2	c_3	c_4
$\mu_1 - \mu_2$	1	-1	0	0
$\mu_1 - \mu_3$	1	0	-1	0
$\mu_1 - \mu_4$	1	0	0	-1
$\mu_2 - \mu_3$	0	1	-1	0
$\mu_2 - \mu_4$	0	1	0	-1
$\mu_3 - \mu_4$	0	0	1	-1

Suppose investigators want to estimate paired differences in means for all possible pairings of the populations. If there are a factor levels, then there will be $a(a-1)/2$ paired differences. Table 3.2 gives the contrast coefficients for all possible pairing of means when $a = 4$. Let's focus on $\mu_i - \mu_j$. This is a linear combination of the means for categories i and j. The corresponding point estimate is

$$\bar{Y}_{i.} - \bar{Y}_{j.}.$$

The variance of this linear combination (assuming equal variances σ^2) is

$$\text{Var}(\bar{Y}_{i.}) + \text{Var}(\bar{Y}_{j.}) = \frac{\sigma^2}{n_i} + \frac{\sigma^2}{n_j},$$

which is estimated as

$$s^2 \left(\frac{1}{n_i} + \frac{1}{n_j} \right).$$

Note that when the n_i are not equal, the estimated standard errors can be large for small sample sizes; in these situations, it is possible that the sample means are quite far apart but the population means cannot be declared statistically unequal. If the sample sizes in the two groups are equal (to n), then the variance estimate reduces to $2s^2/n$. The estimated standard error is the square root of the variance estimate.

Example. Suppose we want to estimate the differences in means and their corresponding estimated standard errors for the six possible pairs of smoking categories. The sample means are given in Table 3.1. Because the sample sizes are constant, the estimated standard errors of the differences in sample means are all equal to $\sqrt{2s^2/n} = \sqrt{2 \times 0.34/6} = \sqrt{0.11} = 0.34$. The point estimates and estimated standard errors for all possible paired differences are given in Table 3.3.

Table 3.3   Paired Differences for Mean FEV1: Parameters, Point Estimates, Standard Errors

Smoking Categories	Parameter	Point Estimate	Standard Error
Nonsmokers − early smokers	$\mu_1 - \mu_2$	0.28	0.34
Nonsmokers − recent smokers	$\mu_1 - \mu_3$	0.76	0.34
Nonsmokers − current smokers	$\mu_1 - \mu_4$	1.00	0.34
Early smokers − recent smokers	$\mu_2 - \mu_3$	0.48	0.34
Early smokers − current smokers	$\mu_2 - \mu_4$	0.72	0.34
Recent smokers − current smokers	$\mu_3 - \mu_4$	0.24	0.34

3.2.2   General Contrasts for Two or More Means

In some investigations, there are contrasts that are of greater interest or appropriateness than paired differences. For example, suppose there are $a = 4$ factor levels in an experiment with the first level corresponding to a control and the three other levels corresponding to three different treatments. Interest may be in determining whether there is any difference in the mean response for the control versus the other three treatments. About which linear combination of means would inference be made? An appropriate linear contrast is $\mu_1 - (\mu_2 + \mu_3 + \mu_4)/3$; here, the coefficients are $c_1 = 1$, $c_2 = -\frac{1}{3}$, $c_3 = -\frac{1}{3}$, $c_4 = -\frac{1}{3}$, which sum to zero. A confidence interval for this contrast, which does not cover 0, would indicate that the mean response for the control was not equal to the mean response of the three treatments.

The general contrast of a population means, $c_1\mu_1 + c_2\mu_2 + \cdots + c_a\mu_a$, is estimated by the contrast of the sample means,

$$c_1 \bar{Y}_{1.} + c_2 \bar{Y}_{2.} + \cdots + c_a \bar{Y}_{a.}. \tag{3.8}$$

The variance of this general contrast of sample means is

$$c_1^2 \frac{\sigma^2}{n_1} + c_2^2 \frac{\sigma^2}{n_2} + \cdots + c_a^2 \frac{\sigma^2}{n_a} = \sigma^2 \sum_{i=1}^{a} \frac{c_i^2}{n_i}. \tag{3.9}$$

Note that when the sample sizes are all equal to n, the variance reduces simply to $\sum_{i=1}^{a} c_i^2 \sigma^2 / n$.

The estimated variance is obtained by replacing the unknown variance σ^2 by its estimate MS_r, or s^2:

$$c_1^2 \frac{s^2}{n_1} + c_2^2 \frac{s^2}{n_2} + \cdots + c_a^2 \frac{s^2}{n_a} = s^2 \sum_{i=1}^{a} \frac{c_i^2}{n_i} \tag{3.10}$$

The estimated standard error is the square root of the variance estimate given in Equation 3.10. Throughout the rest of this chapter, the estimated standard error for a linear combination is expressed as

$$\text{se}\left(\sum_{i=1}^{a} c_i \bar{Y}_{i.}\right) = s\sqrt{\sum_{i=1}^{a} \frac{c_i^2}{n_i}}. \qquad (3.11)$$

3.2.3   General Contrasts for Trends

Alternatively, suppose a factor is a continuous variable but it is categorized when the investigator selects fixed levels. Examples include age groupings, dosages of a single drug, levels of insecticide. In this situation, we may wish to investigate the relationship between the factor levels and the mean response. One frequently used approach to describe the relationship between mean response and the ordered categories is to consider various polynomial relationships. Is there a linear relation between the ordered factor levels and mean responses? What about quadratic or cubic relationships? When $a = 4$, we can consider $a - 1 = 3$ trends: linear, quadratic, and cubic. The coefficients that are used for contrasts which define trends are examples of *orthogonal coefficients*. They depend on a and have the characteristic that for any two of the contrasts, the sum of the products of the c_i's is 0. This characteristic implies that the estimated contrasts are uncorrelated. When there is an *equal interval* between the levels of the factor and the sample sizes are equal for each level, the coefficients are integers; Table 3.4 gives these coefficients for $a = 4$. Note that there is a constant difference (of two) between the coefficients -3, -1, 1, 3 and there is one change in their sign. Similarly, the sign of the coefficients changes twice for the quadratic trend, and three times for the cubic trend [14]. We can verify that the contrasts for linear and quadratic trends are orthogonal by computing the sum of the products: $(-3)(1) + (-1)(-1) + (1)(-1) + (3)(1) = 0$. Coefficients for a between 2 and 5 are provided in Table 9.5. Since not all statistical packages will routinely estimate these trends and their estimated standard errors, the user may have to supply these coefficients in order to obtain the desired contrasts.

Table 3.4 Orthogonal Contrasts for Assessing Polynomial Relationships between Mean Response and $a = 4$ Ordered Levels of a Factor

Trend	c_1	c_2	c_3	c_4
Linear	-3	-1	1	3
Quadratic	1	-1	-1	1
Cubic	-1	3	-3	1

As an example of a contrast that is not a difference in two means, let's consider the estimation of a linear trend for $a = 4$ factor levels in detail. Here, we assume that the factor levels are interval data (continuous data with equal intervals). Examples are ages, temperature, and doses. To make an inference about a linear trend, which linear combination of means should be used? A frequently specified linear contrast is $-3\mu_1 - \mu_2 + \mu_3 + 3\mu_4$; that is, a contrast with coefficients $c_1 = -3$, $c_2 = -1$, $c_3 = 1$, $c_4 = 3$, which sum to zero. The linear contrast of sample means is $-3\bar{Y}_1. - \bar{Y}_2. + \bar{Y}_3. + 3\bar{Y}_4.$. Suppose the sample means in the four groups are all the same; the calculated value of the contrast is then 0. Suppose all the sample means are positive and there is a trend of higher sample mean response associated with higher levels of the factor. The calculated value of the contrast will tend to be positive, and a confidence interval will tend to be above 0. Similarly, suppose all the same means are positive and there is a trend of lower sample mean response associated with higher levels of the factor. The calculated value of the contrast will tend to be negative and a confidence interval will tend to fall below 0. Thus, for making inferences about a linear trend, the linear contrast of population means $-3\mu_1 - \mu_2 + \mu_3 + 3\mu_4$ is reasonable. The estimated contrast will tend to be close to zero when there is no linear trend and to be away from 0 when there is a linear trend. A confidence interval for the contrast of population means which does not cover 0 would be indicative of a linear trend. The estimated variance associated with this estimate, applying Equation 3.10, is $s^2[(-3)^2/n + (-1)^2/n + 1^2/n + 3^2/n]$. The estimated standard error is the square root of this estimated variance.

If the absolute value of the contrast relative to its standard error is large, we conclude that a linear trend is apparent. If a confidence interval for the population contrast does not include 0, this also implies the presence of a linear trend. The same statement applies for quadratic and cubic trends. We discuss inferences about population contrasts in Section 3.3.

Using similar reasoning, we can also explain why using the contrast $\mu_1 - \mu_2 - \mu_3 + \mu_4$ is appropriate for quadratic trends and why the contrast $-\mu_1 + 3\mu_2 - 3\mu_3 + \mu_4$ is appropriate for cubic trends. We will return to orthogonal contrasts in Chapter 9.

3.3 SIMULTANEOUS STATISTICAL INFERENCE

The primary ways to go about making statistical inferences for contrasts of population means involve performing hypothesis tests and constructing confidence intervals. Frequently we want to make inferences about multiple contrasts. The procedure of making multiple contrasts can be referred to as *simultaneous statistical inference*. There have been numerous procedures proposed for doing this, and equally numerous recommendations about what an analyst should or should not do. In this book, we will give some of the alternatives which have been proposed and give some notion of what the problems are.

Most statistical software packages will perform many of the proposed techniques. Indeed, software documentation can be an excellent resource [11]. The book by Milliken and Johnson [10] also provides a good summary. Thoughtful discussions of the subject can also be found in [1, 2, 4, 5, 8, 12], among many others.

None of the multiple comparison procedures described in this chapter depends on a significant F test from the ANOVA. (This is not true in general; some multiple comparison procedures are used only if a significant F is observed.) Even if the F test from the ANOVA table leads an investigator not to reject the null hypothesis of equality of population means, it is still advantageous to make confidence intervals for interesting contrasts. The location and length of an interval in which a contrast lies is of interest, even if it covers zero. For example, a very short interval containing zero tells us that the difference between these means is probably very small; an interval from a small negative number to a large positive one tells us that if the difference is negative, its magnitude is probably small.

3.3.1 Straightforward Approach to Inference

In the context of constructing a confidence interval for $\sum_{i=1}^{a} c_i \mu_i$, the most straightforward approach is to calculate

$$\sum_{i=1}^{a} c_i \bar{Y}_{i.} \pm t_{(1-\alpha/2;\nu)} \text{ se} \left(\sum_{i=1}^{a} c_i \bar{Y}_{i.} \right). \tag{3.12}$$

That is, take the point estimate, then add or subtract the product of the $100(1 - \alpha/2)$ percentage point of a t distribution with ν degrees of freedom and the estimated standard error. The degrees of freedom are those that are used in the determination of MS_r, or s^2, from the ANOVA table used to test equality of population means. In the context of one-way ANOVA, $\nu = N - a$.

Similarly, to make a hypothesis test for a contrast, $H_0 : \sum_{i=1}^{a} c_i \mu_i = 0$, the most straightforward approach involves taking the ratio of the point estimate to its estimated standard error:

$$t = \frac{\sum_{i=1}^{a} c_i \bar{Y}_{i.} - 0}{\text{se}(\sum_{i=1}^{a} c_i \bar{Y}_{i.})}. \tag{3.13}$$

We assume that when H_0 is true (i.e., the contrast of population means is 0), the test statistic follows a t distribution with ν degrees of freedom. If the absolute value of the test statistic is greater than $t_{1-\alpha/2;\nu}$ or, equivalently, if the associated p value is less than the specified level of significance α, the null hypothesis rejected. In the context of one-way ANOVA, the number of degrees of freedom is $\nu = N - a$.

Suppose we wish to make hypothesis tests for all pairwise comparisons of a populations. This procedure would be equivalent to making $\binom{a}{2} = a(a - 1)/2$ two-sample t tests, while using the s^2 estimated from all a populations as the estimate of σ^2 and its corresponding number of degrees of freedom, ν. For one-way ANOVA, the s^2, or MS_r, and its number of degrees of freedom, $\nu = N - a$, can be read directly from the ANOVA table.

When analysts perform these procedures for obtaining confidence intervals or making hypothesis tests, they will sometimes describe their work with the statement "No adjustment was made for multiple comparisons", or they will say they used the unprotected or unrestricted least significant difference (LSD) method,. The LSD corresponds to the product of the critical t value $t_{(1-\alpha/2;\nu)}$ and the estimated standard error for a contrast. If the absolute value of the estimated contrast exceeds the LSD, it is concluded that the contrast of population means is not equal to 0 (see Equation 3.12).

Example. First, consider all possible pairwise comparisons of mean FEV1 for the four different smoking history groupings. See Table 3.5 for the six 95% confidence intervals. These intervals were obtained using SAS software; as before, the critical value of t is $t_{(0.975;20)} = 2.086$. From examining the confidence intervals in the table, we conclude that nonsmokers have significantly greater FEV1 than either recent or current smokers; the lower limits of these confidence limits exceed 0. On average, the FEV1 of nonsmokers is 0.76 liters greater than that of recent smokers and 1.00 liters greater than that of current smokers. Similarly, early smokers have greater FEV1 than recent smokers. However, there is no evidence that the mean FEV1 is different between nonsmokers and early smokers, or between early and recent smokers, or between recent and current smokers. Thus, there is some inconsistency in the findings, which can make interpretation difficult.

3.3.2   Motivation for Multiple Comparison Procedures and Terminology

These procedures, as described, may, or may not be a problem, depending on one's objectives. When making statistical inferences, we seek to control the Type I, or α, errors. Recall that a Type I error is the error of rejecting a null hypothesis which is true or of constructing a confidence interval which fails to cover its population parameter. The chance of making a Type I error is referred to as an *error rate*.

We now define two different Type I error rates:

(1) The *comparisonwise error rate* is the error rate associated with each comparison.

(2) The *experimentwise error rate* is the error rate associated with all comparisons that are made in a study. It is the probability of incorrectly rejecting at least one null hypothesis when making numerous comparisons. This is also called the overall error rate.

The confidence intervals and hypothesis tests described in Section 3.3.1 are based on a comparisonwise error rate controlled at level α. The comparison-

Table 3.5 All Pairwise Comparisons for Mean FEV1 among Smoking Groups: 95% Confidence Intervals with No Adjustments

Smoking Groups	Mean Difference	95% Confidence Limits Lower	Upper
Nonsmokers − early smokers	0.28	−0.42	0.98
Nonsmokers − recent smokers	0.76	0.06	1.46
Nonsmokers − current smokers	1.00	0.30	1.70
Early smokers − recent smokers	0.48	−0.22	1.18
Early smokers − current smokers	0.72	0.02	1.42
Recent smokers − current smokers	0.24	−0.46	0.94

wise error rate can be set by the researcher, say, at $\alpha = 0.05$. This means that each hypothesis test is performed at $\alpha = 0.05$ and each confidence interval has level of confidence 0.95.

The disadvantage of controlling the comparisonwise error rate is that the experimentwise error rate is increased. That is, the chance of making a Type I error somewhere among all the comparisons that are made is higher. For example, if we make six two-sample t tests at say $\alpha = 0.05$ each, then our chance of making an error in at least one of the six tests is higher. Also, if we compute six confidence limits, we cannot expect that all the intervals will cover their parameters 95% of the time. If we decide to make $m = 6$ statistically independent tests, then the chance of incorrectly rejecting at least one test is

$$1 - (1 - \alpha)^m = 1 - (1 - 0.05)^6 = 1 - 0.735 = 0.265. \tag{3.14}$$

The experimentwise error rate is 0.265. Note that as m gets larger, the chance of making an error gets larger.

This is not something to be concerned about if not too many comparisons are made. For example, if someone is interested in making limited contrasts, such as between a control group and $a - 1$ treatment groups, or in evaluating linear, quadratic, or cubic trends, the problem of multiple testing is generally ignored.

However, there can be legitimate concerns about making many comparisons, for example, making all possible paired comparisons. Also, researchers may get ideas about comparisons to make after looking at their data. In these situations, analysts may wish to consider applying a multiple comparison procedure. Multiple comparison procedures are concerned with controlling the experimentwise error rate. This means that the probability of making a Type I error among all the comparisons has an upper bound.

The method of choosing which means to compare can be done in two ways. The first way is to decide which means to compare *before* seeing the results of the test. For example, suppose one of the treatments is a control and we know that we shall want to compare each treatment with the control. The second way is to decide which means to compare *after* we see the summary statistics and the results of the ANOVA. For example, we may get a significant F value when we test for equality of the a means and note that the first mean is much larger than the second mean. We then might want to test if it is significantly larger. Such tests are called *post hoc* tests, since the decision to make them is made after seeing the results.

In this chapter, three different multiple comparison procedures are introduced: the Bonferroni method in Section 3.3.3, the Tukey method in Section 3.3.4, and the Scheffé method in Section 3.3.5. These methods can be used to either make multiple hypothesis tests or make multiple confidence intervals. They can be applied regardless of whether or not the ANOVA test for equality of population means is rejected. Finally, software packages such as SAS have options to easily request all possible pairwise comparisons or all pairwise comparisons with a control. These tests appear together with the ANOVA tests. Keep in mind that what a software package does may or may not correspond with what a user wants to do. To get what is wanted, it may be easier to use the computer to generate the estimates that go into a particular confidence interval or hypothesis test and then to perform the simultaneous inferences by hand.

3.3.3   The Bonferroni Multiple Comparison Method

We can construct m intervals for m linear contrasts of population means using the same t statistic as in Section 3.3.1 and simply adjust the level of the percentile that is determined from the t distribution. If, in place of the $1 - \alpha/2$ point of the t distribution, we use the $1 - \alpha/(2m)$ point, we obtain a set of m confidence intervals such that, in repeated experimentation, the proportion of such sets of m intervals that cover all m contrasts of means is greater than or equal to $1 - \alpha$.

This method is an example of the kind in which the number of inferences is specified prior to looking at the data. The investigators must have specified their research hypotheses, collected data, and then performed the analyses which can answer the research question.

To introduce the idea behind the use of the Bonferroni method, we suppose that m confidence intervals are planned. The intervals will be constructed such that each has probability $1 - \alpha$ of covering a contrast of population means, and probability α of not doing so. The question is asked: What is the probability that the first interval, and the second interval, and ..., and the mth interval will cover their respective contrasts of population means simultaneously? Or, conversely, what is the experimentwise error rate for these m intervals?

In this context, the Bonferroni inequality states that the probability that the intervals will each simultaneously cover their respective contrasts of the population means is greater than or equal to one minus the the sum (over the m intervals) of the probability that each interval will not cover its contrast of population mean. The experimentwise coverage rate is at least $1 - \sum_{i=1}^{m} \alpha = 1 - m\alpha$. The experimentwise error rate is at most $m\alpha$. This tells us that one way to control the experimentwise error rate to a value $\leq \alpha$ is to decrease the error rate for each interval from α to α/m. This is the Bonferroni method of multiple comparisons [6, 7].

To summarize, the Bonferroni method allows us to construct m planned confidence intervals that will simultaneously cover their respective contrasts of population means at least $100(1-\alpha)\%$ of the time. For the contrast $\sum_{i=1}^{a} c_i \mu_i$, a confidence interval is calculated:

$$\sum_{i=1}^{a} c_i \bar{Y}_{i.} \pm t_{(1-\alpha/(2m));N-a} \text{ se} \left(\sum_{i=1}^{a} c_i \bar{Y}_{i.} \right). \tag{3.15}$$

Note that the point estimate and the estimated standard error are the same estimates that were obtained in Section 3.3.1. The only thing that is different is that the comparisonwise level of confidence has been changed from $1 - \alpha$ to $1 - \alpha/m$.

Similarly, in the context of hypothesis testing, the test statistic is the same as that given in Equation 3.13, namely,

$$t = \frac{\sum_{i=1}^{a} c_i \bar{Y}_{i.} - 0}{\text{se}(\sum_{i=1}^{a} c_i \bar{Y}_{i.})}.$$

The hypothesis that $\sum_{i=1}^{a} c_i \mu_i = 0$ is rejected when $|t| > t_{[1-\alpha/2m]}$.

As mentioned earlier, the investigators decide what is appropriate to estimate before looking at the data. The set of confidence intervals to be estimated should be completely planned in advance. Otherwise, the investigators could look at the data, notice a contrast that seemed interesting, and estimate it with a single confidence interval (i.e., with $m = 1$). In this way, they would obtain a shorter interval than if they had decided to form numerous intervals. The confidence level for such an interval becomes meaningless.

Investigators pay for a multiple confidence level by having longer intervals. However, beyond very small values of m, $t_{[1-\alpha/(2m);\nu]}$ increases very slowly with m; therefore, it is just as well to plan to have a large number of confidence intervals with a multiple confidence level. Then, if examination of the data shows that some of the intervals are uninteresting, the calculations for all m intervals need not actually be made. However, $t_{[1-\alpha/(2m);\nu]}$ is used for any intervals that are calculated. If, after planning the analysis, examination of the data discloses an interesting contrast that the investigators failed to anticipate, they note this result. They do not, however, claim to have established it by means of a confidence interval.

This method works particularly well when the number of contrasts is not too large. Its disadvantages are that the number of contrasts must be specified before looking at the results of the analyses and that if large numbers of intervals are specified, they can become so wide as to be uninformative.

Example. Suppose we had planned to make all possible pairwise comparisons using the Bonferroni method for mean FEV1 among the four smoking categories in the example (Table 3.6). Thus, we planned to make $m = 6$ comparisons. To make these six comparisons with experimentwise 95% level of confidence, the critical value of t is $t_{(1-0.05/12;20)} = 2.927$.

With the higher t value of 2.927, compared with $t = 2.086$ when no adjustments for multiple comparisons were made, the confidence intervals are wider. Here, there is only one interval that does not include 0; we conclude that mean lung function is greater for nonsmokers than for current smokers. There isn't evidence to conclude that mean FEV1 is different between early and recent smokers. Furthermore, no significant differences were found between each of these groups and either nonsmokers or smokers. In this particular example, there is some inconsistency in the results, which can make interpretation difficult.

3.3.4   The Tukey Multiple Comparison Method

The Tukey comparison method is an example of a post hoc method, that is, it can be used after the analyst looks at the data.

For the contrast $\sum_{i=1}^{a} c_i \mu_i$, a confidence interval is calculated using the Tukey method as

$$\sum_{i=1}^{a} c_i \bar{Y}_{i.} \pm q_{(1-\alpha, a, N-a)} \text{ se} \left(\sum_{i=1}^{a} c_i \bar{Y}_{i.} \right). \tag{3.16}$$

Here q has a distribution which is called the Studentized range distribution. For a set of a populations, the Studentized range is the largest difference in sample means divided by the estimated standard error of a sample mean. The Studentized range distribution depends on two parameters: the number of populations being compared, a, and the number of degrees of freedom associated with s^2, ν. See Appendix B.6 for a table containing the 95th percentiles of Studentized range distributions.

Hypothesis tests performed using Tukey's method tend to have greater power than those performed using either Bonferroni's or Scheffé's method.

Example. The six confidence intervals corresponding to all pairwise comparisons for mean FEV1 among the four smoking categories are shown in Table 3.7. Since we want the experimentwise error rate to be ≤ 0.05, we select the 95th percentile of the Studentized range distribution, with parameters $a = 4$ and $\nu = 20$. The critical value of the distribution is 3.958. Using these intervals, we reach the same conclusions that were made when the Bonferroni

Table 3.6 All Pairwise Comparisons for Mean FEV1 among Four Groups of Smokers: Confidence Intervals Computed Using the Bonferroni Method

Smoking Comparison	Mean Difference	95% Confidence Limits	
		Lower	Upper
Nonsmokers − early smokers	0.28	−0.70	1.26
Nonsmokers − recent smokers	0.76	−0.22	1.74
Nonsmokers − current smokers	1.00	0.02	1.98
Early smokers − recent smokers	0.48	−0.51	1.46
Early smokers − current smokers	0.72	−0.26	1.70
Recent smokers − current smokers	0.24	−0.74	1.22

method was used: there are significant differences in mean FEV1 between nonsmokers and current smokers. However, note that these intervals are not as wide as those obtained using the Bonferroni method.

3.3.5 The Scheffé Multiple Comparison Method

The Scheffé method is a very general method for obtaining multiple confidence intervals or multiple hypothesis tests for contrasts of population means; like the Tukey procedure, it is a post hoc method. There are an infinite number of contrasts that could be defined. Scheffé's method has the property that the experimentwise error rate for this infinite set of contrasts is α.

For the contrast $\sum_{i=1}^{a} c_i \mu_i$, a confidence interval is calculated as

$$\sum_{i=1}^{a} c_i \bar{Y}_{i.} \pm \sqrt{(a-1)F_{1-\alpha,\nu_1,\nu_2}s^2 \sum_{i=1}^{a} c_i^2 \frac{1}{n_i}} \tag{3.17}$$

As with the Bonferroni and Tukey methods, the point estimate and estimated standard error are the same as those given in Section 3.3.1. In the context of one-way ANOVA, a is the number of populations compared, and the $1 - \alpha$ percentile of an F distribution with $\nu_1 = a - 1$ and $\nu_2 = N - a$ degrees of freedom is the critical value.

The main advantage of the Scheffé procedure is that it can be applied for virtually any contrast; it isn't necessary to plan ahead for specific contrasts as with the Bonferroni procedure. If an analyst examines the data and sees something that looks interesting, there is no reason not to compute the confidence interval or make the hypothesis test.

The main disadvantage to the procedure is that the intervals are wide. It allows for the calculation of an infinite number of contrasts. While some analysts want to make what seem like many contrasts, their number falls far short of infinity. The experimentwise error rate is likely something far less

Table 3.7 All Pairwise Comparisons for Mean FEV1 among Four Groups of Smokers: Confidence Intervals Computed Using the Tukey Method

Smoking Comparison	Mean Difference	95% Confidence Limits Lower	Upper
Nonsmokers − early smokers	0.28	−0.66	1.22
Nonsmokers − recent smokers	0.76	−0.18	1.70
Nonsmokers − current smokers	1.00	0.06	1.94
Early smokers − recent smokers	0.48	−0.46	1.42
Early smokers − current smokers	0.72	−0.22	1.66
Recent smokers − current smokers	0.24	−0.70	1.18

than α; the smaller actual experimentwise error rate for a subset of possible contrasts for this method compared with most other methods is consistent with the wider intervals for this procedure. This method will never find a significant contrast at an experimentwise error rate of α if the ANOVA F test for equality of means is not rejected (i.e., $p > \alpha$); that isn't true for the Bonferroni or Tukey methods.

Example. For the lung function study, confidence intervals for the six possible pairwise comparisons are shown in Table 3.8. The critical value of $F = F_{0.95,3,20}$ is 3.098. To compute each confidence interval, the estimated standard error of the contrast, 0.34, is multiplied by $\sqrt{3 \times 3.098} = 3.049$.

These intervals are quite a bit wider than either the Bonferroni or Tukey intervals. In this case, no statistically significant differences between any of the smoking categories are found.

Table 3.8 All Pairwise Comparisons for Mean FEV1 among Four Groups of Smokers: Confidence Intervals Computed Using the Scheffé Method

Smoking Comparison	Mean Difference	95% Confidence Limits Lower	Upper
Nonsmokers − early smokers	0.28	−0.74	1.31
Nonsmokers − recent smokers	0.76	−0.27	1.79
Nonsmokers − current smokers	1.00	−0.03	2.02
Early smokers − recent smokers	0.48	−0.54	1.50
Early smokers − current smokers	0.72	−0.31	1.74
Recent smokers − current smokers	0.24	−0.79	1.26

There are many other methods for making multiple comparisons, and many are available in the statistical packages. Fisher's protected least significant difference, the Student–Newman–Keuls procedure, and Duncan's multiple range are other procedures that are widely used. These do not control the experimentwise error rate [5].

3.4 INFERENCE FOR VARIANCE COMPONENTS

In Chapter 2, we described point estimation of σ^2 and σ_a^2. Now, we want to consider interval estimation of the two parameters. We may be interested in determining a confidence interval for σ^2, regardless of whether the effects are fixed or random.

A $1 - \alpha$ level confidence interval for σ^2 is

$$0 \leq \sigma^2 \leq \frac{a(n-1)s^2}{\chi^2_{\alpha;a(n-1)}}. \tag{3.18}$$

Interval estimation for σ_a^2 is only of interest when the effects are random. Alternatively, interval estimates of the ratio σ_a^2/σ^2 or of the intraclass correlation ρ may be of greater interest. We do not present these intervals here, but information can be found in other sources, such as [11] and [14].

3.5 PRESENTATION AND INTERPRETATION OF RESULTS

Generally, multiple confidence intervals or multiple tests appear together with results of the ANOVA tests; much of what was written in Section 2.6 is applicable here as well. Investigators have the choice of using multiple confidence intervals or multiple hypothesis tests, although the confidence intervals tend to be preferred because they contain more information.

Whether or not confidence intervals or significance tests were made with adjustment for multiple comparisons should be stated. If adjustment was made, the actual procedure used should also be specified along with the experimentwise or overall error rate. If the Bonferroni procedure is used, the number of preplanned comparisons, m, should also be identified.

When results of multiple comparisons procedures are made in terms of hypothesis tests, different letters (e.g., a, b, c) may be used to indicate which population means are different. Confidence intervals are generally preferred, so that readers can get an idea of how far apart the population means really are.

It is straightforward to report the results of multiple tests or confidence intervals when there is a clear interpretation of the results. For example, suppose the means of three populations are compared and we find that the confidence intervals for $\mu_1 - \mu_3$ and $\mu_2 - \mu_3$ do not include 0, but that the interval for $\mu_1 - \mu_2$ does. From the three intervals, we can conclude that μ_1 and μ_2 may be equal and μ_3 is unequal to the other two means.

It is a bit messier to summarize the results when the findings are not clear cut. Suppose again that we are comparing the means of three populations and we find that the confidence interval for $\mu_1 - \mu_3$ does not cover 0, but that the intervals for $\mu_1 - \mu_2$ and $\mu_2 - \mu_3$ do. In this case, we conclude that μ_1 is not equal to μ_3, but that μ_1 may be equal to μ_2 and that μ_2 may be equal to μ_3. Or we could say that μ_1 is unequal to μ_3 but we don't have evidence that the mean of population 2 is unequal to the means of populations 1 and 3.

3.6 SUMMARY

In Chapter 2 we focused on whether or not the means of a set of populations are equal. In this chapter, we have continued our discussion of analyses applicable to designs with a single factor and directed attention to investigating which means may be equal to each other and which are unequal. We have focused on identifying which populations have means which are unequal or equal.

We first addressed estimation of population means, their estimated standard errors, and confidence intervals for a single population mean and cautioned against using the overlap between these confidence intervals as a decision rule for whether or not two means are equal. The intervals are of interest in themselves, as they provide an indication of a plausible range of values that a population mean can assume.

Next, we considered estimation of linear combinations of population means, called contrasts, and showed how to estimate these contrasts, their estimated standard errors, and confidence intervals. Simple contrasts, such as the difference between two population means, as well as more complex ones, such as a those for examining linear trends across the population, were described.

We noted that typically, investigators are interested in evaluating multiple contrasts. We cautioned against estimating many confidence intervals without making any adjustment for these multiple comparisons. We contrasted the overall or experimentwise error rate with the comparisonwise error rates. When 95% confidence intervals are made for each contrast, the comparisonwise error rate is 0.05, but the experimentwise error rate (the chance of estimating a confidence interval that does not cover the true contrast in population means for the multiple estimated intervals) can become greater than 0.05.

We discussed controlling the experimentwise error rate (for example, fixing it at 0.05) as a technique for adjusting for the multiple comparisons made. These methods are referred to as multiple comparison procedures. While many specific methods have been proposed, we focused on three commonly used procedures: the Bonferroni, Tukey, and Scheffé.

This chapter was written for the special case of a single factor design, but the techniques discussed are much more widely applicable. We will be referring to this chapter repeatedly throughout the book and will illustrate these procedures in a variety of contexts.

Problems

3.1   Using the data from Problem 2.3 (dose $= 0$) in the previous chapter, estimate the population means and standard errors for the four populations. Compute confidence intervals for all paired differences in means, using no adjustment for multiple comparisons, the Bonferroni method, the Tukey method, and the Scheffé method. What are your conclusions about the equality of the population means for each method? Which method would you choose to report? Why?

3.2   Still using the data from Problem 2.3, investigate whether there is any difference between the standard rat chow and the the modified diets, that is, whether $\mu_1 - (\mu_2/3 + \mu_3/3 + \mu_4/3) = 0$. Determine the point estimate, estimated standard error, and 95% confidence interval for this contrast. Explain how to interpret your interval.

3.3   Using the data from Problem 2.4 (dose $= 50$) in the previous chapter, estimate the population means and standard errors for the four populations. Compute confidence intervals for all paired differences in means, using no adjustment for multiple comparisons, the Bonferroni method, the Tukey method, and the Scheffé method. What are your conclusions about the equality of the population means for each method? Which method would you choose to report? Why?

3.4   Still using the data from Problem 2.4, investigate whether there is any difference between the standard rat chow and the the modified diets, that is, whether $(\mu_1 - \mu_2/3 + \mu_3/3 + \mu_4/3) = 0$. Determine the point estimate, estimated standard error, and 95% confidence interval for this contrast. Explain how to interpret your interval.

REFERENCES

1. Carmer, S.G. and Swanson, M.R. [1973]. An Evaluation of Ten Pairwise Multiple Comparison Procedures by Monte Carlo Methods, *Journal of the American Statistical Association*, 68, 66–74.

2. Carmer, S.G. and Walker, W.M. [1982]. Baby Bear's Dilemma: A Statistical Tale. *Agronomy Journal*, 74, 122–124.

3. Cole, S.R. and Blair, R.C. [1999]. Overlapping Confidence Intervals, *Journal of the American Academy of Dermatology*, 41, 1051–1052.

4. Chew, V. [1976]. Comparing Treatment Means: A Compendium, *Horticultural Science*, 11, 348–357

5. Dean, A. and Voss, D. [1999]. *Design and Analysis of Experiments*, New York: Springer-Verlag, 67–97.

6. Dunn, O.J. [1961]. Multiple Comparisons among Means, *Journal of the American Statistical Association*, 56, 52–64.

7. Dunn, O.J. [1958]. Estimation of the Means of Dependent Variables, *Annals of Mathematical Statistics*, 29, 1095–1111.

8. Hochberg, Y. and Tamhane, A.C. [1987]. *Multiple Comparison Procedures*, New York: John Wiley & Sons, 72–109.

9. Hsu, J.C. [1996]. *Multiple Comparisons: Theory and Methods.* London: Chapman and Hall.

10. Milliken, G.A. and Johnson, D.E. [1984]. *Analysis of Messy Data, Volume 1: Designed Experiments*, Belmont, CA: Wadsworth, Inc., 29–45.

11. SAS Institute Inc. [1999]. *SAS Online Documentation, Version 8*, Cary, NC: SAS Institute Inc.

12. Saville, D.J. [1990]. Multiple Comparison Procedures: The Practical Solution, *The American Statistician*, 44, 174–180.

13. Schenker, N. and Gentleman, J. [2001]. On Judging the Significance of Differences by Examining the Overlap between Confidence Intervals, *The American Statistician*, 55, 182–186.

14. Winer, B.J. [1971]. *Statistical Principles in Experimental Design*, New York: McGraw Hill, 177–185, 244–250.

4

Hierarchical or Nested Design

It is often necessary to measure the response to a treatment on each individual of a subsample of a unit rather than on the entire unit to which the treatment is applied. In a fertilizer experiment, for example, the treatment may have been applied to plots of ground; from each plot several plants can be picked at random and the response (perhaps weight) of each plant can be measured. This experiment has what is called a *hierarchical* or *nested* design.

It is convenient to introduce the term *experimental unit*, which designates the unit to which the treatment is applied. In a fertilizer experiment, the experimental unit is the plot of ground to which the fertilizer is applied. When drugs are given to patients, the experimental unit is the individual patient. When a single factor such as fertilizer level is studied, if the response is measured on the entire experimental unit, a simple one-way classification is appropriate. For example, if the yield of the entire plot is measured, the model of Chapter 2 is appropriate. If, however, we draw a random sample (called a *subsample*) from each of the experimental units and measure the response from the observations of the subsamples, a hierarchical design is used. For example, in a study on dyes, the experimental unit might be the batch of wool; from each large batch we might choose several small batches at random and measure some response such as resistance to fading. When response to several drugs is measured on animals, the experimental unit is the animal. However, if the investigator wished to have several chemical determinations or take several biopsies from each animal, those would constitute the subsample.

Hierarchical designs are also applicable in observational studies. In these studies, the term *sampling unit* is used instead of experimental unit. For example, in a survey of residences in a city, the city may be subdivided into blocks, a sample of blocks drawn, and then a subsample of residences on the selected blocks obtained. In this case, the block would be considered the sampling unit, and measurements would be taken from a subsample of residences. Or, in a survey of beetles in a large geographic area, the area might first be divided into subareas defined by elevation (high, medium, and low). Within each subarea, circles of area one square meter could be randomly selected, and all the beetles within the circles counted. Here the three elevations areas are the sampling units, and the subsamples are the counts of beetles within the circles.

ANOVA designs where subsamples of the experimental or sampling units are analyzed are referred to either as nested or as hierarchical designs. This chapter is devoted to such designs and their analyses. In Section 4.1, an example of a nested design is given; this will be used to illustrate many of the design and analysis procedures discussed in the chapter. In Section 4.2, nested models are defined, and the concept of a nested factor is introduced. The following three sections address statistical inference. Hypothesis testing (analysis of variance F tests) is covered in Section 4.3, and estimation for balanced studies (i.e. equal sample sizes) in Section 4.4. Section 4.5 addresses inference when sample sizes are unequal; unlike the one-way classification, hypothesis testing is modified for unequal sample sizes with the nested design. (This section can be skipped on a first reading of the chapter.) How to tell if the model assumptions are satisfied is addressed in Section 4.6, and suggestions of what to do if they aren't are given in Section 4.7. Section 4.8 is a discussion of points to consider when designing a nested study. The chapter is summarized in Section 4.9.

4.1 EXAMPLE

As an example of subsampling, we consider a hypothetical study of three different sprays used on trees. Each of the three sprays was applied to four different trees. After one week the concentration of nitrogen was measured in each of six leaves picked in a random way from each tree. Here the experimental units are the 12 trees; we consider them to have been chosen at random from a large (infinite) population of trees. The leaves thus form 12 subsamples, each consisting of six leaves from a large (infinite) population of leaves on the particular tree. Table 4.1 presents the data and preliminary calculations. Note that in this experiment 12 trees were sprayed and 72 leaves were picked.

In this example, the response variable, Y is the nitrogen concentration in a leaf. Each observation, Y_{ijk} is identified by three subscripts: i indicates the spray, j the tree, and k the leaf. So for example, Y_{111}, the nitrogen content of the first leaf taken from the first tree exposed to the first spray is 4.50 (Table 4.1). From the far right column of Table 4.1, we can see that the overall mean concentration of nitrogen is $\bar{Y}_{...} = 9.79$. The highest sample

EXAMPLE   97

Table 4.1 Data and Summary Statistics for Nitrogen Concentrations with Three Types of Spray

Spray, i	Leaf, k	Tree, j, Exposed to Spray i				
		1	2	3	4	
1	1	4.50	5.78	13.32	11.59	
	2	7.04	7.69	15.05	8.96	
	3	4.98	12.68	12.67	10.95	
	4	5.48	5.89	12.42	9.87	
	5	6.54	4.07	10.03	10.48	
	6	7.20	4.08	13.50	12.79	
	$\bar{Y}_{1j.}$	5.96	6.70	12.83	10.77	
						$\bar{Y}_{1..} = 9.07$
2	1	15.32	14.53	10.89	15.12	
	2	14.97	14.51	10.27	13.79	
	3	14.81	12.61	12.21	15.32	
	4	14.26	16.13	12.77	11.95	
	5	15.88	13.65	10.45	12.56	
	6	16.01	14.78	11.44	15.31	
	$\bar{Y}_{2j.}$	15.21	14.37	11.34	14.01	
						$\bar{Y}_{2..} = 13.73$
3	1	7.18	6.70	5.94	4.08	
	2	7.98	8.28	5.78	5.46	
	3	5.51	6.99	7.59	5.40	
	4	7.48	6.40	7.21	6.85	
	5	7.55	4.96	6.12	7.74	
	6	5.64	7.03	7.13	6.81	
	$\bar{Y}_{3j.}$	6.89	6.73	6.63	6.06	
						$\bar{Y}_{3..} = 6.58$
						$\bar{Y}_{...} = 9.79$

mean concentration is associated with spray 2 ($\bar{Y}_{2..} = 13.73$), and the lowest is associated with spray 3 ($\bar{Y}_{3..} = 6.58$). Taking a look at the individual trees, the highest sample means appear with spray 2; for example, $\bar{Y}_{21.}$, the sample mean for the first tree exposed to spray 2, is equal of 15.21. There is also variation among the leaves selected from a particular tree. Still looking at the first tree receiving spray 2, the sampled leaves vary in their nitrogen concentration from 14.26 to 16.01.

In this example, we are still interested in only one factor — spray — so that the main questions we want to ask is about the effect of spray on nitrogen concentration in the leaves. Is mean nitrogen concentration the same, regardless of which of the three sprays is used? If the means are unequal, we want to identify differences among the sprays. We will answer these questions using ANOVA and multiple comparison procedures.

While our main focus is upon the effects of the sprays upon the trees, we might also want to know something about the variation among the trees. Using available techniques for spraying, is there variation in nitrogen content among the trees? If so, how do we quantify this information? We will use ANOVA to determine the significance of variation and estimate the amount of variation in terms of variance components.

4.2   THE MODEL

Each measurement of nitrogen concentration is denoted by Y_{ijk}, where i, the number of the treatment, runs from 1 to $a = 3$; j, the number of the experimental unit for the ith treatment, runs from 1 to $b = 4$; and k, the observation number from the jth experimental unit on the ith treatment, runs from 1 to $n = 6$. Thus, Y_{ijk} is the nitrogen concentration of the kth leaf from the jth tree that received spray i. In this example, all sample sizes are equal; the same number of experimental units were randomized to each treatment, and the same number of subsamples were drawn from each experimental unit. That is, this is an example of a balanced study.

The general model, for balanced studies, each response can be written

$$Y_{ijk} = \mu + \alpha_i + \beta_{(i)j} + \varepsilon_{(ij)k},$$
$$i = 1, \ldots, a, \quad j = 1, \ldots, b, \quad k = 1, \ldots, n, \tag{4.1}$$

where

$$\sum_{i=1}^{a} \alpha_i = 0, \qquad \beta_{(i)j} \sim \mathrm{IND}(0, \sigma_b^2), \qquad \varepsilon_{(ij)k} \sim \mathrm{IND}(0, \sigma^2),$$

and the $\beta_{(i)j}$'s and $\varepsilon_{(ij)k}$'s are mutually independent — in other words, the ab β's and abn ε's are all independent of one another. We define σ_a^2 to be $\sum_{i=1}^{a} \alpha_i^2/(a-1)$.

In Equation 4.1 we have divided a nitrogen concentration measurement into four parts. The first is the overall mean μ, which is the mean nitrogen concentration for all three sprays. The second is α_i, the part due to the particular spray; if α_i is positive, the ith spray produces a higher nitrogen concentration than the average. The third part, $\beta_{(i)j}$, is due to the particular tree that was used as the jth tree for the ith spray. The fourth part, $\varepsilon_{(ij)k}$, represents the contribution of the particular leaf that we happened to pick.

Here α_i, the effect of the ith spray, is a fixed effect; only a sprays are being considered. The trees are considered to be a random sample from an infinite population of trees, so that $\beta_{(i)j}$ is a random effect. With the α_i fixed and the $\beta_{(i)j}$ random, the nested model can be called a *mixed* model. Mixed models are discussed in Chapter 8.

The notation $\beta_{(i)j}$ signifies that trees (j) are *nested* within sprays (i); $\beta_{(i)j}$ is called a *nested factor*. This means that a tree receives only one spray. Similarly, $\varepsilon_{(ij)k}$ implies that leaves (k) are nested within sprays (i) and trees (j). Leaves can only come from one tree, which can only be exposed to one spray. In the nested design, the effects of an experimental unit $\beta_{(i)j}$ only appear with one level of treatment, α_i. Similarly, the effects of a subunit $\varepsilon_{(ij)k}$ only appear with one treatment, α_i, and one experimental unit, $\beta_{(i)j}$.

The following assumptions are implied by the model:

(1) The ab $\beta_{i(j)}$'s are independently normally distributed; the abn ε_{ijk}'s are also independently normally distributed.

(2) All the $\beta_{(i)j}$'s come from distributions having the same variance; that is, the distribution of the $\beta_{1(j)}$'s has the same variance as the distribution of the $\beta_{2(j)}$'s. Similarly, all the ε's come from distributions having the same variance.

(3) The β's and the ε's are independent of one another.

The statement that the mean of the distribution of the β's is zero is not an assumption, inasmuch as we can make the mean zero by a proper choice of μ and α_i's. Nor is it an assumption to say that the mean of the distribution of the ε's is zero. Assumptions 1 and 2, plus the fact that the mean of the β's is zero, are equivalent to the statement that the β's form a random sample of size ab from a single normally distributed population. Similarly, the ε's form a random sample of size abn from a single normally distributed population. The two random samples are independent of each other, from assumption 3.

With respect to our particular example, the assumptions imply the following statements. We assume that the variation in nitrogen concentration from one tree to another is the same no matter which spray we use. This clearly is an assumption, for it is quite possible that the effects of one spray might vary considerably from tree to tree, whereas there might be little variation among trees when another spray is used. We also assume that the variation in nitrogen from leaf to leaf is the same, no matter which spray and which tree we consider. These are the implications of Assumption 2.

Assumption 3 tells us that any knowledge we have concerning the β's gives us no information concerning the ε's. Knowing that the first tree for which the second spray is used has a particularly high nitrogen concentration tells us nothing about whether the third leaf we examine will have a concentration that is high or low for that particular tree. All the assumptions implied by the model seem to be quite reasonable for the spray example.

We specified the model above with treatment fixed, but it is also possible to have treatment be a random effect. Equation 4.1 would still hold, but instead of the constraint $\sum_{i=1}^{a} \alpha_i = 0$, we assume $\alpha_i \sim \text{IND}(0, \sigma_a^2)$. Since all effects are random, this particular nested model would be an example of a random effects or variance components model.

4.3   ANALYSIS OF VARIANCE TABLE AND F TESTS

4.3.1   Analysis of Variance Table

We now divide the basic sum of squares into three meaningful parts and make an ANOVA table. The difference $Y_{ijk} - \bar{Y}_{...}$ can be expressed as the sum of three parts:

$$ Y_{ijk} - \bar{Y}_{...} = (\bar{Y}_{i..} - \bar{Y}_{...}) + (\bar{Y}_{ij.} - \bar{Y}_{i..}) + (Y_{ijk} - \bar{Y}_{ij.}). \qquad (4.2) $$

Note that Equation 4.2 is an algebraic identity. Further, the three quantities in parentheses on its right-hand side provide estimates of α_i, $\beta_{(i)j}$, and $\varepsilon_{(ij)k}$, respectively; $\bar{Y}_{...}$ furnishes an estimate of μ. Thus we have in Equation 4.2 a sample estimate of the terms in

$$ Y_{ijk} - \mu = \alpha_i + \beta_{i(j)} + \varepsilon_{(ij)k}, $$

which is obtained by subtracting μ from both sides of Equation 4.1.

As before, we now square both sides of Equation 4.2. When we sum over all the observations, the cross-product terms sum to zero, leaving

$$ \sum_{i=1}^{a}\sum_{j=1}^{b}\sum_{k=1}^{n}(Y_{ijk} - \bar{Y}_{...})^2 \;=\; bn\sum_{i=1}^{a}(\bar{Y}_{i..} - \bar{Y}_{...})^2 + n\sum_{i=1}^{a}\sum_{j=1}^{b}(\bar{Y}_{ij.} - \bar{Y}_{i..})^2 $$

$$ + \sum_{i=1}^{a}\sum_{j=1}^{b}\sum_{k=1}^{n}(Y_{ijk} - \bar{Y}_{ij.})^2. \qquad (4.3) $$

This, then, is the basic sum of squares. The total sum of squares, SS_t, has been broken into three parts. The first sum on the right-hand side of the Equation 4.3 is the treatment sum of squares (in the example, the treatment is spray; it is denoted by SS_a. The second sum is said to be samples nested within treatment, generally called "sample(treatment)" or, in our example, "tree(spray)"; it is denoted as SS_b. The third sum is called the residual sum of squares and is denoted by SS_r; it is within treatment and within sample but among subsamples, or "within spray within tree among leaves."

In Table 4.2, we have the ANOVA table for the nested design. The sum of squares column in Table 4.2 is taken from Equation 4.3 and does not need discussion. The degrees of freedom for the total sum of squares are 1 less than the total number of observations — in this case, $abn - 1$. The residual or among-subsample sum of squares is simply the sum that would be used in a pooled estimate of the variance in which ab samples of size n are pooled; there are $n - 1$ degrees of freedom from each of the ab samples, and therefore the degrees of freedom for SS_a are $ab(n - 1)$. The among-sample sum of squares SS_b uses a sums of squares, each with $b-1$ degrees of freedom; thus the degrees of freedom for this sum of squares are $a(b - 1)$. With a treatments, the due treatment sum of squares SS_a has $a-1$ degrees of freedom. Again, the various numbers of degrees of freedom, when added, equal the total number of degrees of freedom. The mean squares are, as before, calculated as the ratio of a sum of squares to the corresponding degrees of freedom. The mean squares are denoted MS_a, MS_b, and s^2 or MS_r, for between treatments, within treatment among samples, and residual, respectively.

In the EMS column we find that the residual mean square s^2 is used as an estimate of σ^2; this mean square measures the variability in nitrogen from leaf to leaf and nothing else. The among-samples mean square MS_b reflects variation of two types: first, differences between one leaf and another, and second, differences among trees. These two sources of variation appear in the EMS column, where σ^2 has coefficient one (every Y_{ijk} is based on one observation) and σ_b^2 is multiplied by n (every $\bar{Y}_{ij.}$ is based on n observations). Similarly, the size of the due treatment mean square depends on three considerations — variation among leaves, variation among trees, and the differences among nitrogen levels — and we find three terms in the expected value of the mean square. (The $\phi(\alpha)$ in the EMS for treatment corresponds to $\sum_{i=1}^{a} \alpha_i^2/(a-1)$.)

4.3.2 F Tests

First we test the null hypothesis that there are no differences among the treatment means (Table 4.3). This hypothesis can be expressed in terms of the means for each treatment group:

$$H_0 : \mu_1 = \cdots = \mu_a,$$

or in terms of the treatment effects

$$H_0 : \alpha_1 = \cdots = \alpha_a = 0.$$

From the EMS column we see that if the null hypothesis is true, MS_a and MS_b are both estimates of $\sigma^2 + 6\sigma_b^2$. Therefore, the test statistic is $F = MS_a/MS_b$, which is calculated to be 11.54. The corresponding p value is 0.0033. At an $\alpha = .05$ level of significance, the hypothesis of equal nitrogen content using the three sprays is rejected; we conclude that nitrogen concentration differs among the sprays.

It is also possible to make a second F test from Table 4.3. We might wonder whether differences really exist from tree to tree; perhaps all the sampling variation seen in the data is actually from leaf to leaf. In this case,

Table 4.2 Analysis of Variance Table for One-Way Classification: Nested Design, Equal Numbers of Observations, Mixed Model

Source of Variation	SS	df	MS	EMS	F
Treatment	SS_a	$a-1$	MS_a	$\sigma^2 + n\sigma_b^2 + bn\phi(\alpha)$	MS_a/MS_b
Samples(Treatment)	SS_b	$a(b-1)$	MS_b	$\sigma^2 + n\sigma_b^2$	MS_b/s^2
Residual	SS_r	$ab(n-1)$	s^2	σ^2	
Total	SS_t	$abn-1$			

the null hypothesis to be tested is $H_0 : \sigma_b^2 = 0$, and again from the EMS column we can find an appropriate F test. If H_0 is true and $\sigma_b^2 = 0$, we have two independent estimates of σ^2 (viz., MS_b and s^2). The appropriate statistic is therefore MS_b/s^2. In our example, $MS_b/s^2 = 12.75$, with $p < 0.0001$. We reject the null hypothesis and conclude that there is a variation among trees in nitrogen concentration.

4.3.3 Pooling

Sometimes (usually when the available degrees of freedom for the denominator of an F statistic are few), an investigator is tempted to obtain a more sensitive F test by a process called *pooling*. Testing for equality of treatment means with a balanced nested design is one such case when this is considered. The numerator degrees of freedom are, in general, $\nu_1 = a-1$, and the denominator degrees of freedom $\nu_2 = a(b-1)$.

This situation arises when the test of $H_0 : \sigma_b^2 = 0$ is not rejected. If we really believe σ_b^2 is zero, or that it is of negligible size, then σ_b^2 can be canceled in the EMS columns of Table 4.2 from both the due treatment row and the within-treatment among-sample row. Since the within-treatment mean square then

Table 4.3 Analysis of Variance Table for Nitrogen Content of Leaves

Source of Variation	Sum of Squares	df	Mean Square	EMS	F	p Value
Sprays	633.34	2	316.67	$\sigma^2 + 6\sigma_b^2 + 24\sigma_a^2$	11.54	0.0033
Tree(Spray)	246.93	9	27.43	$\sigma^2 + 6\sigma_b^2$	12.75	< 0.0001
Residual	129.16	60	2.15	σ^2		
Total	1009.43	71				

becomes an estimate of σ^2, it can be pooled with the residual mean square to obtain a combined estimate of σ^2. This estimate of σ^2 can be determined by summing the appropriate sums of squares and dividing by the summed number of degrees of freedom. For example, if MS_b had been 3.0 instead of 27.43, the pooled residual estimate would be $s^2 = (9 \times 3.00 + 60 \times 2.15)/(9 + 60) = 2.48$ with 69 degrees of freedom. The within-treatment and residual sums of squares have been *pooled*. Using statistical software, this is equivalent to specifying a one-way ANOVA, ignoring the nesting factor.

In pooling one hopes to make a more powerful test and at the same time to keep the level of significance at the stated value, say $\alpha = 0.05$. If there is no variation among samples ($\sigma_b^2 = 0$), these objectives are attained; $\alpha = .05$, and if among-treatment differences exist, they are more likely to be detected with $a(b-1) + ab(n-1) = a(bn-1)$ degrees of freedom in the denominator than with just $a(b-1)$. On the other hand, if σ_b^2 is actually sizable, the calculated F statistic does not have an F distribution with $a-1$ and $a(bn-1)$ degrees of freedom, and the actual significance level of the test may be much larger than .05.

Often the statistician has no reason to believe, before examining the data, that σ_b^2 is zero or close to zero. If the test of $H_0 : \sigma_b^2 = 0$ fails to reject the null hypothesis, should a pooled test of $H_0 : \sigma_a^2 = 0$ be made? Research has shown that this is not a good idea [2]. The procedure almost never helps when the nested factor has few degrees of freedom. Similarly, for more degrees of freedom (say, 15) the increase in degrees of freedom obtained by pooling doesn't make much of a difference to the critical F value. In the absence of knowledge, either theoretical or from experience that the variance σ_b^2 is zero, pooling is not recommended.

Pooling after examination of the data is usually done when the degrees of freedom for the denominator of the F statistic are very few, so that a very large calculated value of F is needed to reject the null hypothesis. Sometimes the experiment can be redesigned in such a way that the denominator degrees of freedom are more for the tests considered most important. For example, if a study is designed with $a = 3$, $b = 2$, and $n = 5$, there are 3 degrees of freedom for the within-treatment among-sample mean square. Redesigning the study with $a = 3$, $b = 5$, and $n = 2$ would result in 12 degrees of freedom associated with this mean square. (Designing a nested study is considered in more detail in Section 4.8.) When practical considerations necessitate a small number of denominator degrees of freedom, pooling can be termed a desperation move, and the stated F levels must be viewed with skepticism.

4.4   ESTIMATION OF PARAMETERS

In addition to the hypothesis tests, we are also interested in estimating various parameters. The various treatment means or linear combinations of treatment means we may wish to estimate appear in Table 4.4, column 1, with the statistics used to estimate them in column 2, their variances in column 3, and their estimated variances in column 4. This table is for the special case of equal sample sizes n in each subsample.

Of particular interest are the treatment means $\mu + \alpha_i = \mu_i$ and the differences of the means, $\mu_i - \mu_{i'}$, or some other contrasts of means, $\sum_{i=1}^{a} c_i \mu_i$. The unbiased estimate of the ith mean is $\bar{Y}_{i..}$, the unbiased estimate of the difference in means between the ith and i'th treatments is $\bar{Y}_{i..} - \bar{Y}_{i'..}$, and for the general contrast of means, $\sum_{i=1}^{a} c_i \mu_i$, the unbiased estimate is $\sum_{i=1}^{a} c_i \bar{Y}_{i..}$.

Since these estimates are linear combinations of the Y_{ijk}, it is straightforward to determine standard errors using the same procedures that were used in Chapter 3. However, for our nested design, the variation in $\bar{Y}_{i..}$ incorporates variation of the experimental units within a particular treatment, or σ_b^2, as well as the residual variation σ^2. The variance of $\bar{Y}_{i..}$ is equal to

$$\frac{\sigma_b^2}{b} + \frac{\sigma^2}{bn} = \frac{n\sigma_b^2 + \sigma^2}{bn}.$$

Note that the numerator of this expression is the expected mean square associated with variation due to samples within treatments and is estimated by MS_b. The estimated standard error of $\bar{Y}_{i..}$ is then equal to

$$\mathrm{se}(\bar{Y}_{i..}) = \sqrt{\frac{\mathrm{MS}_b}{bn}}.$$

The $100(1 - \alpha)\%$ confidence interval for a difference of two means, $\mu_i - \mu_{i'}$, is determined as

$$\bar{Y}_{i..} - \bar{Y}_{i'..} \pm t_{1-\alpha/2;a(b-1)} \sqrt{\frac{2\mathrm{MS}_b}{bn}}.$$

The number of degrees of freedom to be used in entering the t table for corresponding confidence intervals is that of MS_b, the estimate of $\sigma^2 + n\sigma_b^2$; from the ANOVA table presented in Table 4.2, we find it to be $a(b - 1)$. Multiple comparison procedures, as discussed in Chapter 3, could also be applied.

We now need estimates of the two variance components σ^2 and σ_b^2; these also can be found from Table 4.4. For σ^2 we have the point estimate s^2; for $\sigma^2 + n\sigma_b^2$ we have the estimate MS_b. Subtracting s^2 from MS_b and dividing by n, we estimate the variance component σ_b^2 by

$$s_b^2 = \frac{\mathrm{MS}_b - s^2}{n}. \tag{4.4}$$

From the general rule for obtaining χ^2 variables from the mean square, we have as a $1 - \alpha$ level confidence interval for σ^2

$$0 < \sigma^2 < \frac{ab(n-1)s^2}{\chi^2_{\alpha;ab(n-1)}}. \tag{4.5}$$

Table 4.4 Parameters and Their Estimates for a Nested One-Way Mixed Effects Design with Equal Sample Sizes n

Parameter	Point Estimate	Variance of Estimate	Estimated Variance
μ	$\bar{Y}_{...}$	$(\sigma^2 + n\sigma_b^2)/abn$	MS_f/abn
μ_i	$\bar{Y}_{i..}$	$(\sigma^2 + n\sigma_b^2)/bn$	MS_f/bn
α_i	$\bar{Y}_{i..} - \bar{Y}_{...}$	$(\sigma^2 + n\sigma_b^2)(a-1)/abn$	$\mathrm{MS}_f(a-1)/abn$
$\mu_i - \mu_{i'}$	$\bar{Y}_{i..} - \bar{Y}_{i'..}$	$2(\sigma^2 + n\sigma_b^2)/bn$	$2\,\mathrm{MS}_b/bn$
$\sum_{i=1}^{a} c_i(\mu_i)$	$\sum_{i=1}^{a} c_i \bar{Y}_{i..}$	$(\sigma^2 + n\sigma_b^2)(\sum_{i=1}^{a} c_i^2)/bn$	$\mathrm{MS}_b(\sum_{i=1}^{a} c_i^2)/bn$
σ^2	s^2		
σ_b^2	$(\mathrm{MS}_b - s^2)/n$		

Similarly, a $100(1 - \alpha)\%$ confidence interval for $\sigma^2 + n\sigma_b^2$ is

$$0 < \sigma^2 + n\sigma_b^2 < \frac{a(b-1)\mathrm{MS}_b}{\chi^2_{\alpha;a(b-1)}}. \tag{4.6}$$

From the interval given in Equation 4.6, we can write down the following interval for σ_b^2, with confidence level $\geq$ to $1 - \alpha$:

$$0 < \sigma_b^2 < \frac{a(b-1)\mathrm{MS}_b}{n\chi^2_{\alpha;a(b-1)}}. \tag{4.7}$$

Each term of the inequality has been divided by n, and σ^2/n has been replaced by its lower bound, 0. Greater details and alternative variance component estimation procedures can be found in [1, 3, 5].

Example. For the spray example, the estimates of the sample mean nitrogen concentrations on spray 1, spray 2, and spray 3 were 9.07, 13.73, and 6.58, as presented in Table 4.1. It was determined from the ANOVA that the mean nitrogen concentrations of leaves exposed to the three different sprays were unequal. We wish to investigate which means are unequal. Let's use the Tukey procedure (Section 3.3.4) to get confidence intervals for the three paired differences, $\mu_1 - \mu_2$, $\mu_1 - \mu_3$, and $\mu_2 - \mu_3$.

For a nested design such as this one, the general expression for the overall $100(1 - \alpha)\%$ confidence intervals using the Tukey procedure is

$$\mu_i - \mu_{i'} \pm q_{1-\alpha;a,a(b-1)} \sqrt{\mathrm{MS}_b/bn}. \tag{4.8}$$

As we saw in Chapter 3, the distribution of the Studentized range depends on two parameters: the number of treatment groups, a, and the number of degrees of freedom associated with the appropriate variance estimate. In our case, $a = 3$ treatments, and the number of degrees of freedom used in the calculation of MS_b is $\nu = 9$. For 95% confidence intervals, the value of q that is used is $q_{.95;3,9} = 3.95$, which can be determined from the table in Appendix B.6. Since $MS_b = 27.43$ (see Table 4.3) and $bn = 4 \times 6 = 24$, the quantity $3.95\sqrt{27.43/24} = 4.22$ is added to and subtracted from each mean difference. The three differences in population means, corresponding point estimates, and interval estimates are presented in Table 4.5. From examining the three intervals, we conclude that the mean nitrogen concentration when spray 2 is applied is significantly higher than when either spray 1 or 3 is applied; no significant differences were detected between sprays 1 and 3.

Now, let's consider the variance components. The point estimate of σ^2 is $s^2 = 2.15$. The 95% confidence interval for σ^2 is

$$0 < \sigma^2 < 2.99.$$

Similarly, the point estimate of σ_b^2 is 4.21. The corresponding 95% confidence interval for σ_b^2 is

$$0 < \sigma_b^2 < 12.38.$$

4.4.1   Comparison with the One-Way ANOVA Model of Chapter 2

Data of the type just analyzed could have been handled by using the methods of Chapter 2. The measurements on the six leaves from each tree could have been averaged to obtain a single measure of nitrogen concentration for that tree. We then would have a simple one-way ANOVA problem. For each $Y_{ijk} = \mu + \alpha_i + \beta_{(i)j} + \varepsilon_{(ij)k}$ as in Equation 4.1, the mean for the jth tree on the ith spray is then $\bar{Y}_{ij.} = \mu + \alpha_i + \beta_{(i)j} + \bar{\varepsilon}_{(ij).}$. If we now denote $\bar{Y}_{ij.}$ by Z_{ij} and $\beta_{(i)j} + \bar{\varepsilon}_{(ij).}$ by η_{ij}, we have

$$Z_{ij} = \mu + \alpha_i + \eta_{ij}. \tag{4.9}$$

Table 4.5 Comparisons of Mean Nitrogen Concentrations from the Spray Study Using the Tukey Procedure

Parameter	Point Estimate	Interval Estimate
$\mu_1 - \mu_2$	−4.67	$-8.89 \le \mu_1 - \mu_2 \le -0.44$
$\mu_1 - \mu_3$	2.49	$-1.73 \le \mu_1 - \mu_3 \le 6.71$
$\mu_2 - \mu_3$	7.16	$2.93 \le \mu_2 - \mu_3 \le 11.38$

Because the variance of $\beta_{(i)j}$ is σ_b^2 and the variance of $\varepsilon_{(ij)k}$ is σ^2, we obtain the variance σ_η^2 of η_{ij} as $\sigma_b^2 + (\sigma^2/n)$. So η_{ij} is normally distributed with mean 0 and variance $\sigma_b^2 + (\sigma^2/n)$, and we have exactly the model of Chapter 2.

The confidence intervals for μ_i, $\mu_i - \mu_{i'}$, and so on, will be exactly the same when the determinations are averaged this way. The test of $H_0 : \mu_1 = \cdots = \mu_a$ is precisely the same.

The advantage in analyzing the data as a nested design is that we obtain both an estimate of the variance among leaves and an estimate of the variance among trees.

4.5 INFERENCES WITH UNEQUAL SAMPLE SIZES

4.5.1 Hypothesis Testing

In Sections 4.3 and 4.4, we addressed analyses when sample sizes were equal, that is, the number of experimental units, b, was the same for all treatments, and the number of subsamples, n, was the same for each experimental unit subsampled. This was the easiest case. With unequal sample sizes, we can still break the total sums of squares into distinct parts, which sum to the total. However, hypothesis testing is more complex; we shall see what the problem is by examining the EMSs. This problem is not unsurmountable, and statistical packages can make the adjustments with ease. ANOVA can be used to estimate variance components, but these estimates tend to be biased. Thus, some of the conventional analysis strategies have limitations, which the analyst needs to be aware of. Alternatives to the procedures discussed here, which have more desirable properties, will be described in Chapter 8.

We are still interested in testing the same hypotheses that were tested in Section 4.3 ($H_0 : \mu_1 = \cdots = \mu_a$ and $H_0 : \sigma_b^2 = 0$) and in estimating population means and variance components.

We will illustrate the procedures in terms of an example. As an illustration, let's go back to the spray example, only modify it so that, for spray 3, data were obtained from the first three trees, and also for spray 3, only the first four observations were used in the analysis. The data are presented in Table 4.6.

The ANOVA table is presented in Table 4.7. We can see from this table that there is no problem with the test of $H_0 : \sigma_b^2 = 0$; no modifications to the test statistic need to be made. The calculated F is $\mathrm{MS}_b/\mathrm{MS}_r = 30.63/2.33 = 13.16$, with $p < 0.0001$.

However, it is clear from this table that there is no simple F test of $H_0 : \alpha_i = 0$, $i = 1, \ldots, a$. The problem can be seen by looking at the EMS column. Under the null hypothesis, we do not have two mean squares in the ANOVA table which estimate the same quantity. The EMS associated with spray is $\sigma^2 + 5.2\sigma_b^2 + \phi(\alpha)$, (where $\phi(\alpha) = [\sum_{i=1}^a n_i\alpha_i^2 - (\sum_{i=1}^a n_i\alpha_i)^2/N]/(a-1)$ with n_i is the sample size for treatment i and $N = \sum_{i=1}^a n_i$ is the total sample size) while the EMS associated with tree(spray) is $\sigma^2 + 5.5\sigma_b^2$. We can't simply take

Table 4.6 Data and Summary Statistics for Nitrogen Concentrations With Three Types of Spray — Unequal Sample Sizes

Spray, i	Leaf, k	Tree, j, Exposed to Spray i				
		1	2	3	4	
1	1	4.50	5.78	13.32	11.59	
	2	7.04	7.69	15.05	8.96	
	3	4.98	12.68	12.67	10.95	
	4	5.48	5.89	12.42	9.87	
	5	6.54	4.07	10.03	10.48	
	6	7.20	4.08	13.50	12.79	
	$\bar{Y}_{1j.}$	5.96	6.70	12.83	10.77	
						$\bar{Y}_{1..} = 9.07$
2	1	15.32	14.53	10.89	15.12	
	2	14.97	14.51	10.27	13.79	
	3	14.81	12.61	12.21	15.32	
	4	14.26	16.13	12.77	11.95	
	5	15.88	13.65	10.45	12.56	
	6	16.01	14.78	11.44	15.31	
	$\bar{Y}_{2j.}$	15.21	14.37	11.34	14.01	
						$\bar{Y}_{2..} = 13.73$
3	1	7.18	6.70	5.94		
	2	7.98	8.28	5.78		
	3	5.51	6.99	7.59		
	4	7.48	6.40	7.21		
	$\bar{Y}_{3j.}$	7.04	7.09	6.63		
						$\bar{Y}_{3..} = 6.92$
						$\bar{Y}_{...} = 10.50$

the ratio of the two mean squares to test for no effect of spray, because the two EMS differ by something that depends on σ_b^2 when there is no spray effect. We must work with the EMSs associated with trees(spray) and with the residual to get $\sigma^2 + 5.5\sigma_b^2$.

First, the EMS for tree(spray) can be multiplied by $5.2/5.5 = 0.9455$. This will give $0.9455\sigma^2 + 5.2\sigma_b^2$. Now, the term involving σ_b^2 is correct, but there is a discrepancy in the coefficient associated with σ^2. To correct this, we add $(1 - 0.9455)\sigma^2 = 0.0545\sigma^2$ to σ^2. Thus, the coefficient of σ^2 is 1.

An ANOVA table appropriate for testing $H_0 : \alpha_i = 0$ is shown in Table 4.8. To test for no effect of spray, the mean square for trees(spray) is estimated as

$$MS_b' = 0.0545MS_r + 0.9455MS_b = (0.0545)(2.33) + (0.9455)30.63 = 29.09.$$

This is a linear combination of two mean squares, $c_1MS_r + c_2MS_b$, where $c_1 = 0.0545$ and $c_2 = 0.9455$. We need MS_a/MS_b' to follow an F distribution with the appropriate degrees of freedom when there is no effect of spray on mean nitrogen content of the leaves, and to follow a noncentral F distribution when there is an effect of spray on mean nitrogen. The quantity $(a-1)MS_a/EMS_a$ is distributed as χ^2 or as a noncentral χ^2 with $a-1$ degrees of freedom, depending on whether or not there is an effect of spray. However, we must modify the degrees of freedom ν_2 associated with MS_b' so that $\nu_2 MS_b'/EMS_b'$ approximates that of a χ^2 distribution with ν_2 degrees of freedom. One commonly used approach to determine ν_2 is to use Satterthwaite's approximation [4]. For a general linear combination of mean squares, $\widetilde{MS} = c_1MS_1 + c_2MS_2$, with corresponding numbers of degrees of freedom df_1 and df_2, the number of degrees of freedom for $\widetilde{MS}$ are chosen as

$$\nu_2 = \frac{\widetilde{MS}}{(c_1MS_1)^2/df_1 + (c_2MS_2)^2/df_2}. \tag{4.10}$$

Applying this approximation to our example, let the subscript 1 correspond to residual and the subscript 2 correspond to tree(spray). Then for the contribution of the mean square residual we have $c_1 = 0.0545$, $MS_1 = MS_r = 2.33$, and $df_1 = 49$, and for the contribution of the mean square trees(spray) we have $c_2 = 0.9455$, $MS_2 = MS_b = 30.63$, and $df_2 = 8$. Then $\widetilde{MS} = MS_b' = 29.09$ and the corresponding degrees of freedom are

$$\nu_2 = \frac{29.09^2}{(0.0545 \times 2.33)^2/49 + (0.9455 \times 30.63)^2/8} = 8.07.$$

Table 4.7 Analysis of Variance Table for Nitrogen Content of Leaves: Unequal Sample Sizes

Source of Variation	SS	df	MS	EMS	F	p
Sprays	453.74	2	226.87	$\sigma^2 + 5.2\sigma_b^2 + \phi(\alpha)$	—	—
Trees(spray)	245.07	8	30.63	$\sigma^2 + 5.5\sigma_b^2$	13.16	< 0.0001
Residual	114.07	49	2.33	σ^2		
Total	812.88	59				

Thus, when there is no effect of spray, we assume that $\nu_2 MS_b/EMS_b$ approximately follows a χ^2 distribution with $\nu_2 = 8.07$ and the F statistic MS_a/MS_b' approximately follows an F distribution with 2 and 8.07 degrees of freedom. In our example, $F = 226.87/29.09 = 7.80$ and $p = 0.013$ (Table 4.8).

4.5.2 Estimation

Once MS_b' has been determined, the variance components can be computed in the same way presented for estimation when the sample sizes are all equal. For the spray example, the two variance components are estimated as $s_b^2 = 5.15$ and $s^2 = 2.33$. Confidence intervals of the variance components can be found in [3].

   As we indicated at the beginning of this section, the main objective in going over the case of unequal sample sizes is to illustrate some of the difficulties than can arise. With newer programs, alternative methods for hypothesis testing and estimation are utilized. The greatest problem with the approach described here is in the variance components; they tend to be biased. We will discuss some alternative approaches when we come back to mixed models in Chapter 8.

4.6 CHECKING IF THE DATA FIT THE MODEL

There is nothing new in checking model assumptions. To investigate the assumption of normality, plots of sample means versus sample variances or sample standard deviations can be made. However, with nested designs, there may be more points to plot because a sample mean and sample variance can be computed for each of the subsamples. For balanced studies, there are samples for ab populations. Normality can also be assessed using normal quantile plots of residuals.

Example. For the spray example, there are three treatments, each applied to four different trees, with measurements taken on six leaves. In this case, there are 12 samples from which means, variances, and standard deviations can be estimated. Figure 4.1a is a plot of the 12 sample variances versus the same means, and Figure 4.1b is a plot of the 12 sample standard deviations versus the sample means. No particular trends are apparent from these graphs, so that we don't see any indication that the nitrogen concentration in the leaves is not normally distributed.

Table 4.8 Analysis of Variance Table for Nitrogen Content of Leaves: Testing No Effect of Spray with Unequal Sample Sizes

Source of Variation	SS	df	MS	EMS	F	p Value
Sprays	453.74	2	226.87	$\sigma^2 + 5.2\sigma_b^2 + \phi(\alpha)$	7.80	0.013
Tree(spray)	234.76	8.07	29.09	$\sigma^2 + 5.2\sigma_b^2$		

4.7 WHAT TO DO IF THE DATA DON'T FIT THE MODEL

If there are concerns about violations of any of the assumptions, it is appropriate to consider transforming the observations, as discussed in Chapter 2.

There isn't a well-established distribution free alternative to the nested ANOVA test as there is for the completely randomized design discussed in Chapter 2 (Kruskal-Wallis test).

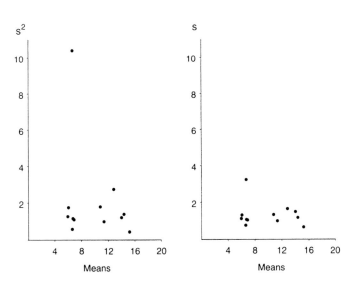

Fig. 4.1 Assessment of normality of nitrogen concentration in leaves: (a) sample variances versus sample means; (b) sample standard deviations versus sample means.

4.8   DESIGNING A STUDY

In experiments involving subsampling, it is preferable if possible to keep the sizes of the subsamples equal. This makes sample size calculations and data analyses much simpler. However, it is not always possible. It may be that the study is designed to have equal subsamples but it is impossible to include all subsampled units in the data analysis. For example, it may not be possible to measure response, the measured response may be in error and have to be discarded, or the like.

Two of the most important decisions to make when using a nested design are (1) how many experimental units to sample and (2) how many subunits to sample. Here is where knowing something about the variance components, σ_b^2 and σ^2, is especially important. We focus on the variance of a treatment mean, and illustrate how the variance is influenced by both the number of experimental units (b) and the number of subunits (n) sampled.

4.8.1   Relative Efficiency

The efficiency of an experimental design is often judged in terms of the variance of a treatment mean. The smaller the variance of the treatment mean, the more *efficient* is the design.

In the example on spray, the variance of a treatment mean is

$$\text{Var}(\bar{Y}_{i..}) = \frac{\sigma^2 + n\sigma_b^2}{bn}.$$

After the experiment has been performed, the variance components can be estimated from the ANOVA table. From Table 4.3, σ^2 is estimated by $s^2 = 2.152$ and σ_b^2 by $s_b^2 = (\text{MS}_b - s^2)/n = (27.434 - 2.152)/6 = 4.214$. We may now wonder if it would have been better to have used five trees and four leaves from each tree instead of four trees and six leaves. (Possibly these two designs would be approximately equal in difficulty.)

With $b = 5, n = 4$, we estimate the variance of a treatment mean by

$$\text{Var}(\bar{Y}_{i..}) = \frac{2.152 + 4 \times 4.214}{4 \times 5} = 0.1076 + 0.8428 = 0.9504.$$

With $b = 4$ and $n = 6$, our estimate is

$$\text{Var}(\bar{Y}_{i..}) = \frac{2.152 + 6 \times 4.214}{6 \times 4} = 0.0897 + 1.0535 = 1.1432.$$

Other things being equal, we would prefer four leaves from each of five trees to six leaves from each of four trees. We consider four leaves from five trees to be a more efficient design because the variance of the treatment mean has been estimated to be smaller in that case. The variance is smaller when the total sample size is 20 rather than 24.

Usually, we think of larger sample sizes as better because we tend to associate them with smaller variances and narrower confidence intervals. This example illustrates an important point about how to select sample sizes when we are using a nested design. The residual error is divided by the total sample size, but the variation between experimental units is divided by the number of experimental units sampled. From the example, we can see that the variation between experimental units contributed much more than the residual variation. To get the variance down, it tends to be more important to take more experimental units than to take more subunits. Here, it was more efficient to sample more trees. However, in some cases this may require greater work or expense, so cost considerations may limit the number of experimental units that can be used. Furthermore, it may not be possible to use more units — for example, if the researcher is limited by available equipment.

It is important to keep in mind that what we did here was replace variance components by their point estimates. There is clearly variability in these estimates.

4.9 SUMMARY

In this chapter, we introduced the idea of a nested factor, which is usually assumed to be random, in the context of the nested design. This design is appropriate when determinations are not made on an entire unit but on subsamples of one. The model was reviewed, as well as hypothesis testing and point and interval estimation. We indicated that comparisons of population means were appropriate for fixed effects, but for the random nested effects, interest is in variance components. Inference for the straightforward case of equal sample sizes was discussed in detail, and modifications for unequal sample sizes were considered. Since inferences about treatment means are based on the number of units rather than the number of subunits sampled, we stressed the importance of having a large number of units to increase the power of tests of equality of treatment means and to shorten the lengths of confidence intervals. Using a balanced design (with equal numbers of experimental units per treatment and equal numbers of subsamples per experimental unit) was encouraged. Most statistical packages will handle nested designs, whether balanced or unbalanced; the use of procedures which fit a general linear model or mixed model will handle either one.

We have considered the nested design as an extension of one-way ANOVA. However, nested factors can be used in more complex ANOVA. We will illustrate the use of nested factors in repeated measures analysis in Chapter 9.

Problems

4.1 Three diets were given to a group of adult volunteers to assess their effects on serum cholesterol levels. The 12 volunteers were randomly assigned to the three diets, and there were four volunteers for each diet. Duplicate determinations of cholesterol level were made at the laboratory on each individual. The data were as follows:

Diet	Individual			
	1	2	3	4
1	273	302	247	228
	266	287	235	237
2	240	221	244	238
	234	228	250	245
3	205	223	233	210
	211	230	224	217

a)   State the model in terms of this problem.

b)   Test whether the mean cholesterol level is equal for the three diets.

c)   Obtain confidence intervals with overall 95% level for the mean cholesterol level for each of the diets and for the contrast $\mu_3 - (\mu_1 + \mu_2)/2$.

d)   Determine the sample mean cholesterol level for each of the 12 volunteers. Using one-way ANOVA, test whether diet affects mean cholesterol level. Compare the computer output obtained here with that obtained from part(b) and verify that the results are the same.

4.2   A plant scientist is interested in investigating the relationship between the percentage of fungal spores that germinate and temperature. He selects $a = 4$ temperatures (15, 20, 25, and 30° Celsius) and incubates $b = 4$ microscopic slides at each of the four temperatures. He selects $n = 10$ locations on each slide and determines the percentage of spores germinated. The data are available on the Wiley web site.

a)   State the model, and explain why a nested model is appropriate.

b)   Explain why microscopic slide is a random effect.

c)   For each of the 16 slides, determine the sample mean, sample variance, and sample standard deviation. Plot sample variance versus sample mean, and sample standard deviation versus sample mean. On the basis of these plots, do the data appear normally distributed? Repeat using log transformed and square root transformed data. Do any transformations seem to better satisfy the assumptions for the nested model?

d)   Once you have made the transformations, use your ANOVA table to test whether there is any variation among microscopic slides nested within temperature. Estimate the variance components for slide(temperature) and residual, and get 95% confidence intervals for them. Estimate the intraclass correlation.

e)   Test for equality of germination percentage across the four temperatures. What do you conclude about mean germination percentage of mold spores incubated at the four different temperatures?

f)   Determine the mean germination percentage for the 16 slides. Perform a one-way ANOVA using the 16 means and verify that the test is equivalent to the test you performed when you fitted the nested model.

g)   For the contrast $-3\mu_{15} - \mu_{20} + \mu_{25} + 3\mu_{30}$, determine the point estimate, and estimate its standard error. Would you conclude there is evidence for a linear trend in mean germination percentage over temperature?

h)   For the contrast $\mu_{15} - \mu_{20} - \mu_{25} + \mu_{30}$, determine the point estimate, and estimate its standard error. Would you conclude there is evidence for a quadratic trend in mean germination percentage over temperature?

REFERENCES

1. Dean, A. and Voss, D. [1999]. *Design and Analysis of Experiments,* New York: Springer-Verlag, 645–673.

2. Janky, D.G. [2000]. Sometimes Pooling for Analysis of Variance Hypothesis Tests: A Review and Study of a Split Plot Model, *The American Statistician,* 54, 269–279.

3. Rao, P.S.R.S. [1997]. *Variance Components Estimation,* New York: Chapman and Hall.

4. Satterthwaite, F.E. [1946]. An Approximate Distribution of Estimates of Variance Components, *Biometrics Bulletin,* 2, 110–114.

5. Searle, S.R. [1971]. *Linear Models,* New York: John Wiley & Sons.

6. Winer, B. J. [1971] *Statistical Principles in Experimental Design,* 2nd ed., New York: McGraw Hill, 359–366, 464–468.

5

Two Crossed Factors: Fixed Effects and Equal Sample Sizes

Often researchers can use single experiments advantageously to study two or more different kinds of treatment. For example, in investigating crop yields for two types of seed, they may also wish to vary the level of fertilizer used during the experiment. If they chose three levels of fertilizer — low, medium, and high — one factor would be type of seed, and the second factor, level of fertilizer. A factorial design, with two factors, would consist of employing all six treatments formed by using each type of seed with each level of fertilizer. Factorial designs can involve more than two factors; in this chapter, we consider first the case of two factors.

A factorial design can also be used in a survey. For example, researchers might wish to compare three methods of teaching grade school mathematics, and at the same time compare the first four grades. They might have records on standardized tests taken before and after the use of the three methods. The change from initial test to final test could be the measure of success. Their data would then consist of changes for each of 12 (3 methods in 4 grades) different treatment combinations.

The characteristic of the factorial design is that the factors are *crossed*, that is, every level of one factor is used in combination with every level of the other factor. The design is effective for studying the two factors in combination.

Some factors can be measured quantitatively, and different levels for them are chosen on an ordered scale; level of fertilizer, dosage level, and temperature are all factors of this type. Other factors involve no obvious underlying continuum and can be said to be qualitative; drug and type of seed are factors of this second type. In a two-way classification, both factors can be quantitative, both qualitative, or one quantitative and one qualitative.

In this chapter, the topic of two-way classification is restricted to the balanced design, that is, there are equal sample sizes for each of the factor combinations. The advantage of considering the balanced case is that the total sum of squares can be broken into parts which can be easily expressed and understood. The unbalanced situation is perhaps a more realistic one, but the breaking apart of the total sums of squares is more complex; this topic is discussed in Chapter 7.

In Section 5.1, an example of a two-way classification with equal sample sizes is introduced. A model is described in Section 5.2, followed by a discussion of the concept of interaction in Section 5.3. Tests for equality of population means are described in Section 5.4, and confidence intervals addressed in Section 5.5. In Section 5.6 we discuss some things to consider when planning a cross-classified design and briefly mention ANOVA with more than two factors. Presentation and interpretation of results are discussed in Section 5.7. The chapter is summarized in Section 5.8.

In this chapter, we don't address checking if the data fit the underlying model. The procedures for that are about the same whether or not a study is balanced, and are taken up in Chapter 7.

5.1 EXAMPLE

As an example of a two-factor design with equal sample sizes, let us take a hypothetical study of rye yields involving two types of seed, each used at three fertilizer levels — low, medium, and high. There are available 24 small plots of ground, and the six treatment combinations are assigned to them at random, four plots receiving each treatment. The data are presented in Table 5.1 and Figure 5.1. A response (in this case yield) is denoted by Y_{ijk}, where i indicates the seed type, j indicates the fertilizer level, and k is the observation number. For example, Y_{213} is the yield in the third of the four plots that used seed type 2 and a low fertilizer level, and is equal to 11.0 bushels/acre. The cell means, denoted by $\bar{Y}_{ij.}$, are the means for each treatment combination. For example, $\bar{Y}_{21.}$, the mean yield for plots of ground exposed to seed type 2 and low levels of fertilizer, is 11.73 bushels/acre. The mean of all 12 observations on the ith seed type is $\bar{Y}_{i..}$; in this case, the means are 16.43 bushels/acre for seed type 1 and 12.84 for seed type 2. The mean of all eight observations on the jth fertilizer is $\bar{Y}_{.j.}$; the means are 12.60 for the low fertilizer, 13.89 for the medium level, and 17.43 for the high level. The overall mean of the 24 observations is $\bar{Y}_{...}$, or 14.64 bushels/acre.

We could use these data to investigate a number of questions. Does the type of seed affect the mean yield of rye? Does the level of fertilizer affect the mean yield of rye? Does the effect of seed type on mean yield of rye depend on the level of fertilizer? Does the effect of level of fertilizer on mean yield of rye depend on the seed type? These questions can be investigated using two-way ANOVA. Furthermore, we may want to determine which means are

Table 5.1   Yields of Rye and Their Means (Bushels/Acre)

Seed Type, i	Fertilizer Level, j			
	1=Low	2=Medium	3=High	
1	14.3	18.1	17.6	
	14.5	17.6	18.2	
	11.5	17.1	18.9	
	13.6	17.6	18.2	
$\bar{Y}_{1j.}$	13.48	17.60	18.23	$\bar{Y}_{1..} = 16.43$
2	12.6	10.5	15.7	
	11.2	12.8	17.5	
	11.0	8.3	16.7	
	12.1	9.1	16.6	
$\bar{Y}_{2j.}$	11.73	10.18	16.63	$\bar{Y}_{2..} = 12.84$
$\bar{Y}_{.j.}$	12.60	13.89	17.43	$\bar{Y}_{...} = 14.64$

different, using multiple-comparison procedures, and to find effective ways to summarize the results.

5.2   THE MODEL

We turn now to an underlying model. We divide each observation Y_{ijk} into four parts, which together form the mean of a population of responses to the ijth treatment combination, and a fifth part, which is the deviation of the particular observation from its population mean. We express each observation as

$$Y_{ijk} = \mu + \alpha_i + \beta_j + (\alpha\beta)_{ij} + \varepsilon_{ijk}, \qquad (5.1)$$

where $i = 1, \ldots, a$, $j = 1, \ldots, b$, $k = 1, \ldots, n$, and

$$\sum_{i=1}^{a} \alpha_i = \sum_{j=1}^{b} \beta_j = \sum_{i=1}^{a} (\alpha\beta)_{ij} = \sum_{j=1}^{b} (\alpha\beta)_{ij} = 0,$$

and we assume $\varepsilon_{ijk} \sim \text{IND}(0, \sigma^2)$. [Equivalently, we could have assumed that $Y_{ijk} \sim \text{IND}(\mu + \alpha_i + \beta_j + (\alpha\beta)_{ij}, \sigma^2)$.] Here a is the number of levels of the first factor ($a = 2$ seed types in the example), b is the number of levels of the second factor ($b = 3$ levels of fertilizer), and n is the number of observations on each treatment combination ($n = 4$ replicates). The population parameters are as follows:

μ = overall mean response; the average of the mean responses for the ab populations;

α_i = effect of the ith level of the first factor, averaged over the b levels of the second factor, (the ith level of the first factor adds α_i to the overall mean μ);

β_j = effect of the jth level of the second factor averaged over the a levels of the first factor;

$(\alpha\beta)_{ij}$ = interaction between the ith level of the first factor and the jth level of the second factor, (the population means for the ijth treatment minus $\mu + \alpha_i + \beta_j$);

ε_{ijk} = deviation of Y_{ijk} from the population mean response for the ijth population.

The terms α_i and β_j are called *main effects*. They are average effects for each type of seed and for each level of fertilizer. The term $(\alpha\beta)_{ij}$ is an interaction. If seed and fertilizer levels behave in a strictly additive way — that is, if a high level of fertilizer adds a certain amount to the average yield, regardless of the seed type — the $(\alpha\beta)_{ij}$'s are all zero. On the other hand, if a high level of fertilizer increases yield more with seed type 1 than with seed type 2, $(\alpha\beta)_{13}$ is positive and $(\alpha\beta)_{23}$ is negative.

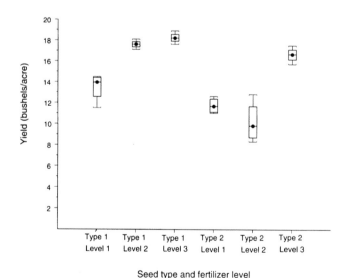

Fig. 5.1 Graphical summarization of rye yields, by seed type and level of fertilizer.

Implicit in the statement of the model are three assumptions.

(1) Responses to the ijth treatment combination, Y_{ijk}, are from a normal distribution (there are ab distributions).

(2) The variances of the ab distributions are all equal. This property is known as *homoscedasticity*. (We might suspect that in the presence of high fertilizer level, the yields will vary more widely from one observation to another; in this case we cannot claim equal variances.)

(3) The ε_{ijk} (deviations from the population means) are statistically independent and are normally distributed. If, for example, several of the plots were planted a month before all the remaining plots, the deviations could not be said to be independent of one another. The several plots planted earlier might all tend to have particularly high yields.

These are the only assumptions we must make for the design. It can be shown that any set of ab population means can be expressed in the form $\mu + \alpha_i + \beta_j + (\alpha\beta)_{ij}$ in such a way that the following conditions are fulfilled: all the α_i sum to zero; all the β_j sum to zero; for each particular j, all the $(\alpha\beta)_{ij}$ sum to zero; and for each fixed i, all the $(\alpha\beta)_{ij}$ sum to zero.

For making inferences about the means of the populations, we introduce some notation that will help focus attention on the means: for example,

$$
\begin{aligned}
\mu_{ij} &= E(\bar{Y}_{ij.}) = \mu + \alpha_i + \beta_j + (\alpha\beta)_{ij}, \\
\mu_{i.} &= E(\bar{Y}_{i.}) = \mu + \alpha_i, \\
\mu_{.j} &= E(\bar{Y}_{.j}) = \mu + \beta_j.
\end{aligned}
$$

5.3 INTERPRETATION OF MODELS AND INTERACTION

To illustrate the interpretation of main effects and interactions, let us consider possible sets of population means, μ_{ij}, with $i = 1,2$ seed types and $j = 1,2,3$ levels of fertilizer. These sets of population means were determined for instructional purposes only — we rarely know population parameters.

Example 1. No effects of seed type or fertilizer level on mean yield. This is the simplest model; the means of all six populations are exactly the same:

Seed	Fertilizer Level				
Type	1	2	3	$\mu + \alpha_i$	α_i
1	15	15	15	15	0
2	15	15	15	15	0
$\mu + \beta_j$	15	15	15		
β_j	0	0	0		

Here, $\mu_{ij} = \mu = 15$. This indicates that neither seed type nor level of fertilizer affects mean yield; all the α_i's and β_j's are 0.

Example 2. Effects of seed type but no effects of fertilizer level on mean yield:

Seed	Fertilizer Level		
Type	1	2	3
1	17	17	17
2	13	13	13

For this table, the means can be written as $\mu_{ij} = \mu + \alpha_i$. Regardless of the level of fertilizer provided, the mean yield is 17 bushels for seed type 1 and 13 bushels for seed type 2. We say there is an effect of seed type but there is no effect of fertilizer. Averaging over all six population means, we determine the overall mean, μ is 15. Averaging over the three populations corresponding to seed type 1, we find $\mu+\alpha_1$ is 17; similarly, averaging over the three populations corresponding to seed type 2, we find $\mu + \alpha_2$ is 13. Thus, we determine that $\alpha_1 = 17 - 15 = 2$ and $\alpha_2 = 13 - 15 = -2$.

Graphs can be useful to illustrate the effects of different factors on mean response. (See Figure 5.2.) Graphing mean yield versus fertilizer level for each

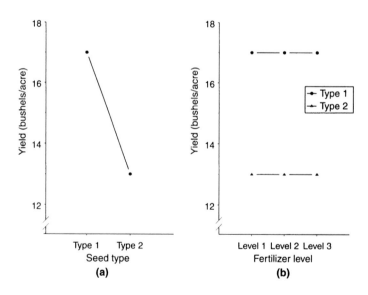

Fig. 5.2 Illustration of effect of seed type but no effect of fertilizer level. Population mean yield versus (a) fertilizer level, by seed type and (b) seed type, by fertilizer level.

seed type (and connecting the points) produces two lines parallel to the X axis — one at 17 and one at 13. Graphing mean yield versus seed type for each fertilizer level produces three overlapping lines, connecting the mean of 17 for seed type 1 with the mean of 13 for seed type 2. The graph illustrates that the difference in mean yield for seed types 1 and 2 is $\alpha_1 - \alpha_2 = 4$ bushels/acre.

Example 3. Effects of fertilizer level but no effects of seed type on mean yield:

Seed Type	Fertilizer Level 1	2	3
1	13	14	18
2	13	14	18

This example is quite similar to the previous one. The means could be expressed as $\mu_{ij} = \mu + \beta_j$. Regardless of the seed type, the mean yield is 13 bushels/acre for the low level of fertilizer, 14 for the medium level of fertilizer, and 18 for the high level of fertilizer. Averaging over the appropriate populations and with the constraints put on the terms of the model, we determine $\mu = 15$, $\beta_1 = 13 - 15 = -2$, $\beta_2 = 14 - 15 = -1$, and $\beta_3 = 18 - 15 = 3$.

Plotting mean yield versus fertilizer level, and connecting the means, produces two overlapping lines. (See Figure 5.3a.) Plotting mean yield versus seed type provides three lines, all parallel to the X axis — one at mean yield 13, one at 14, and one at 18 (Figure 5.3b). The figure shows that the difference in mean yield between medium and low fertilizer is $\beta_2 - \beta_1 = -1 - (-2) = 1$ bushel/acre, the difference between high and low fertilizer is $\beta_3 - \beta_1 = 3 - (-2) = 5$, and the difference between high and medium fertilizer is $\beta_3 - \beta_2 = 3 - (-1) = 4$.

Example 4. Main effects of seed type and fertilizer level on mean yield — the model of *additivity* or *no interaction* between seed type and level of fertilizer:

Seed Type	Fertilizer Level 1	2	3	$\mu + \alpha_i$	α_i
1	15	16	20	17	2
2	11	12	16	13	-2
$\mu + \beta_j$	13	14	18		
β_j	-2	-1	3		

In this example, there is an effect of seed type on mean yield, but the effect does not depend on level of fertilizer. Similarly, there is an effect of fertilizer level, but the effect does not depend on seed type. The population means can be expressed as $\mu_{ij} = \mu + \alpha_i + \beta_j$. The means in the table are said to be additive. We determine $\mu = 15$, $\alpha_1 = 17 - 15 = 2$, $\alpha_2 = 13 - 15 = -2$,

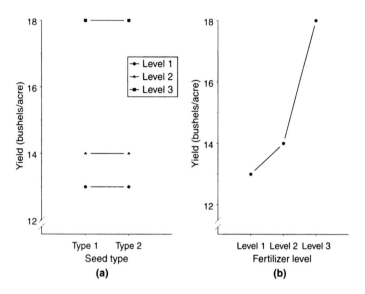

Fig. 5.3 Illustration of no effect of seed type but effect of fertilizer level. Population mean yield versus (a) fertilizer level, by seed type, and (b) seed type, by fertilizer level.

$\beta_1 = 13 - 15 = -2$, $\beta_2 = 14 - 15 = -1$ and $\beta_3 = 18 - 15 = 3$. For example, $\mu_{11} = 15 + 2 - 2 = 15$.

The plots of the means in Figure 5.4 now show lines that are parallel to each other, but not to the X axis. We can clearly see that mean yield depends on both seed type and fertilizer level. The effect of seed type is the same regardless of fertilizer level; the distance between any two means, $\mu_{11} - \mu_{21} = \mu_{12} - \mu_{22} = \mu_{13} - \mu_{23}$, is always 4 bushels/acre. Similarly, the effect of fertilizer level is the same regardless of seed type. The difference in mean yield between medium and low levels of fertilizer is $\mu_{12} - \mu_{11} = \mu_{22} - \mu_{21} = -1 - (-2) = 1$ bushel/acre; the difference does not depend on seed type.

Example 5. Interaction between seed type and fertilizer level on mean yield. This final example of the section illustrates *interaction* between two factors. Interaction indicates a lack of additivity, or that the effect of one factor on the mean response depends on the level of the other factor,. The interaction could represent synergistic effects, in which the effects of levels of two factors produce a mean that is higher than the sum of the effects by themselves. Or the interaction could represent antagonistic effects, that is, the effects of levels of two factors might be producing a mean response that is lower than the sum

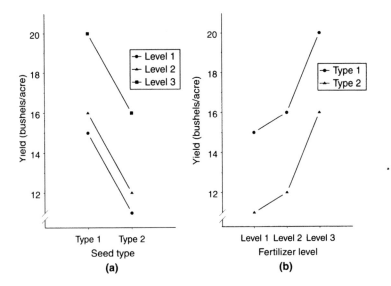

Fig. 5.4 Illustration of effect of seed type and effect of fertilizer level, with no interaction between seed type and fertilizer level. Population mean yield versus (a) fertilizer level, by seed type, and (b) seed type, by fertilizer level.

of the effects by themselves (see Figure 5.5). Consider the following table of six population means:

Seed	Fertilizer Level				
Type	1	2	3	$\mu + \alpha_i$	α_i
1	14	18	19	17	2
2	12	10	17	13	-2
$\mu + \beta_j$	13	14	18		
β_j	-2	-1	3		

As before, averaging the mean response of all six populations, we obtain the overall mean, $\mu = 15$. Averaging over the mean response of all three populations that correspond to seed type 1 we obtain $\mu + \alpha_1 = 17$ bushels/acre, so that $\alpha_1 = 17 - 15 = 2$; averaging over the mean response of the two populations that correspond to low fertilizer level, we obtain $\mu + \beta_1 = 13$ and $\beta_1 = -2$. But now $\mu_{11} = 14 \neq \mu + \alpha_1 + \beta_1 = 15$. The difference is the interaction between seed type 1 and low level of fertilizer on mean yield. It is denoted by $\alpha\beta_{11}$, which is equal to $14 - 15 = -1$ in this case. That is, the combination of low fertilizer and seed type 1 produces one bushel/acre less than we would have expected if fertilizer and seed type had additive effects on yield. Here, the main effects of fertilizer and seed type (α_i and β_j) are of less interest in themselves, because the effect of fertilizer level depends on seed type and the effect of seed type depends on the fertilizer level.

The plots of the mean yield versus level of fertilizer by seed type and versus seed type by level of fertilizer are also instructive; see Figure 5.5. We note that the difference in yield between the two seed types is larger for the middle level of fertilizer than for the low and high levels ($18 - 10$ versus $14 - 12$ and $19 - 17$). We see also that the differences between any two fertilizer levels differ for the two seed types ($18 - 14$, $10 - 12$, etc.).

5.4 ANALYSIS OF VARIANCE AND F TESTS

In order to analyze the variance, we apply methods similar to those used in Chapter 2. We divide $Y_{ijk} - \bar{Y}_{...}$, the deviation of each observation from the overall mean, into meaningful parts. We do so with the following equation in mind:

$$Y_{ijk} - \mu = \alpha_i + \beta_j + (\alpha\beta)_{ij} + \varepsilon_{ijk}. \tag{5.2}$$

The left-hand side of Equation 5.2 is clearly to be estimated by $Y_{ijk} - \bar{Y}_{...}$. On the right-hand side, α_i should be estimated by $\bar{Y}_{i..} - \bar{Y}_{...}$, and β_j by $\bar{Y}_{.j.} - \bar{Y}_{...}$. Because we have made no assumptions at all concerning the population means, ε_{ijk} is estimated by $Y_{ijk} - \bar{Y}_{ij.}$. By subtracting the estimates of α_i, β_j, and ε_{ijk} from the estimate of $Y_{ijk} - \mu$, we obtain $\bar{Y}_{ij.} - \bar{Y}_{i..} - \bar{Y}_{.j.} + \bar{Y}_{...}$ as an estimate of $(\alpha\beta)_{ij}$. Thus we have

$$Y_{ijk} - \bar{Y}_{...} = (\bar{Y}_{i..} - \bar{Y}_{...}) + (\bar{Y}_{.j.} - \bar{Y}_{...}) + (\bar{Y}_{ij.} - \bar{Y}_{i..} - \bar{Y}_{.j.} + \bar{Y}_{...}) + (Y_{ijk} - \bar{Y}_{ij.}). \tag{5.3}$$

If we express each deviation $Y_{ijk} - \bar{Y}_{...}$ in this way, square both sides, and sum over all the observations, the cross product terms add to zero and we have

$$\sum_{i=1}^{a}\sum_{j=1}^{b}\sum_{k=1}^{n}(Y_{ijk} - \bar{Y}_{...})^2 = bn\sum_{i=1}^{a}(\bar{Y}_{i..} - \bar{Y}_{...})^2$$
$$+ an\sum_{j=1}^{b}(\bar{Y}_{.j.} - \bar{Y}_{...})^2$$
$$+ n\sum_{i=1}^{a}\sum_{j=1}^{b}(\bar{Y}_{ij.} - \bar{Y}_{i..} - \bar{Y}_{.j.} + \bar{Y}_{...})^2$$
$$+ \sum_{i=1}^{a}\sum_{j=1}^{b}\sum_{k=1}^{n}(Y_{ijk} - \bar{Y}_{ij.})^2. \tag{5.4}$$

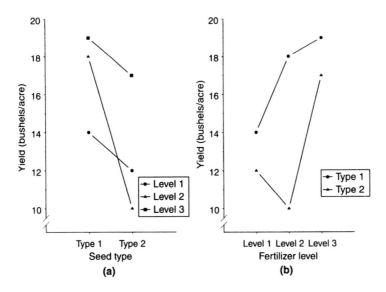

Fig. 5.5 Illustration of interaction between seed type and fertilizer level: population mean yield versus (a) fertilizer level, by seed type, and (b) seed type, by fertilizer level.

The first term on the right-hand side of Equation 5.4 is said to be *variation due to the first factor*, or the *main effect* of the first factor. We often call it the *factor A* sum of squares, or the *A effect* The second term, similarly, is the *factor B* sum of squares or the *B effect*. The third term is called the *interaction* between factors A and B or the *AB effect*. The last term is the residual.

Thus, the total sum of squares, $SS_t = \sum_{i=1}^{a}\sum_{b=1}^{j}\sum_{k=1}^{n}(Y_{ijk} - \bar{Y}_{...})^2$, is broken down into four parts. The first is $SS_a = bn\sum_{i=1}^{a}(\bar{Y}_{i..} - \bar{Y}_{...})^2$, the second is $SS_b = an\sum_{j=1}^{b}(\bar{Y}_{.j.} - \bar{Y}_{...})^2$, the third is $SS_{ab} = n\sum_{i=1}^{a}\sum_{j=1}^{b}(\bar{Y}_{ij.} - \bar{Y}_{i..} - \bar{Y}_{.j.} + \bar{Y}_{...})^2$, and the fourth is $SS_r = \sum_{i=1}^{a}\sum_{j=1}^{b}\sum_{k=1}^{n}(Y_{ijk} - \bar{Y}_{ij.})^2$. These sums of squares are expressed in these terms in Table 5.2, which gives the ANOVA table for the balanced two-way classification, fixed effects model.

The numbers of degrees of freedom for the A sum of squares, the B sum of squares, and the total sum of squares are easily obtained as $a - 1$, $b - 1$, and $abn - 1$. The residual sum of squares is simply the pooled estimate of the variance from ab independent samples, and thus its degrees of freedom are $abn - ab = ab(n - 1)$. By subtracting $a - 1$, $b - 1$, and $ab(n - 1)$ from the total number of degrees of freedom $abn - 1$, we obtain $(a - 1)(b - 1)$ as the number of degrees of freedom for the interaction term, the only remaining sum of squares.

The mean square and EMS columns of Table 5.2 have the same forms as in the one-way classification fixed effects model of Chapter 2. Now $MS_a = SS_a/(a-1)$ estimates $\sigma^2 + bn\phi(\alpha)$, where $\phi(\alpha) = \sum_{i=1}^{a} \alpha_i^2/(a-1)$ and bn is the number of observations on which a single $\bar{Y}_{i..}$ is based. Similarly, $MS_b = SS_b/(b-1)$ estimates $\sigma^2 + an\phi(\beta)$, where $\phi(\beta) = \sum_{i=1}^{b} \beta_j^2/(b-1)$ and an is the number of observations on which a single $\bar{Y}_{.j.}$ is based. The interaction mean square $MS_{ab} = SS_{ab}/(a-1)(b-1)$ estimates $\sigma^2 + n\phi(\alpha\beta)$, where $\phi(\alpha\beta) = \sum_{i=1}^{a} \sum_{j=1}^{b} (\alpha\beta)_{ij}^2/(a-1)(b-1)$ and n is the number of observations on which each $\bar{Y}_{ij.}$ is based. The quantity MS_r, or s^2, provides an estimate of σ^2.

By considering the EMS column, we see that it is possible to make three tests. First we want to test whether interaction exists between the two factors. If there is interaction, then we conclude that the effects of A and B are not additive and tests for the main effects of the two factors are less meaningful, as it isn't clear how to interpret main effects in the presence of interaction. In this case, we recommend plotting the means for each factor on a single graph, as illustrated in Figure 5.5. The null hypothesis of no interaction is

$$H_0 : (\alpha\beta)_{ij} = 0, \qquad i = 1,\ldots,a, \quad j = 1,\ldots,b,$$

or, expressed in terms of the population means,

$$H_0 : \mu_{ij} = \mu + \alpha_i + \beta_j.$$

If H_0 is true, MS_{ab} and s^2 are two independent estimates of σ^2. Therefore, the test statistic MS_{ab}/s^2 is compared with $F[1-\alpha; (a-1)(b-1), ab(n-1)]$.

If there is no interaction, then we are interested in testing for main effects of the two factors. The null hypothesis for no main effects of factor A is

$$H_0 : \alpha_i = 0, \qquad i = 1,\ldots,a,$$

or, expressed in terms of the population means,

Table 5.2 Analysis of Variance, Two-Way Cross Classification, Fixed Effects Model, with Equal Sample Sizes

Source of Variation	Sums of Squares	df	MS	EMS	F
Factor A	SS_a	$a-1$	MS_a	$\sigma^2 + bn\phi(\alpha)$	MS_a/s^2
Factor B	SS_b	$b-1$	MS_b	$\sigma^2 + an\phi(\beta)$	MS_b/s^2
Interaction of A and B	SS_{ab}	$(a-1)(b-1)$	MS_{ab}	$\sigma^2 + n\phi(\alpha\beta)$	MS_{ab}/s^2
Residual	SS_r	$ab(n-1)$	MS_r	σ^2	
Total	SS_t	$abn-1$			

$$H_0 : \mu_{i.} = \mu + \alpha_i.$$

This is tested by comparing MS_a/s^2 with $F_{[1-\alpha;a-1,ab(n-1)]}$.
The null hypothesis for no main effects of factor B is

$$H_0 : \beta_j = 0, \qquad j = 1, \ldots, b,$$

or, expressed in terms of population means,

$$H_0 : \mu_{.j} = \mu + \beta_j,$$

which is tested by comparing MS_b/s^2 with $F_{[1-\alpha;b-1,ab(n-1)]}$.

Example. In Table 5.3, the ANOVA table for the data of Table 5.1 is presented. The sums of squares obtained for each of the four sources of variation add up to SS_t. From the columns of Table 5.3, we conclude that interactions exist between seed type and fertilizer level ($p < 0.0001$). Thus certain (seed type, fertilizer level) combinations give higher yields than would be expected on the basis of the seed type and the fertilizer level; certain combinations perform worse than would be expected. Plots of the sample means are shown in Figure 5.6. Level of fertilizer is shown on the X axis and mean yield on the Y axis. Lines connecting the means for each seed type separately are clearly nonparallel, which is suggestive of the presence of interaction.

Similarly, we reject the hypotheses concerning the main effects of seed type and level of fertilizer. We conclude that there is an effect of seed type on mean yield when averaging is done over the three levels of fertilizer ($p < 0.0001$), and that there is an effect of level of fertilizer on mean yield when averaging is done over the two seed types ($p < 0.0001$).

In some situations, the sample size from each of the ab populations is $n = 1$. The SS_r is 0 in this case. If it is desired to test for the main effects of the two factors, then the MS_{ab} term is used in the denominator in the computation of the F tests. If there is no interaction between the two factors, there is no problem in doing this, as $\phi(\alpha\beta) = 0$ and MS_{ab} estimates σ^2. However, if there is interaction between the two factors, MS_{ab} estimates σ^2 plus something more. The ratio of a main effect to interaction mean squares does not follow an F distribution when there is interaction.

5.5   ESTIMATES OF PARAMETERS AND CONFIDENCE INTERVALS

It is unsatisfactory to perform a two-way ANOVA, find significant results, and stop there. If differences are detected, investigators want to know something more — how the means differ. These questions can better be answered in terms of estimation.

Table 5.3 Analysis of Variance Table for Experiment on Two Types of Seed with Three Fertilizer Levels

Source of Variation	SS	df	MS	EMS	Computed F	p Value
Seeds	77.4	1	77.4	$\sigma^2 + 12\phi(\alpha)$	63.3	0.0001
Fertilizer level	99.9	2	49.9	$\sigma^2 + 8\phi(\beta)$	40.9	0.0001
Seed by Fertilizer interaction	44.1	2	22.1	$\sigma^2 + 4\phi(\alpha\beta)$	18.0	0.0001
Residual	22.0	18	1.2	σ^2		
Total	243.4	23				

Since all of the point estimates are linear combinations of the Y_{ijk}, their expected values and variances can be verified by applying the rules for obtaining expected values and variances of linear combinations, as given in Appendix A. The estimate for σ^2 and its confidence interval follow as usual from the ANOVA table.

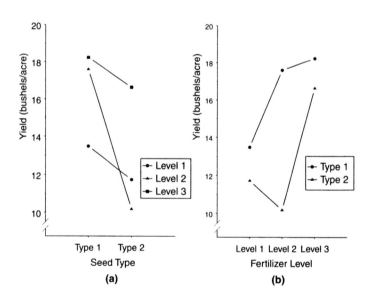

Fig. 5.6 Data example: plot of sample mean yield versus level of fertilizer, by seed type.

Table 5.4 Two-Way Classification, Fixed Effects Model, Equal Sample Sizes: Estimates of Parameters and Their Estimated Variances

Parameter	Point Estimate	Estimated Variance of Estimate
μ	$\bar{Y}_{...}$	$s^2/(abn)$
$\mu_{i.}$	$\bar{Y}_{i..}$	$s^2/(bn)$
$\mu_{.j}$	$\bar{Y}_{.j.}$	$s^2/(an)$
μ_{ij}	$\bar{Y}_{ij.}$	s^2/n
α_i	$\bar{Y}_{i..} - \bar{Y}_{...}$	$s^2(1 - \frac{1}{a})/bn$
β_j	$\bar{Y}_{.j.} - \bar{Y}_{...}$	$s^2(1 - \frac{1}{b})/an$
$(\alpha\beta)_{ij}$	$\bar{Y}_{ij.} - \bar{Y}_{i..} - \bar{Y}_{.j.} + \bar{Y}_{...}$	$s^2(1 - \frac{1}{a})(1 - \frac{1}{b})/n$
$\mu_{i.} - \mu_{i'.}$	$\bar{Y}_{i..} - \bar{Y}_{i'..}$	$2s^2/(bn)$
$\mu_{.j} - \mu_{.j'}$	$\bar{Y}_{.j.} - \bar{Y}_{.j'.}$	$2s^2/(an)$
$\sum_{i=1}^{a} c_i\mu_{i.}$	$\sum_{i=1}^{a} c_i\bar{Y}_{i..}$	$s^2[\sum_{i=1}^{a} c_i^2/(bn)]$
$\sum_{j=1}^{b} c_j\mu_{.j})$	$\sum_{j=1}^{b} c_j\bar{Y}_{.j.}$	$s^2[\sum_{j=1}^{b} c_j^2/(an)]$
σ^2	s^2	

Our primary interest involves estimating means. For the two-way classification, there are different means that could be considered. Possible parameters, corresponding point estimates, and estimated variances of the point estimates are shown in Table 5.4, along with some other parameters that are potentially of interest. For example, suppose we are interested in the effect of factor A on the response Y. One approach would be to *average* over factor B, in which case the parameters to be estimated are $\mu_{i.} = E(\bar{Y}_{i..}) = \mu + \alpha_i$, $i = 1, \ldots, a$. The point estimates are $\bar{Y}_{i..}$, $i = 1, \ldots, a$. This is one way of adjusting for factor B. Similarly, if interest is in the effect of factor B on Y, we could average over all levels of factor A, so that the parameters we wish to estimate are $\bar{\mu}_{.j} = E(\bar{Y}_{.j}) = \mu_{.j}$, $j = 1, \ldots, b$, and the corresponding point estimates are $\bar{Y}_{.j.}$, $j = 1,\ldots, b$. These means provide useful summaries, regardless of the presence or absence of interaction.

An alternative way to adjust for a second factor B is to restrict estimation to a specific value of B. In this case, the parameters are the means of the cross classified groupings, $\mu_{ij} = \mu + \alpha_i + \beta_j + (\alpha\beta)_{ij}$, $i = 1,\ldots, a$, $j = 1,\ldots, b$. The corresponding point estimates are the group-specific means, $\bar{Y}_{ij.}$. This method of adjusting for the second factor may be of particular interest in the presence of interaction, since, as discussed earlier in Section 5.3, the effect of one factor depends on the level of the second factor in this situation.

Instead of individual means, the investigator may wish to consider paired differences or some other linear combination of means. Again, these linear combinations can be obtained by averaging over the other factor or by restricting the other factor to a specific level. Paired differences such as $\mu_{i.} - \mu_{i'.}$, or general linear combinations of the form $\sum_{i=1}^{a} c_i(\mu_{i.})$, are applicable when someone wants to average over the levels of the B. Paired differences such as $\mu_{ij} - \mu_{ij'}$, or general linear combinations of the form $\sum_{j=1}^{b} c_j \mu_{ij}$, are applicable when someone wants to compare means across levels of B when A is restricted to level i.

Since all of the point estimates are linear combinations of the Y_{ijk}, their expected values and variances can be verified by applying the rules for obtaining expected values and variances of linear combinations, as applied in Chapter 3 and as given in Appendix A. The estimate for σ^2 and its confidence interval follow as usual from the ANOVA table.

Confidence intervals are computed in the same way as in Chapter 3. In general, a $100(1 - \alpha)\%$ confidence interval is computed as

$$(\text{point estimate}) \pm t_{1-\alpha/2;\nu} \times (\text{ standard error}) \tag{5.5}$$

where ν is the number of degrees of freedom used in the estimation of σ^2, here $ab(n - 1)$, and the standard error is the estimated standard error of the corresponding point estimate. (Or a t test can be made, where the t statistic is calculated as the ratio of the point estimate to the estimated standard error; the value of the t statistic is then compared with the $t_{1-\alpha/2,\nu}$ when making a two-sided test.)

Typically, we are interested in obtaining more than one confidence interval, so some multiple comparison procedure would be warranted. There are numerous multiple comparison procedures available, and the ones that were considered in Chapter 3 could similarly be applied for the two-way cross-classification. The same discussion of appropriateness of a given procedure applies here as well. See Chapter 3 for details of multiple comparison procedures, and [4] for further examples.

Example. For the agricultural data example considered in this section, significant interactions and main effects were obtained. Suppose we are interested in two contrasts. We want to estimate the difference in mean yields for seed 1 versus seed 2, averaging over level of fertilizer. Second, we want to investigate whether there is a linear trend in mean yield as level of fertilizer is increased, averaging over type of seed. Here we are assuming that the levels of fertilizer are equally spaced; the difference between low and medium amounts of fertilizer is the same as the difference between medium and high amounts.

For the difference in mean yield from seed 1 versus seed 2, the parameter we wish to estimate is $\mu_{1.} - \mu_{2.}$. The point estimate is $\bar{Y}_{1..} - \bar{Y}_{2..} = 16.43 - 12.84 = 3.59$, and the estimated standard error is $\sqrt{2s^2/(bn)} = \sqrt{2 \times 1.2/(3 \times 4)} = 0.45$.

For a linear trend in mean yield as the level of fertilizer is increased, the linear combination is $1 \cdot \mu_{.1} + 0 \cdot \mu_{.2} - 1 \cdot \mu_{.3}$. The point estimate is $\bar{Y}_{.1.} - \bar{Y}_{.3.} = 12.60 - 17.43 = -4.83$, and the standard error is $\sqrt{2s^2/(an)} = 0.55$.

If we were using the Bonferroni method (see Section 3.3.3), we would have decided we were interested in making these $m = 2$ comparisons, so that the value of t that would be used in constructing the intervals is $t_{[1-\alpha/4;\nu=18]}$. If we want the experimentwise error rate to be 0.05, the value of t is $t_{[0.9875,18]} = 2.445$. The first confidence interval is

$$2.50 \leq \mu_{1.} - \mu_{2.} \leq 4.68.$$

This indicates that we are 95% confident that the difference in mean yields for the two seed types, when we average over level of fertilizer, is between 2.50 and 4.68. If we were using this interval for hypothesis testing, we would conclude that the mean yield for seed type 1 is higher than the mean yield for seed type 2 (averaging over levels of fertilizer used).

Similarly, the second confidence interval is

$$-6.16 \leq \mu_{.1} - \mu_{.3} \leq -3.49.$$

Because this interval does not cover 0, the conclusion is made that there is a linear trend; that is, as the level of fertilizer is increased, the mean yield is increased, when we average over seed type.

The advantages of averaging over the levels of a second factor are that the presentation of the findings is simple (the number of intervals to report is not too large) and, if you are only looking at paired comparisons, it is easy to perform the calculations using standard statistical software. The disadvantages are that the procedure is incomplete and may not answer the questions that were asked.

Alternatively, suppose the investigator desires to summarize the experiment by constructing confidence intervals for paired differences in mean yield for one factor when the level of the second factor is restricted. For example, to compare the two seed types at low, medium, and high levels of fertilizer, the parameters that need to be estimated are $\mu_{11} - \mu_{21}$, $\mu_{12} - \mu_{22}$, and $\mu_{13} - \mu_{23}$.

In this example, interest would be in three pairwise comparisons of the means of the six different populations. Since the sample sizes are all equal, Tukey intervals for these comparisons are made, as described in Section 3.3.4.

Because $a = 6$ means are being compared and the number of error degrees of freedom is $\nu = 18$, the 95th percentile of the Studentized range statistic is 4.49 (see Table B.6). Using this value allows us to construct intervals with an experimentwise error rate of 0.05. See Table 5.5 for the intervals.

Examination of these intervals in Table 5.5 suggests that mean yield is higher for seed type 1 when a medium level of fertilizer is applied because the interval is above 0; no differences are apparent at low or high levels, as the confidence intervals include 0.

5.6   DESIGNING A STUDY

In this section, we first consider the advantages of designing a study with two-way cross-classification as opposed to the one-way design [2]. While we focus on experiments, the same advantages apply to surveys.

Suppose an investigator wishes to study the distribution of labeled cholesterol in tissues of rats following various diets. To assess cholesterol levels in the plasma, liver, and other locations, rats are fed one of three diets, and additional dosages of cholesterol are administered within 24 hours of sacrifice. The investigator assigns the treatments to the following numbers of rats using a two-way fixed effects ANOVA design with equal sample size, as follows:

		Additional Dosage of Cholesterol		
Basic Diet		None	One Large Dose	Four Equal Small Doses
1.	Standard + no fat	n rats	n rats	n rats
2.	Standard + saturated fat	n rats	n rats	n rats
3.	Standard + unsaturated fat	n rats	n rats	n rats

In a single experiment, the investigator is able to assess the main effects of three diets, the main effects of the three additional dosages of cholesterol prior to sacrifice, and the interactions between diet and cholesterol dosage. The ANOVA table for for the effect of any one measure — say, cholesterol level in the liver — is as follows:

Table 5.5   All Pairwise Comparisons for Population Means — Rye Yield Example

Difference of Population Means	Difference of Sample Means	Lower Limit of CI	Upper Limit of CI
$\mu_{seed1,high} - \mu_{seed2,high}$	1.60	−0.88	4.08
$\mu_{seed1,med} - \mu_{seed2,med}$	7.43	4.94	9.91
$\mu_{seed1,low} - \mu_{seed2,low}$	1.75	−0.73	4.23

	df	EMS
Diet	2	$\sigma^2 + 3n\phi(diet)$
Cholesterol	2	$\sigma^2 + 3n\phi(chol)$
Interaction	4	$\sigma^2 + n\phi(diet \times chol)$
Residual	$9(n-1)$	σ^2
Total	$9n - 1$	

An investigator unfamiliar with the two-way ANOVA may plan to experiment with diets using just two diets at a time. A procedure that is still widely used consists of several experiments, each comparing one treatment with a standard treatment. As the first experiment two diets, (1) standard + no fat and (2) standard + saturated fat, might be used; from this the effect of the addition of saturated fat to the standard diet can be assessed. The one-way ANOVA table is as follows:

	df	EMS
Due diet	1	$\sigma^2 + n\phi(diet)$
Residual	$2(n-1)$	σ^2
Total	$2n - 1$	

After the first one-way ANOVA, the investigator can perform a similar experiment to compare (1) standard diet with (2) standard diet + unsaturated fat, and can then make statements comparing these two diets relative to the control diet.

It is extremely important that, with a given number of rats, the experimental result produces as reliable an estimate of σ^2 (s^2) as possible. The estimate of σ^2 tends to be quite variable for small numbers of degrees of freedom (the variance of s^2 is $2\sigma^4/\mathrm{df}$). Since it is highly desirable to have a stable estimate of σ^2, the investigator in our example wishes to use a limited number of rats to achieve as many degrees of freedom as possible for the mean square residual.

In the two-way design, with five rats assigned to each diet, 45 rats are used and there are $9(5 - 1) = 36$ degrees of freedom for σ^2, which measures the basic variation in liver cholesterol of rats fed the same diet. If, on the other hand, five rats are used in each of the one-way experiments, then the degrees of freedom available from each experiment are only $2(5 - 1) = 8$. To obtain more sensitive F tests, more accurate estimates of σ^2, and shorter confidence intervals, the investigator may increase the number of rats on each treatment. With 10 rats on each treatment, there are 18 degrees of freedom in each of the two experiments; 40 rats (only five less than in the two-way analysis of variance) have already been used, and the investigator still has no information on the effect of additional cholesterol or on the interaction of diet and cholesterol.

The importance of having many degrees of freedom for s^2 cannot be overstated. We have seen the usefulness of s^2 in making confidence intervals and in computing F test statistics. In addition, s^2 is useful in determining sample size for future experiments. From the two-way experiment, the investigator might focus on the length of a confidence interval for $\mu_{ij.}$, and select a sample size n so that $2t_{1-\alpha/2;ab(n-1)}\sqrt{s^2/n}$ (with s^2 from the previous experiment) equals approximately the length desired in the next experiment.

The calculated s^2 value should always be carefully considered. All too often it is ignored as the researcher concentrates on various contrasts and on F tests. If s^2 is much higher than in past experiments, the discrepancy may indicate a loss in accuracy in the present study that should be investigated before further analyses are made on the data.

We also notice in comparing the several one-way experiments with the two-way design that the due diet mean square estimates $\sigma^2 + n\phi(diet)$ in the one-way, whereas in the two-way it estimates $\sigma^2 + 3n\phi(diet)$. The parameter σ^2 is not necessarily the same quantity in the two designs; nevertheless, if the same n is used in the same designs, we expect that $\sigma^2 + n\phi(diet)$ will usually be smaller than $\sigma^2 + 3n\phi(diet)$. The due diet mean square appears in the numerator of the F statistic for testing differences among diets; therefore, it seems reasonable to suggest that the F test is usually less sensitive in the one-way analysis to differences among the diets.

Another advantage of the two-way design over the one-way design is that the investigators are able to make wider inferences. This is because they are varying a second factor.

The two-way ANOVA is among the most widely used approaches, particularly in laboratory work. If investigators wish to examine several factors, they can obtain more information from a given number of observations than from successive one-way ANOVA experiments. Furthermore, since these designs are relatively simple, analysis and interpretation are not too difficult. After investigators have learned to interpret data in their field from these designs, they find them to be a big help in their research.

In defense of the one-way ANOVA approach of comparing two treatments at a time, it should be noted that there are situations in which performing one small experiment after another has advantages. For example, if the second factor (instead of cholesterol dosage) is dosage of a chemical that may or may not be lethal, it may be better to begin with several small one-way experiments, each comparing just two dosage levels. Sometimes a series of small one-way experiments is advantageous when little is known about the response being measured and the investigator does not at first know how to pick levels or sample sizes.

The two-way cross-classification can easily be generalized to three-way or higher cross-classifications. Suppose there are three factors of interest, A, B, and C. When specifying the underlying model, we will want to consider main effects, two-way interactions, and three-way interactions. The model is specified as follows:

$$
\begin{aligned}
Y_{ijkl} \; = \; & \mu + \alpha_i + \beta_j + \gamma_k \\
& + (\alpha\beta)_{ij} + (\alpha\gamma)_{ik} + (\beta\gamma)_{jk} \\
& + (\alpha\beta\gamma)_{ijk} + \varepsilon_{ijkl},
\end{aligned}
$$

where $i = 1, \ldots, a$, $j = 1, \ldots, b$, $k = 1, \ldots, c$, $l = 1, \ldots, n_{ijkl}$, and ε_{ijkl} are independent and normally distributed with mean 0 and variance σ^2. When summed over all levels of a factor specified by its subscript, each parameter in the model must sum to zero.

The two- and three-way ANOVA designs are among the most widely used designs. They possess a happy degree of complexity, combining ease in interpretation with the ability to study several factors simultaneously. Further discussion on designing experiments can be found elsewhere [1, 3].

5.7   PRESENTATION AND INTERPRETATION OF RESULTS

When communicating the statistical methods for a study, it is important to specify how the data were generated (for example, from a two-way cross classification) and how many levels are associated with each factor. The clearest way to communicate this is to state specifically what model was fitted to the data. Anything that was done to check the appropriateness of the model, and any modifications that were made, should be indicated. For example, if the data were transformed, the transformation should be identified. How the analyses are to be presented should also be given. Whether or not comparisons among means were adjusted for multiple comparisons should be stated and, if so, which method was selected. If multiple-comparison procedures were applied, the method needs to be identified.

Regardless of what was done, summary statistics or graphs are useful for each group sampled; at a minimum, the mean, standard deviation, and sample sizes should be presented. This information will provide a good initial summary and will be important preliminary data for the planning of future investigations.

Sometimes, investigators get so focused on the hypothesis tests that the only information that gets presented is in the ANOVA tables. (It may not even be necessary, when a p value would suffice.) The ANOVA is only part of the analysis.

Which population parameters should be estimated depends on whether or not the interaction is present and what the objectives of the analysis are. In some situations, interest is in the means from each of the ab populations; this is particularly the case when there is interaction and how the two factors interact is important. Whether or not there is synergy or antagonism and what combination of factors yields a "best" or "worst" response may be the focus of the research. Otherwise, these means are computed by averaging over the levels of the second factor (in the case of equal sample sizes) or by taking some other linear combination. Such means are simpler, but they may or may not have a meaningful interpretation.

Finally, when ANOVA tests indicate that the means of the populations are unequal, the researcher generally wants to find out which means are different. The comparisons which are made should reflect the objectives of the study. These might include all pairwise comparisons of means, comparisons with a baseline or control combination, assessment of linear trend, and so on.

5.8 SUMMARY

In this chapter, the one-way classification introduced in Chapters 2 and 3 was generalized to the two-way classification. The idea of breaking the total variation into four parts — a first factor, a second factor, the interaction between the two, and the residual — was illustrated for the simplest case, that of equal sample sizes from each population. How to interpret main effects and interactions was also addressed. The ANOVA tests were presented. We considered point and interval estimates of parameters. We also went over determining whether the two-way ANOVA is an appropriate procedure and if not, what some alternatives are. We considered advantages of this design over the one-way classification and other things to consider when planning a cross-classification study.

In this chapter, all effects were assumed to have fixed effects, that is, conclusions were intended to apply only to the populations that were actually sampled. In the following three chapters, we introduce other examples of two way cross classifications. In Chapter 6, we discuss the randomized block design. In Chapter 7, we consider the unbalanced two-way cross-classification with fixed effects, and in Chapter 8 we address balanced two-way cross-classifications where one factor has fixed effects and the other factor's effects are random.

In the next chapter, we will illustrate the two way cross classification with fixed effects but unequal sample sizes from each population.

Problems

5.1 Eighteen adult males were used in a study to compare the sphygmo-manometers from three manufacturers. The subjects were assigned at random into six groups of three each. Three groups had systolic blood pressure measurements (mm Hg) made at entry to the experiment; the other three groups were measured after resting 10 minutes. (The investigators were interested in making inferences only with respect to these two resting time periods and these three manufacturers.) The data were as follows:

Resting	Manufacturer		
	I	II	III
No	147	156	127
	124	127	122
	113	155	153
Yes	140	100	114
	130	140	139
	112	105	126

a) State the model.

b) Perform a two-way ANOVA. Test whether there are differences in mean blood pressure measurements among the three manufacturers. Test whether there is a difference in mean blood pressure between resting time periods.

c) Give confidence intervals for $\mu_{1.} - \mu_{2.}$, $\mu_{.1} - \mu_{.2}$, $\mu_{.1} - \mu_{.3}$, and $\mu_{.2} - \mu_{.3}$, using an overall level of 0.95.

d) Perform a one-way ANOVA only testing if there is a difference in manufacturers. Compare your results with those in b).

e) Test for equality of variances in the three manufacturing groups using the Levene's test.

f) Perform a one-way ANOVA only testing if there is a difference in resting or not resting. Compare the results from this analysis and d) with the results from b).

5.2 Brain weights measured on 28 individuals were as follows:

Age (years)	Weight (g) Men	Weight (g) Women
50–80	1312	1211
	1323	1196
	1325	1207
	1318	1198
	1319	1204
	1342	1191
	1309	1205
20–49	1331	1234
	1330	1204
	1335	1222
	1327	1211
	1338	1228
	1338	1217
	1335	1223

a) Determine sample means and sample standard deviations for the four groups.

b) What assumptions are implicit in the model, in terms of the problem?

c) Generate an ANOVA table.

d) Test ($\alpha = .05$) for no interaction between age and gender. What is your conclusion?

e) Test ($\alpha = .05$) for no effect of age and no effect of gender. What are your conclusions?

f) Determine 95% confidence intervals for the mean difference in age ($\mu_{1.} - \mu_{2.}$) and for the difference in gender ($\mu_{.1} - \mu_{.2}$). Interpret these intervals.

5.3 Four levels of fertilizer were used in a field experiment, with and without irrigation. The eight treatment combinations were assigned at random to eight plots. Barley yields, in bushels per acre, were

Irrigation	Level of Fertilizer None	Low	Medium	High
No	317	341	354	329
Yes	275	304	334	380

a) State the appropriate model.

b) Obtain a two-way ANOVA table. Test whether fertilizers make any difference.

c) Estimate the overall difference in yield due to irrigation, in terms of a point estimate and a confidence interval estimate.

d) Estimate the mean difference in yield between no fertilizer and fertilizer at a low level (point estimate and confidence interval estimate).

5.4 Thirty-six adults — 18 males (M) and 18 females (F) — were used in a study to compare the sphygmomanometers from three manufacturers. Subjects from each sex were assigned at random into six groups of three each. Three groups from each sex had systolic blood pressure measurements made at entry to the experiment; the other three groups were measured after resting 10 minutes. The data were as follows:

| | | Manufacturer | | | | |
| | I | | II | | III | |
Resting	M	F	M	F	M	F
No	147	122	156	131	127	110
	124	142	127	133	122	115
	113	136	155	146	153	105
Yes	140	108	100	141	114	103
	130	151	140	125	139	135
	112	138	105	139	126	114

a) State the model and appropriate assumptions.

b) Make an ANOVA table.

c) Test H_0 : No interaction in blood pressure between resting and sex.

d) Test whether there are differences in blood pressure measurement among the three manufacturers.

e) Test whether there is a difference in blood pressure between resting and no resting.

f) Test whether there is a difference in blood pressure between males and females.

5.5 An experiment was performed in order to study the effects of temperature, concentration of a chemical, and length of mixing time on yield. Two observations were taken for each treatment combination. The following data were obtained:

Concentration (%)	Time (min)	Temperature		
		5^0C	10^0C	15^0C
30	5	10.1, 12.1	9.9, 8.3	11.2, 12.4
	10	8.3, 10.1	10.7, 8.5	12.3, 13.2
	15	8.9, 10.2	11.5, 10.5	11.2, 10.7
35	5	11.3, 11.8	11.3, 12.0	13.8, 12.8
	10	12.4, 11.4	13.4, 11.5	14.5, 14.4
	15	14.3, 12.2	12.2, 13.7	15.2, 14.6

a)   State the model.

b)   Obtain an ANOVA table.

c)   State any conclusions that can be drawn from this experiment (assume that a high yield is preferable to a low yield).

REFERENCES

1. Box, G.E.P., Hunter, W.G., and Hunter, J.S. [1978]. *Statistics for Experimenters,* New York: John Wiley & Sons, 306–351.

2. Czitrom, V. [1999]. One Factor at a Time versus Designed Experiments, *The American Statistician,* 53, 126–131.

3. Dean, A. and Voss, D. [1999]. *Design and Analysis of Experiments,* Springer-Verlag, 135–191.

4. Milliken, G.A. and Johnson, D.E. [1984]. *Analysis of Messy Data, Volume 1: Designed Experiments,* Belmont, CA: Wadsworth, Inc., 116–125.

6

Randomized Complete Block Design

There are many instances in which an investigator wishes to study the effect of a single factor such as economic level or type of fertilizer, but a design that is more complicated than that given in Chapter 2 is either required or desired. In this chapter, we explore one alternative: the randomized complete block design. This design deals with factors that are known to be important, in that they affect the response, and that the investigator wishes to eliminate rather than study. Practical problems may dictate that this design be used, or it may be selected for its own advantages. While we will consider it in terms of an experiment, the design applies equally well in nonexperimental situations. For this chapter, the factor that we wish to study will be referred to as the *treatment* factor, and the factor we wish to eliminate will be referred to as the *blocking* factor.

In Chapter 5, the cross-classified design was introduced. The randomized complete block design is an example of a cross-classification. In the previous chapter, however, we were interested in making inferences about the two factors. Now, we have one factor which we are interested in and a blocking factor whose effects we wish to remove.

In Section 6.1, we introduce an example in which the randomized complete block design was used. This will be followed in Section 6.2 by some general comments about the randomized complete block design. The model will be presented in Section 6.3. The design we are considering is a cross-classification of treatment and block with sample size $n = 1$ for each treatment and block combination; it is based on the assumption of no interaction between the effects of treatment and block. Inference will be discussed in terms of hypothesis testing in Section 6.4 and estimation in Section 6.5. Checking whether the data fit the model is covered in Section 6.6, and recommendations concerning what to do if they don't are presented in Section 6.7. General comments about designing a randomized complete block study are provided in Section 6.8; this is followed by a brief consideration of its extensions in Section 6.9. The chapter is summarized in Section 6.10.

6.1 EXAMPLE

Pest management is one of the problems facing those who maintain fruit orchards. One approach to dealing with the problem is to develop trees that are resistant to pests or disease. For example, the Liberty apple tree is resistant to the fungal disease scab. Studies have suggested that, compared with some other cultivars (varieties) of apple trees, Liberty trees need less fungicide in order to maintain tree health without affecting the apple crop. While these trees are resistant to scab, they are not resistant to other other fungal diseases, such as sooty blotch and fly speck.

In an apple orchard at the University of Vermont Horticulture Research Center, an experiment was performed to evaluate the long-term (four year) effects of fungicide versus no fungicide applications on tree vigor, productivity, and fruit quality of Liberty apple trees grown in Vermont.

The motivation for performing this study was that an earlier study, conducted in the Hudson River Valley of New York, found detrimental effects on tree vigor and productivity when no fungicide was used [8]. More recent results are summarized in [5]. The trees used in that study were of rootstock Malling (M) M.9. In Vermont and in other areas of New England, the more vigorous rootstock M.7 is planted and accepted. The question was whether Liberty trees from a more vigorous rootstock would see the same detrimental effects.

Measures of tree vigor include such quantities as trunk cross-sectional area, tree height, shoot length, and time of leaf abscission. Total yield (weight of crop) is an example of productivity. Fruit quality involves assessment of fruit diameters, firmness, disorders, and so on.

Eight blocks of Liberty trees were identified. A block of trees consisted of two sets of three adjacent trees. Outcomes for the three trees were averaged, and analyses performed on these averages. The investigators chose to block on (mean) trunk cross-sectional area prior to randomization. Thus, the sets of trees within a block should have similar trunk cross-sectional areas before being randomized to receive or not to receive fungicide applications. Trunk cross-sectional area is a measure of tree vigor; trees that were larger before the study would be larger at the end of the study and would have the capacity to yield more fruit. By blocking on trunk cross-sectional area prior to randomization, we hope that the trees will be similar before treatment is applied. Thus, any differences in tree vigor or productivity can be explained by the treatment.

Numerous measures of tree vigor, productivity, and fruit quality were observed. We will focus on two outcomes: tree height and fruit size. (Other outcomes are considered in the homework problems.) The tree heights, in meters, were measured, and their means determined. At harvest, 20 apples were sampled from the trees, their diameters, in centimeters, measured, and the mean of the 20 diameters calculated. Tree heights are shown in Table 6.1 and fruit diameters are shown in Table 6.2. Data are classified by treatment group and block. Details of how to measure these and other outcomes are described in [1, 7].

The primary questions we want to investigate concern the treatment means. Is the mean height the same for Liberty apple trees that are treated and not treated with fungicide? Is the mean fruit diameter the same? A question of secondary interest would be, was it worthwhile to block on initial trunk cross-sectional area?

We use the notation Y_{ij} to denote the observation obtained from the ith treatment and jth block. For tree height, $Y_{12} = 2.85$. $\bar{Y}_{i.}$ denotes the mean for the ith treatment, computed over all blocks. So, for example, $\bar{Y}_{1.} = 3.10$ meters is the mean height for all trees which received the fungicide. Similarly, $\bar{Y}_{2.} = 3.19$ is the mean height for all trees which did not receive the fungicide. $\bar{Y}_{.j}$ denotes the mean for the jth block, averaged over all treatments. So, for example, $\bar{Y}_{.2} = 2.70$ is the mean for all trees in the second block. Finally, $\bar{Y}_{..}$ denotes the overall mean, obtained by averaging over all treatments and blocks. Again for tree height, $\bar{Y}_{..} = 3.15$.

The mean diameter of apples obtained from all trees receiving fungicide is $\bar{Y}_{1.} = 7.07$, and the mean diameter of apples not receiving fungicide is $\bar{Y}_{2.} = 7.26$; the mean diameter of all apples obtained from all trees is $\bar{Y}_{..} = 7.17$.

6.2 THE RANDOMIZED COMPLETE BLOCK DESIGN

In this section, we clarify what identifies a randomized complete block design and how it differs from the completely randomized design discussed in Chapter 2. We first state the meaning of the first three words in "randomized complete block design":

(1) *Block.* All units included in a block are homogeneous with respect the level of a (blocking) factor that is thought to affect the outcome.

(2) *Complete.* All treatments are administered to units that are included in the block. (Another design, the *randomized incomplete block*, is one in which not all treatments are administered in each block; this design is not covered in this text.)

(3) *Randomized.* To avoid subjective allocation of units to treatment and to equalize other influences on outcome that have not been blocked, the

Table 6.1   Observed Data for Tree Height, in Meters

Fungicide i	Block j								Means
	1	2	3	4	5	6	7	8	
Yes	2.59	2.85	3.15	3.10	2.54	3.25	3.81	3.51	3.10
No	2.59	2.54	3.61	3.66	3.05	3.40	3.35	3.35	3.19
Means	2.59	2.70	3.38	3.38	2.80	3.30	3.58	3.43	3.15

units that are included in the block are assigned at random to receive one of the treatments.

In terms of the Liberty apple study, "randomized complete block" means the following:

(1) *Block.* Two sets of trees with similar trunk cross-sectional areas at the start of the study defined the block. The size of a tree, as measured by its trunk cross-sectional area, was known to be related to other measures of tree vigor. There were eight blocks in this study.

(2) *Complete.* Each set of trees in the block received one of the two possible treatments: fungicide or no fungicide. That is, two treatments were being compared. One set of trees in a block received the fungicide and the other set did not.

(3) *Randomized.* The plots of trees in each block were randomly assigned to receive reduced fungicide or no fungicide.

This design is an example of a *cross-classified* design. This means that every level of the treatment factor appears with every level of the blocking factor. Having complete blocks is what makes this a cross-classification.

This example, like all the randomized complete block designs considered in this chapter, is a *balanced* design. This means that the sample size is the same for each of the factor combinations. (Here, that sample size is one.)

This study could have been designed as a completely randomized design. The sets of apple trees would have been selected at random, with half randomized to receive fungicide and half no fungicide. What was the advantage

Table 6.2   Observed Data for Fruit Diameter, in Centimeters

Fungicide i	Block j								Means
	1	2	3	4	5	6	7	8	
Yes	7.14	7.21	7.10	7.17	6.43	7.21	7.37	6.95	7.07
No	7.49	7.13	7.48	7.33	7.10	7.08	7.14	7.33	7.26
Means	7.32	7.17	7.29	7.25	6.77	7.15	7.26	7.14	7.17

of the randomized block design? The investigators believed that tree vigor at the start of the study (as measured by trunk cross-sectional area) could affect tree vigor and productivity. They wanted to control, or remove the effect of, baseline vigor. In a completely randomized design, it is *hoped* that randomization will average out effects of initial tree vigor; in a randomized block design, it is *assured*. Furthermore, in a completely randomized design, variation in responses that can be explained by initial tree vigor is part of the residual variation. With a randomized block design, baseline tree vigor is identified as a unique source of variation. For both designs, it is hoped that randomization will equalize other effects that could affect outcome (for example, exposure to other pests) across the treatment groups.

We will come back to the advantages and disadvantages of the randomized complete block design in Section 6.8, after we have identified the appropriate model and have discussed hypothesis testing and construction of confidence intervals.

6.3   THE MODEL

In Chapter 2, where the completely randomized design was introduced, the effect of a factor was considered to be either fixed or random. There were some small differences in the specification of the model to reflect whether fixed or random effects were assumed. Similarly, for the randomized complete block design, the model is specified to reflect whether effects are fixed or random.

In this chapter, we assume that the effect of treatment is a fixed effect but that the effect of the block may be fixed or random. In the case of the apple tree experiment, the treatment factor is clearly fixed; the investigators were interested in the effects of application of the specified level of fungicide or of no fungicide; they wanted to make inferences about only the two levels of treatment. The blocking factor — initial tree vigor — is likely random. The researchers wanted to make inferences about Liberty apple trees of rootstock M.7 grown in Vermont. They did not select trees with specific trunk cross-sectional areas and did not want to generalize their results to trees with the chosen measurements. The two models (treatment and block fixed, treatment fixed and block random) are summarized below.

In Chapter 2, we expressed the mean of a population as $\mu_i = \mu + \alpha_i$, where the subscript i identified the factor level. For the randomized complete block design, we use the second subscript, j, to identify the block, and include a term for the effect of block on the mean: $\mu_{ij} = \mu + \alpha_i + \beta_j$. The treatment factor has a levels and the blocking factor has b levels. There is a sample of size $n = 1$ from each of the ab populations.

We assume that each observation can be described as follows:

$$Y_{ij} = \mu + \alpha_i + \beta_j + \varepsilon_{ij}, \qquad i = 1, \ldots, a, \quad j = 1, \ldots, b. \qquad (6.1)$$

For *fixed* block effects, we further assume:

$$\sum_{i=1}^{a} \alpha_i = 0, \qquad \sum_{j=1}^{b} \beta_j = 0, \quad \text{and} \quad \varepsilon_{ij} \sim \text{IND}(0, \sigma^2).$$

The assumptions could also be written as $Y_{ij} \sim \text{IND}(\mu + \alpha_i + \beta_j, \sigma^2)$. The mean can also be expressed as μ_{ij}.

For *random* block effects, we further assume:

$$\sum_{i=1}^{a} \alpha_i = 0, \qquad \beta_j \sim \text{IND}(0, \sigma_b^2), \quad \text{and} \quad \varepsilon_{ij} \sim \text{IND}(0, \sigma^2).$$

Here α_i is the mean effect of the ith level of the factor, and β_j is the mean effect of the jth block. That is, α_i is the effect of the ith level of the factor, averaged over all b levels of the block. Similarly, β_j is the effect of the jth level of the block, averaged over all a levels of the factor.

In words rather than symbols, the following assumptions are made for the randomized complete block model:

(1) The response to the ith factor level in the jth block Y_{ij} is from a normal distribution. (There are ab distributions.)

(2) The means of these ab normal distributions can be expressed in the form $\mu_{ij} = \mu + \alpha_i + \beta_j$. The effects of the treatment and the block are simply added to the overall mean effect to get the means of the ab populations. This property is often called *additivity*, or alternatively, *no interaction*.

(3) The variances of the ab populations are all equal.

(4) The ε_{ij} (deviations from the means) are statistically independent and normally distributed. If we know that ε_{11} is large, we have no reason to expect ε_{12} to be small (or large, for that matter). With random block effects, we also assume β_j are statistically independent and that the β_j are independent of the ε_{ij}.

Whether the model with the fixed or random block effects is assumed, the hypothesis testing is the same. The distinction between the two does become important when the sample sizes from the ab populations are greater than one. The two-way ANOVA model with fixed effects, described in Chapter 5 is applicable when the design is balanced and the blocking factor is fixed. The material in Chapter 7 can be applied when the design is unbalanced and the blocking factor is fixed. The methods discussed in Chapter 8 are appropriate when the blocking factor is random.

6.4   ANALYSIS OF VARIANCE TABLE AND F TESTS

For hypothesis testing, our primary interest is in testing whether or not there is an effect of treatment. The null hypothesis of no treatment effect can be expressed in a variety of ways, such as in terms of the model

$$H_0 : Y_{ij} = \mu + \beta_j + \varepsilon_{ij}$$

or, in terms of the treatment effects, as

$$H_0 : \alpha_1 = \cdots = \alpha_a = 0.$$

There is generally less interest in testing the block effects, because when an investigator uses a randomized block design, it is usually because a significant block effect is expected. However, the null hypothesis of no block effect could be stated in the same ways that were used for testing of no treatment effect, for example, $H_0 : \beta_1 = \cdots = \beta_b = 0$ or $H_0 : \sigma_b^2 = 0$.

As in Chapter 5, we proceed now to divide the basic sum of squares into meaningful parts and to make an ANOVA table. From this, we will see how to perform the hypothesis tests. Corresponding to

$$Y_{ij} - \mu = \alpha_i + \beta_j + \varepsilon_{ij}, \tag{6.2}$$

we can express the difference $Y_{ij} - \bar{Y}_{..}$ as the sum of three terms:

$$Y_{ij} - \bar{Y}_{..} = (\bar{Y}_{i.} - \bar{Y}_{..}) + (\bar{Y}_{.j} - \bar{Y}_{..}) + (Y_{ij} - \bar{Y}_{i.} - \bar{Y}_{.j} + \bar{Y}_{..}). \tag{6.3}$$

Note that Equation 6.3 is an algebraic identity. Note also that $\bar{Y}_{i.} - \bar{Y}_{..}$ provides an estimate of α_i and that $\bar{Y}_{.j} - \bar{Y}_{..}$ provides an estimate of β_j. The third term on the right-hand side of Equation 6.3 must estimate ε_{ij}.

As in Chapter 5, we now square both sides of Equation 6.3. If we do this for every observation and sum over the entire set of data, the cross-product terms again sum to zero. The basic sums of squares is thus expressed as the sum of three terms:

$$\sum_{i=1}^{a} \sum_{j=1}^{b} (Y_{ij} - \bar{Y}_{..})^2 = b \sum_{i=1}^{a} (\bar{Y}_{i.} - \bar{Y}_{..})^2 + a \sum_{j=1}^{b} (\bar{Y}_{.j} - \bar{Y}_{..})^2$$

$$+ \sum_{i=1}^{a} \sum_{j=1}^{b} (Y_{ij} - \bar{Y}_{i.} - \bar{Y}_{.j} + \bar{Y}_{..})^2. \tag{6.4}$$

We recognize the first term on the right-hand side of Equation 6.4 as the sum of squares among treatments; the second term, of similar form, is the sum of squares among blocks. The third term represents the residual variation, after variation due to blocks and to treatments has been removed. Thus, for this randomized complete block design, we have divided the total variation (the term on the left) into three parts: variation due to treatments, variation due to blocks, and residual variation. Under the assumption of no interaction, the residual term provides an estimate of σ^2. Note that the residual sum of squares is the same as the interaction sum of squares for a two-way ANOVA with $n = 1$.

Table 6.3 is the ANOVA table. The total sum of squares, SS_t, has been subdivided into three parts: sums of squares due treatment SS_a, due block SS_b, and residual variation SS_r.

The number of degrees of freedom associated with the treatment, block, and total sums of squares are what we expected from the two-way ANOVA model described in Chapter 5; the number of degrees of freedom for the residual sum of squares can be obtained by subtraction; thus we have

$$(a - 1)(b - 1) = (ab - 1) - (b - 1) - (a - 1).$$

The mean squares are computed as the ratios of the sums of squares to the numbers of degrees of freedom, and are denoted MS_a, MS_b, and MS_r or s^2. The EMS column needs little explanation; the due treatment and due block EMS are exactly what we would expect. The symbols $\phi(\alpha)$ and $\phi(\beta)$ are defined by

$$\phi(\alpha) = \sum_{i=1}^{a} \frac{\alpha_i^2}{a - 1} \qquad \text{and} \qquad \phi(\beta) = \sum_{j=1}^{b} \frac{\beta_i^2}{b - 1},$$

respectively, when treatment and block effects are fixed. For random effects, they represent variance components. Under the assumption of no interaction, the EMS associated with residual variation is σ^2.

Example. The results of the analyses of variance are shown in Tables 6.4 and 6.5. The main interest is in whether or not there is any effect of treatment on mean tree height and mean fruit diameter. For tree height, the ratio of the fungicide mean square to the residual mean square is $0.035/0.077 = F = 0.46$. Observing a value of F of 0.46 or greater would not be particularly unusual if there were no effect of fungicide treatment on this measure of tree vigor ($p = 0.52$, see Table 6.4). Thus, the hypothesis of no treatment effect is not rejected, and we conclude that the mean tree height may be the same in both groups. Similarly, the hypothesis of no effect of treatment on mean fruit diameter is not rejected; the calculated F statistic is 2.89, and the corresponding p value is 0.13 (Table 6.5). The null hypothesis of no effect of fungicide on mean fruit diameter is not rejected, and we conclude that the mean fruit diameter may be the same in the two groups.

There is generally less interest in whether or not there is an effect of block (tree vigor at baseline) on mean outcomes. For tree height, there is an effect

Table 6.3 Analysis of Variance Table: Randomized Complete Block Design

Source of Variation	SS	df	MS	EMS	Computed F
Treatments	SS_a	$a-1$	MS_a	$\sigma^2 + b\phi(\alpha)$	MS_a/s^2
Blocks	SS_b	$b-1$	MS_b	$\sigma^2 + \phi(\beta)$	MS_b/s^2
Residual	SS_r	$(a-1)(b-1)$	s^2	σ^2	
Total	SS_t	$ab-1$			

of block ($p = 0.046$). However, no effect of block was found for mean fruit diameter ($p = 0.38$).

Since tree height is also a measure of tree vigor, it may not be surprising that blocking on an initial measurement of tree vigor results in a significant block effect. On the basis of this small example here, we don't have any evidence that baseline tree vigor is related to diameter of apples harvested three years later.

In this particular example, with two treatment groups, the test for no effect of fungicide is equivalent to the paired t test. There are $n = 8$ differences of tree height with fungicide minus tree height without fungicide. The paired t test has $n - 1 = (a - 1)(b - 1) = 7$ degrees of freedom, the same as the residual number for the ANOVA test. The value of the calculated statistic for difference (fungicide minus no fungicide) in mean tree height is $t = -0.68$ with $p = 0.520$. Similarly, for the mean difference in fruit diameter, the calculated test statistic is $t = -1.70$ with $p = 0.313$. Note that the square of the t statistic is equal to the F statistic [e.g., $(-1.70)^2 = 2.89$], and the p values obtained from the t test are equivalent to those from the F test.

One interesting result in the ANOVA table for tree height is that the computed F value is less than one. Note that since EMS_a for the fungicide effect is equal to $\sigma^2 + \phi(\alpha)$ and EMS_r is σ^2, we would expect the computed F to be greater than one. In this case, $F = 0.46$. This result occurs because the two means for fungicide and no fungicide are somewhat closer together than is expected considering the variation in the data. This is usually due simply to chance. However, if the F value is very small, it is recommended that a check be made on how the data were obtained.

6.5 ESTIMATION OF PARAMETERS AND CONFIDENCE INTERVALS

Some of the model parameters that we might be interested in estimating include $\mu_{i.} = \mu + \alpha_i$ (the mean response for the ith level of treatment, when

Table 6.4   Analysis of Variance Table for Tree Height

Source of Variation	SS	df	MS	EMS	Computed F	p Value
Fungicide	0.035	1	0.035	$\sigma^2 + \phi(\alpha)$	0.46	0.52
Blocks	2.093	7	0.299	$\sigma^2 + \phi(\beta)$	3.91	0.046
Residual	0.535	7	0.077	σ^2		
Total	2.663	15				

averaged over all levels of the blocking factor) and $\mu_{ij} = \mu + \alpha_i + \beta_j$ (the response for the combination of the ith treatment and jth block). If blocks are random, an estimate of the variance component can provide information about how variable the blocking effects are. The point estimates and their estimated variances are shown in Table 6.6.

If there are more than two levels of treatment, multiple comparison procedures can be performed to identify which means are different. Confidence intervals or tests, which were described in Chapter 3, can be applied. For a general linear combination $c_i\alpha_i$, the $100(1 - \alpha)\%$ confidence interval has the form

$$\sum_{i=1}^{a} c_i \bar{Y}_{i.} \pm t_{1-\alpha/2,(a-1)(b-1)} \sqrt{s^2 \sum_{i=1}^{a} c_i^2/b}. \tag{6.5}$$

Even when no significant differences are found, or if there are only two treatments being compared, an investigator might still want to construct a confidence interval to get an idea of how precisely a difference in means is estimated. When intervals are computed for the purposes of precision, adjustments for multiple comparisons generally are not made.

Table 6.5   Analysis of Variance Table for Apple Diameter

Source of Variation	SS	df	MS	EMS	Computed F	p Value
Fungicide	0.141	1	0.141	$\sigma^2 + \phi(\alpha)$	2.89	0.13
Blocks	0.429	7	0.061	$\sigma^2 + \phi(\beta)$	1.26	0.38
Residual	0.340	7	0.049	σ^2		
Total	0.910	15				

Table 6.6 Selected Parameters and Their Point Estimates with Estimated Variances for the Randomized Complete Block Design

Parameter	Point Estimate	Estimated Variance of Point Estimate
$\mu_{i.} - \mu_{i'.}$	$\bar{Y}_{i.} - \bar{Y}_{i'.}$	$2s^2/b$
$\sum_{i=1}^{a} c_i \mu_{i.}$	$\sum_{i=1}^{a} c_i \bar{Y}_{i.}$	$s^2 \sum_{i=1}^{a} c_i^2 / b$
σ^2	s^2	$\cdots$
σ_b^2	$(MS_b - s^2)/a$	$\cdots$

Example. For the Liberty apple study, suppose we want to construct a 95% confidence interval for the mean difference in the tree heights. The parameter we wish to make a confidence interval for is $\alpha_1 - \alpha_2$, or $\mu_{1.} - \mu_{2.}$. See Tables 6.1 and 6.4 that present the preliminary calculations. The point estimate from the samples is $\bar{Y}_{1.} - \bar{Y}_{2.} = 3.10 - 3.19 = -0.09$. The estimated variance of this estimate is $2s^2/b = 2(0.077)/8 = 0.019$. The estimated standard error, the square root of the estimated variance, is $\sqrt{0.019} = 0.138$. The appropriate t value for a 95% confidence interval is $t_{0.975,7} = 2.365$. Thus, for the mean difference in tree height, the 95% confidence interval is $-0.09 \pm 2.365 \times 0.138 = -0.09 \pm 0.327$, or $-0.42 \le \alpha_1 - \alpha_2 \le 0.24$. The length of this interval is 0.66 meters. Note that we did find a significant difference in tree heights.

Because the blocking effects were random, we may wish to estimate the variance component associated with it. We denote the estimate of σ_b^2 by s_b^2, which can be estimated as $(MS_b - s^2)/2$, which equals $(0.299 - 0.077)/2 = 0.111$ in this example; the standard deviation is the square root, or 0.33 meters. Further, the proportion of the total variation in tree height (defined as $\sigma^2 + \sigma_b^2$) that is due to the variation in blocking effects (σ_b^2) is estimated as $s_b^2/(s_b^2 + s^2) = 0.111/(0.111 + 0.077) = 0.59$, or 59%.

Repeating the same calculations for apple diameter, the 95% confidence interval is $-0.19 \pm 2.365\sqrt{2 \times 0.049/8} = -0.19 \pm 0.26$, or $-0.45 \le \alpha_1 - \alpha_2 \le 0.07$. The length of this interval is 0.52 cm.

The variance component associated with the blocking factor is $(0.061 - 0.049)/2 = 0.006$; the standard deviation is 0.08. The proportion of the total variation in fruit diameter that is due to variation in blocking effects is estimated as $0.006/(0.006 + 0.049) = 0.11$, or 11%. In comparison with the tree height, we see that the variation in blocking effects accounts for a smaller percentage of the variation in fruit diameters. This is consistent with the nonsignificant blocking effect shown in a previous table. See Tables 6.2 and 6.5 for preliminary calculations.

6.6   CHECKING IF THE DATA FIT THE MODEL

There are four assumptions that are made in the randomized complete block model: normally distributed populations with equal variance, no interaction, and independence of residuals (and, if applicable, random block effects).

The assumption that is easiest to check is that of normality. Estimates of residuals can be computed (i.e., $Y_{ij} - \bar{Y}_{i.} - \bar{Y}_{.j} + \bar{Y}_{..}$), which can be used in normal quantile plotsand formal tests for normality (such as the Shapiro-Wilk test), as described in Chapter 1.

Example. Normal quantile plots for the residuals obtained from the fitting of the randomized complete block model are shown in Figures 6.1 and 6.2. The points for the apple diameter (Figure 6.2) are approximately linear, so there is no major concern about normality here. The points for the tree height appear somewhat S-shaped, indicating the possibility that the assumption that tree height residuals are normally distributed is violated, particularly in the tails of the distribution. However, the calculated test statistics and p values for the Wilk-Shapiro test are $W = 0.97$, $p = 0.17$ for tree height and $W = 0.96$, $p = 0.60$ for fruit diameter. We would expect the residuals to be approximately normally distributed. Recall from the study description that the tree height was the mean height of the three trees in each plot and that the fruit diameter was the mean diameter of 20 apples randomly selected at harvest. Because means tend to be approximately normally distributed (by the central limit theorem) we would expect the assumption of normality to be satisfied. This is particularly true for the apple diameters, since 20 apples were averaged, but less true for the tree height, since only three heights were averaged.

The assumption of equal variance can't be checked when there is only a sample of size one from each of the populations. Whether or not researchers assume no interaction (additivity) frequently depends on their knowledge of the subject matter. Certainly, if there had been belief or concern that this assumption could be violated, the experiment would not have been set up in this manner. Whenever the assumption of no interaction is made, it is, of course, possible that some interaction actually exists. When there is interaction, the residual variance s^2 no longer estimates just σ^2, but σ^2 plus an additional, positive component which reflects the interaction. Thus, s^2 tends to be too large as an estimate of the variance σ^2. Such tests therefore are conservative, for the presence of interaction makes it more difficult to establish differences among the main effects. Confidence intervals, discussed in Section 6.5 are also conservative; they are somewhat longer than necessary. (Note that in the two-way classification in Chapter 5, this additional component was referred to as σ_{ab}^2; it quantifies the interaction between the two factors. Samples of

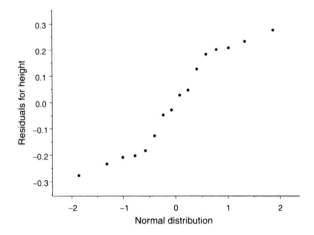

Fig. 6.1 Normal quantile plot of residuals for tree height.

size $n > 1$ are needed to estimate the variation due to the interaction between two factors.)

Similarly, independence of (random) blocking effects and residuals is difficult to verify. The satisfaction of this assumption generally rests with the investigator's knowledge of the conduct of the experiment.

6.7   WHAT TO DO IF THE DATA DON'T FIT THE MODEL

If there are concerns about lack of normality, then transformations can be considered or nonparametric alternatives to the ANOVA test applied. A commonly used nonparametric alternative is Friedman's rank sum test.

6.7.1   Friedman's Rank Sum Test

Friedman's rank sum test is a generalization of the sign test (a non-parametric alternative to the paired t test). Within each block, the observations are ranked from 1 to a. The test statistic can be computed as

$$\frac{12\text{SS}_a}{a(a+1)}, \tag{6.6}$$

where SS_a is the treatment sum of squares when the ranks, rather than the observations, are used. When the means of the a populations are equal, the test statistic follows a χ^2 distribution with $a-1$ degrees of freedom when the number of blocks, b, is sufficiently large. (The χ^2 distribution with $a-1$ degrees of freedom is a large sample approximation to the "exact" distribution of the test statistic.) Details of this test are provided in [2, 6], among others. This test is available in most software packages.

Example. The data for tree height from the Liberty apple project are repeated, with the ranks added, in Table 6.7. Note that the tree heights in the first block are both measured at 2.59 meters. Because the values are tied, the mean rank of $(1+2)/2 = 1.5$ is used for the ranked data. But for the second block, the height of the fungicide sprayed trees is 2.85 meters, which is greater than the paired value 2.54 meters. Thus, for the second block, the rankings are 2 and 1, respectively, for fungicide-exposed and -nonexposed trees. If we were to perform ANOVA on the ranks, we would find $SS_a = 0.0625$, $SS_b = 0$, $SS_r = 3.4375$. Applying Friedman's test, using Equation 6.6, the calculated test statistic is $2(0.0625) = 0.125$ with $p = 0.72$. Similarly, for the fruit diameter variable, the Friedman test statistic is 0.50 with $p = 0.48$. In this example, we reached the same conclusions whether the parametric or non-parametric test was used, although the p values obtained from Friedman's test are higher.

6.7.2 Missing Data

When there is only one observation per cell, the loss of one or more observations complicates the analysis. The missing values can be estimated from

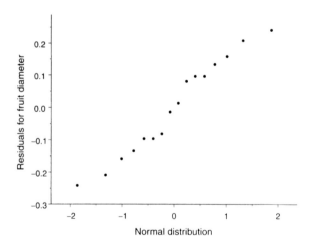

Fig. 6.2 Normal quantile plot of residuals for apple diameter.

Table 6.7 Tree Heights: Observed and Ranked Data

Fungicide	Observed Data, in Meters, by Block								Treatment Means
	1	2	3	4	5	6	7	8	
Yes	2.59	2.85	3.15	3.10	2.54	3.25	3.81	3.51	3.10
No	2.59	2.54	3.61	3.66	3.05	3.40	3.35	3.35	3.19

Fungicide	Ranked Data by Block								Treatment Means
	1	2	3	4	5	6	7	8	
Yes	1.5	2	1	1	1	1	2	2	1.44
No	1.5	1	2	2	2	2	1	1	1.56

the available observations and from the model, and then the analysis can be made using all the data, actual and estimated. An unbiased estimate of σ^2 is obtained (we are assuming $\sigma_{ab}^2 = 0$), but the estimates of σ_a^2 and σ_b^2 are biased. For every missing value estimated, the degrees of freedom for the residual mean square are reduced by 1.

When a single observation is missing, it can be estimated by

$$m_{ij} = \frac{aT_{i.} + bT_{.j} - T_{..}}{(a-1)(b-1)},$$

where $T_{i.}$ denotes the total of $b - 1$ observations in the ith row, $T_{.j}$ denotes the total of $a - 1$ observations in the jth column, and $T_{..}$ denotes the sum of all $ab - 1$ observations. This is described in greater detail in [4].

When more than one observation is missing, then methods described in [4] can be applied. However, it is suggested that appropriate statistical programs be used. This is discussed in greater detail in Chapters 7 and 8.

6.8   DESIGNING A RANDOMIZED COMPLETE BLOCK STUDY

6.8.1   Experimental Studies

In planning an experiment, it is important to identify in advance any factors that may introduce unwanted variation in the response (i.e., variation not due to the treatment effect). Identification of these factors usually comes from an investigator's knowledge of the subject matter. If another factor has a strong association with the response, it can be advantageous to block on that factor. Blocking on the wrong factors can do more harm than good. An investigator may be better off, in terms of power to detect significant treatment effects, if a completely randomized design is used instead of a randomized block design with a poor blocking variable.

Suppose there are ab experimental units available for randomization. The degrees of freedom associated with treatment are $a-1$, regardless of the design. The degrees of freedom associated with the residual are $a(b-1) = ab - a$ for the completely randomized design and $(a-1)(b-1) = ab - a - b + 1$ for the randomized block design. Thus, there are more degrees of freedom associated with the residual variation for the completely randomized design. If you take a look at an F table (see Table B.4) to see what happens to the 95th percentile of the F distributions as the number of denominator degrees of freedom, ν_2, is increased while the number of numerator degrees of freedom, ν_1, is held fixed, you will see that the value of F for the 95th percentile decreases. This would suggest that there is an advantage to using the completely randomized design in that a smaller value of the F statistic is required to reject the hypothesis of no treatment effect.

However, with a completely randomized design, the residual variation may be greater because the residual variation includes all sources of variation other than variation due to treatment. If a large amount of variation in response can be explained by the blocking factor and removed from the residual into a separate source of variation due block, the residual variance for a randomized block design can be smaller than the residual variance in the completely randomized design. The smaller residual variation produced by use of the randomized block design will make it easier to get larger calculated F statistics.

Therefore, for blocking to be effective, the reduction in residual variation must overcome the effects of having fewer degrees of freedom for the residual variation (or higher F values) for assessing statistical significance.. If the decision is made to block on a variable which does not account for a lot of the variation in response, there are fewer degrees of freedom associated with the residual but no offsetting reduction in residual variation. The power to detect an effect of treatment is therefore reduced.

There may be multiple response variables that an investigator wants to study. A variable may be a good blocking factor for one response variable but not for another. This was illustrated in the Liberty apple study, where it appeared that initial tree vigor (as measured by trunk cross-sectional area) was related to subsequent tree height and was therefore an effective variable to block on. In contrast, it appeared that initial tree vigor was not an effective variable to block on for productivity measures, such as apple diameter. Generally, the researcher would identify the response variables that are most important, and make sure there are sufficient numbers of blocks to demonstrate a hypothesized treatment effect. A good discussion of this can be found in [4].

6.8.2 Observational Studies

This chapter has been written in terms of experimental studies, but the model can also be applied to observational studies. In this case, there is no randomization, so the design might be referred to only as a *blocked* design. One would block on factors that are associated with the response variable, for the purpose of removing its effects. Examples of observational studies with blocking are found in the problems at the end of this chapter.

6.9 MODEL EXTENSIONS

In this chapter, we have restricted the sample size to $n = 1$ from each of the treatment-block cross-classifications. In this situation, the assumption of no interaction between treatment and block effects, or additivity, was made. In some situations, only one observation can be taken from a block (for example, an ophthalmology study, in which the block is an individual person and the experimental units are the two eyes). If obtaining the response measurements is very costly, it may be necessary to have no replication.

If it isn't feasible to have randomized complete blocks, it is possible to consider incomplete blocks. This means that all treatments are not administered in the same block. This topic is not addressed in this chapter; information about it can be found in [3, 4].

For many studies, there isn't any reason not to have sample sizes from each treatment-block combination exceed one. This situation is also covered elsewhere in this book in Chapters 5 and 8. For randomized complete block designs with fixed effects for both the treatment and blocking factors, the methods discussed in Chapter 5 are appropriate. If treatment is fixed and block is random, the methods discussed in Chapter 8 are applicable.

6.10 SUMMARY

In this chapter, we have introduced the randomized complete block design for a special case: when an investigator is interested in a single factor and has a sample of size $n = 1$ from each population. This design is applicable when there is another factor, called a blocking factor, which is expected to have an influence on the response; the blocking factor is not of interest but the blocking is done to remove its effect. The model was defined for random blocking effects and fixed blocking effects. Both hypothesis testing and interval estimation were covered. The Friedman test and rank transformations were discussed as nonparametric alternatives to the F test. The randomized complete block design was contrasted with the completely randomized design discussed in Chapter 2. Reference was made to Chapters 5, 7, and 8 for appropriate analyses when there is more than one observation from each population.

Problems

6.1   Three cleansing agents for the skin were used on three persons. For each person, three patches of skin were exposed to a contaminant and subsequently cleansed using each of three cleansing agents, one at each patch. After eight hours, the residual contaminant was measured. The measurements of residual contamination were:

Cleansing Agent	Individual 1	2	3
A	1.25	2.30	1.45
B	0.87	1.45	0.65
C	1.11	1.38	2.99

a)   Write down an appropriate model, and state its necessary assumptions in terms of the problem. Would you expect individual to be a fixed or random factor? Explain.

b)   Obtain the ANOVA table, and test for treatment effects with $\alpha = 0.01$.

c)   Estimate the following by confidence intervals with an overall 95% level: (i) The overall mean. (ii) The population mean difference between residual contaminant using cleansing agents A and B. (iii) The population mean residual contaminant for individual 1 using cleansing agent C.

6.2   Six 4-month-old rats were used to compare the plasma cholesterol for diets involving three levels of butterfat. Two technicians were used. The six rats were assigned at random to the three butterfat levels with two rats at each level. For each butterfat level, the two rats were assigned at random to the two technicians. The data were as follows:

Percent	Technicians I	II
0	69.3	70.3
10	84.8	80.5
20	85.0	72.6

a)   State an appropriate model, including assumptions that must be made.

b)   Make an ANOVA table.

c)   Test with $\alpha = 0.05$ whether there are differences among the three levels of butterfat.

d)   Test with $\alpha = 0.05$ whether there is a difference between the two technicians.

e)   Make confidence intervals for $\alpha_1 - \alpha_2$, $\alpha_1 - \alpha_3$, and $\alpha_1 - (\alpha_2 + \alpha_3)/2$ using an overall level of 0.95. Interpret the intervals.

6.3   Many other response variables were considered for the Liberty apple study. The data for the study can be found on the Wiley ftp site given in the Preface. For the response variable tree spread, do the following:

a)   Obtain the analysis of variable table.

b)   Is the mean tree spread equal for trees which received and which did not receive fungicide application?

c)   Is the mean tree spread equal across blocks?

d)   Does the assumption of normality appear to be satisfied? Justify your answer. Estimate the variance components σ_b^2 and σ^2. What percentage of the variance is explained by the blocks?

e)   Calculate a 95% confidence interval for the difference in means for fungicide- and non-fungicide-treated plots of trees.

6.4   Repeat Problem 6.3 for total yield of apples (in kilograms).

6.5   Repeat Problem 6.3 for the percentage of apples that have a pack-out rating of US No. 1.

6.6   So far, we have discussed designs with factors that are crossed or nested, with effects that are random or fixed. For the descriptions of experiments given below, state an appropriate model, and give sources of variation, numbers of degrees of freedom, and expected mean square columns for an ANOVA table.

a)   Twenty rats are available to study four treatments. The rats are randomly assigned to the four treatments, with five rats on each treatment.

b)   Twenty rats are available to study four treatments. There are five litters, each consisting of four rats. The treatments are assigned at random within each litter; thus one rat in each litter receives each treatment.

c)   Twenty rats are available to study four treatments. The rats are divided into five blocks of four each according to initial weight, with the four lightest rats in one block, and so forth. The four treatments are assigned at random within each block, with one rat receiving each treatment. Why did the experimenter not form four blocks of five rats each, randomly assign the four treatments to the four blocks, and give all rats in a single block the same treatment?

d)   Six litters, each consisting of four rats, were available to study two treatments for two time periods. In each litter, two rats were assigned to each treatment; of the two rats on the same treatment, one was sacrificed after one week and the response measured, and the other rat was sacrificed after one month.

e)   Twelve animals were assigned at random to each of two treatments, with six on each treatment. The animals on each treatment were sacrificed as follows: two after one week, two after two weeks, and two after one month.

f)   Twelve animals were assigned to each of two treatments, with six on each treatment. Three animals on each treatment were sacrificed after one month and three after two months. Two determinations were made on each animal.

g)   Sixteen animals were assigned to two treatments, with eight on each treatment. On each treatment, four were given a low dosage and four a high dosage. Of the four animals on each treatment combination, two were sacrificed after one month, two after two months.

REFERENCES

1. Clements, J.M., Cowgill, W.P., and Costante, J.F. [1994]. UVM Apple Fruit Quality Testing: An Efficient Procedure for Measuring and Recording Data, *Horticultural Science*, 29, 520.

2. Conover, W.J. [1999]. *Practical Nonparametric Statistics*, New York: John Wiley & Sons, 367–373.

3. Dean, A. and Voss, D. [1999]. *Design and Analysis of Experiments*, Springer-Verlag, 339–378.

4. Fleiss, J.L. [1986]. *The Design and Analysis of Clinical Experiments*, New York: John Wiley & Sons, 120–148.

5. Garcia, M.E., Berkett, L.P., Costante, J.F., Clements, J. and Neff, N. [2002]. Productivity and Fruit Quality Evaluation of 'Liberty' (Malus X domestica Borkn.) under a Reduced Fungicide Program. *Acta Horticultureae*, 595, 121–126.

6. Gibbons, J.D. and Chakraborti, S. [1992]. *Nonparametric Statistical Inference*, New York: Marcel Dekker, Inc., 386–396.

7. Lombard, P.B., Callan, N.W., Dennis, F.G., Jr., Looney, N.E., Martin, G.C., Renquist, A.R., and Mielke, E.A. [1988]. Towards a Standardized Nomenclature, Procedures, Values, and Units in Determining Fruit and Nut Tree Yield Performance, *Horticultural Science*, 23, 813–817.

8. Rosenberger, D.A., Engle, C.A., and Meyer, F.W. [1996]. Effects of Management Practices and Fungicides on Sooty Blotch and Flyspeck Diseases and Productivity of Liberty Apples, *Plant Disease*, 80, 798–803.

7

Two Crossed Factors: Fixed Effects and Unequal Sample Sizes

In Chapter 5, we discussed balanced two-way factorial designs with both factors fixed. Not all two-way cross-classifications end up with equal sample sizes across the ab levels of the cross-classification. Sample sizes may be unequal by design. In some experiments, investigators allocate more experimental units to particular treatments. For example, suppose multiple treatments will be compared with a control group. If the new treatments are expensive or if a more precise estimate of the control mean is desired, researchers may want to have more experimental units assigned to the control group. Or, in cross-sectional surveys, investigators decide on the total sample size $\sum_{i=1}^{a} \sum_{j=1}^{b} n_{ij}$ to be obtained from an underlying population; each subject included in the sample is cross-classified into one of the ab groups. The proportions in each group should reflect the proportions in the underlying population; unequal sample sizes are expected.

A study may have been designed to be balanced, but usable data are not collected from all units. Animals may die prior to data collection, or a measuring device may break down at a critical point. In these cases, the study is no longer balanced, due to missing data.

Whether or not a study is balanced, we are still interested in using the two-way classification to investigate the same set of questions as we had in Chapter 5, but there are some technical differences which need to be noted. These involve the sums of squares that go into the ANOVA table, estimation of means, and construction of confidence intervals. Because these differences are important and a user of statistical software may be confused or misled by the computer output, we make special mention of these issues. Computations performed for the analysis of two-way factorial designs with unbalanced data are more complex than those that can be applied with balanced data. Some of the less sophisticated software packages do not include procedures for analyzing unbalanced factorial designs, so the software should be checked prior to its use. If the data are nearly balanced, so that only one or a very few observations are missing, one option is to replace the missing observations by the mean for the particular sample and reduce the residual sum of squares by one for each missing value replaced [1]. For further discussion on missing values in ANOVA, see [9].

In this chapter, we introduce an example of a two-way cross classification with unequal sample sizes in Section 7.1. A model, quite similar to that given in Chapter 5, is presented in Section 7.2. The ANOVA and F tests are discussed in Section 7.3. An important distinction between the sums of squares when designs are and are not balanced is stressed. Estimation of means, standard errors, and confidence intervals is included in Section 7.4. Two ways of estimating means result in unequal values when sample sizes are unequal; these are referred to as means and unadjusted means, and their different interpretations are emphasized in that section. How to tell if the data fit the model is discussed in Section 7.5, and some things to do if they don't are suggested in Section 7.6. The chapter is summarized in Section 7.7.

7.1 EXAMPLE

Persons with a history of coronary heart disease who completed a 3-month cardiac rehabilitation program were identified. Study participants were cross-classified according to gender and age group (< 60 versus ≥ 60 years), so that four groups, with each level of gender appearing with each level of age group, were identified. Here, the outcome we are focusing on is physical functioning. This measure can range from 0 to 100, with higher values indicating better physical functioning. Summary statistics for the four subgroups are found in Table 7.1. A graphical summarization, with sample means and error bars (± 1 standard deviation) is presented in Figure 7.1. The investigator did not specify that the number of subjects in each of the four groups was fixed and the sample sizes were unequal: 45, 13, 63, and 30.

Using these data, we want to ask the following questions:

(1) Is the mean physical function score equal for men and women?

(2) Is the mean physical function score equal for those under age 60 and for those age 60 or older?

(3) Does the effect of gender on mean physical function score depend on age group (i.e., < 60 versus ≥ 60)? Or, does the effect of age group on mean physical function score depend on gender? That is, is there an interaction between age group and gender on mean physical function score?

Table 7.1 Summary Statistics for Subgroups Defined According to Gender and Age Group

	Age < 60 Male	Age < 60 Female	Age ≥ 60 Male	Age ≥ 60 Female
Sample size	45	13	63	30
Mean	74.4	64.6	65.6	57.5
Std. dev.	18.5	26.6	21.6	20.4
Minimum	25	15	0	0
Q_1	65	35	50	45
Median	80	75	70	57.5
Q_3	90	85	85	75
Maximum	100	95	100	90
Skewness	−0.62	−0.59	−0.55	−0.53
W p value	0.028	0.136	0.056	0.400

We will investigate these questions using two-way ANOVA and then construct confidence intervals to aid us in the interpretation of these data, as in Chapter 5. The questions are the same, but the procedures are modified.

7.2 THE MODEL

The appropriate model for the two-way cross-classification is expressed as

$$Y_{ijk} = \mu + \alpha_i + \beta_j + (\alpha\beta)_{ij} + \varepsilon_{ijk} \tag{7.1}$$

for $i = 1, \ldots, a$, $j = 1, \ldots, b$, $k = 1, \ldots, n_{ij}$. As before,

$$\sum_{i=1}^{a} \alpha_i = \sum_{j=1}^{b} \beta_j = \sum_{i=1}^{a}(\alpha\beta)_{ij} = \sum_{j=1}^{b}(\alpha\beta)_{ij} = 0.$$

We assume $\varepsilon_{ijk} \sim \text{IND}(0, \sigma^2)$. [Equivalently, we could assume that $Y_{ijk} \sim \text{IND}(\mu + \alpha_i + \beta_j + (\alpha\beta)_{ij}, \sigma^2)$.] Note that the only difference between this model and the one given in Equation 5.1 is that there is not a constant sample size n for each of the groups. We identify the sample size associated with each group with a doubly subscripted n, n_{ij}, which corresponds to the group with the ith level of factor A and jth level of factor B.

In our example, factor A corresponds to age group and factor B to gender. Each factor assumes two levels, so $a = b = 2$.

7.3 ANALYSIS OF VARIANCE AND F TESTS

One important difference in the analysis of balanced and unbalanced two-way cross-classifications concerns the sums of squares. The total sum of squares is broken into the four distinct parts (due factor A, due factor B, interaction of A and B, and residual), which sum to the total when sample sizes are equal. We need to apply alternative procedures to quantify the four sources of variation when sample sizes are unequal.

There are a variety of ways to define sums of squares. (These are described in [7], [12], and [13], among others.) These sources refer to four types of sums of squares: Type I, Type II, Type III, and Type IV. We have not yet presented the background to fully describe these. Suffice it to say that for all of the models we have considered so far — balanced or unbalanced one-way ANOVA, balanced or unbalanced hierarchical ANOVA, and balanced two-way ANOVA — the four types of sums of squares are equivalent. We have been able to define the sums of squares in terms of specific formulas.

Many statistical software packages have programs that can be used when data are balanced. In this case, the sums of squares are referred to as Type I or there is no type associated with them.

Differences among the four types of sums of squares are found with unbalanced studies with two or more factors. Programs that allow for these

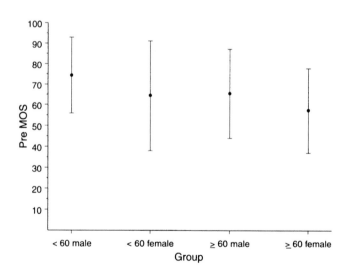

Fig. 7.1 Graphical summarization for physical functioning data by age group and gender.

unbalanced designs routinely print out both Type I and Type III sums of squares,. (Some packages refer to them as sequential and adjusted sums of squares, respectively.) The Type III sums of squares are the ones that are appropriate for most hypothesis tests that investigators wish to perform for ANOVA models. The Type III sums of squares no longer add up to the total sum of squares, although the Type I sums of squares still have that property. If the sample size is 0 for at least one factor combination, the Type IV sums of squares are not equivalent to the others and should be used instead.

Example. The ANOVA table for this example is presented in Table 7.2. The sums of squares obtained for the four different sources of variation (age, gender, age by gender interaction, residual) — that is, the Type III, or adjusted sums of squares — do not add up to the total sum of squares.

From the ANOVA in Table 7.2, we note that the calculated F for the test of no interaction is unusually small: $F = 0.05$. The interaction mean square should be about the same as the residual mean square when there is no interaction (since both mean squares are estimating the same thing, σ^2). We assume here that the small F value is a result of chance and conclude that there is no interaction between age and gender. The p value for the test of no interaction is 0.83.

One interpretation of no interaction is that the difference in mean physical functioning score between men and women is the same if they are younger than 60 or at least 60. The summary statistics given in Table 7.1 are certainly consistent with this. For persons younger than 60, the difference in mean score (male versus female) is $74.4 - 64.6 = 9.8$; for persons at least 60, the difference is $65.6 - 57.5 = 8.1$. Another interpretation of no interaction is that the difference in mean physical functioning score between younger and older persons is the same for men and women. For men, the difference in mean score (< 60 versus ≥ 60) is $74.4 - 65.6 = 8.8$. For women, the difference in mean scores is $64.6 - 57.5 = 7.1$. There isn't much difference between 9.8 and

Table 7.2 Two-Way Analysis of Variance Table for the Physical Functioning Example. Sums of Squares Are Type III or Adjusted.

Source of Variation	Sum of Squares	df	Mean Square	Computed F	p Value
Age	1726.55	1	1726.55	3.93	0.049
Gender	2156.09	1	2156.09	4.91	0.028
Age × Gender	21.20	1	21.20	0.05	0.83
Residual	64527.24	147	438.96		
Total	69899.67	150			

8.1 or between 8.8 and 7.1. Given the summary statistics, it is not surprising that the p value for this test is as high as it is. Another possibility is that there are some outliers in the data set that have inflated the residual sum of squares. (This is discussed further in Section 7.5.)

There is a significant effect of gender ($p = 0.028$) and of age ($p = 0.049$). Although there are only two levels of age and gender, so that we can conclude mean physical functioning is not the same for men and women or for younger and older people, we still would be interested in constructing confidence intervals for the difference in means. The hypothesis tests don't give any indication of the magnitude of the difference. To do this, we want to get point estimates and confidence intervals of means and linear combinations of means.

7.4   ESTIMATION OF PARAMETERS AND CONFIDENCE INTERVALS

7.4.1   Means and Adjusted Means

Another important difference between the balanced and unbalanced two-way ANOVA concerns the estimation of means. Recall that in Section 5.5 we focused on the estimation of two types of means. One choice involved averaging over a second factor, and the second choice involved restriction to a specified level of the second factor.

For the ith level of factor A, when sample sizes were all equal, we used

$$\bar{Y}_{i..} = \hat{\bar{\mu}}_{i.} = \frac{\sum_{j=1}^{b} \sum_{k=1}^{n} Y_{ijk}}{bn} \tag{7.2}$$

$$= \frac{\sum_{j=1}^{b} \bar{Y}_{ij.}}{b} \tag{7.3}$$

as an estimate of its expected value,

$$E(\bar{Y}_{i..}) = \mu + \alpha_i = \bar{\mu}_{i.}$$

However, with unequal sample sizes, there are at least two ways we can average over the second factor. In one approach, the mean of all observations classified at level i is determined. This amounts to taking a weighted average of the $\bar{Y}_{ij.}$ over all levels of j, 1 to b, with weights of $n_{ij}/\sum_{j=1}^{b} n_{ij}$, so that groups with the larger sample sizes are given greater weight. So this mean is calculated as

$$\bar{Y}_{i..} = \frac{\sum_{j=1}^{b} n_{ij} \bar{Y}_{ij.}}{\sum_{j=1}^{b} n_{ij}}. \tag{7.4}$$

Means estimated in this way are usually referred to simply as *means*; we are using $\bar{Y}_{i..}$ to denote the mean for the ith level of the first factor.

An alternative way of averaging over the second factor is to take an unweighted average of the $\bar{Y}_{ij.}$,

$$\hat{\mu}_{i.} = \frac{\sum_{j=1}^{b} \bar{Y}_{ij.}}{b}. \tag{7.5}$$

Means estimated in this way are frequently referred to as *adjusted* or *least square means*. We are using $\hat{\mu}_{i.}$ to denote the least square mean for the ith level of the first factor. The adjusted means are estimated as in Equation 7.5 when the two-way ANOVA model with interaction is fitted. When a model is fitted to the data without some of the terms (for example, without the interaction term), the adjusted means are computed in such a way that there is no interaction among them. We are only considering the estimation of the adjusted means which reflect the possibility of interaction. Note that when the sample sizes are all equal, these adjusted means are equivalent to the means, that is, the means given in Equation 7.4 are equivalent to those in Equation 7.5.

Interpretation of means and adjusted means can be illustrated in terms of a small example [7]. Consider a cross-classified study with two factors, each assuming two levels, so that there are four possible groups. Suppose the sample sizes are $n_{11} = 2$, $n_{12} = 1$, $n_{21} = 1$, and $n_{22} = 2$. The observations can be expressed in terms of the model

$$\begin{array}{|ll|}
\hline
\mu + \alpha_1 + \beta_1 + (\alpha\beta)_{11} + \varepsilon_{111} & \mu + \alpha_1 + \beta_2 + (\alpha\beta)_{12} + \varepsilon_{121} \\
\mu + \alpha_1 + \beta_1 + (\alpha\beta)_{11} + \varepsilon_{112} & \\
\mu + \alpha_2 + \beta_1 + (\alpha\beta)_{21} + \varepsilon_{211} & \mu + \alpha_2 + \beta_2 + (\alpha\beta)_{22} + \varepsilon_{221} \\
& \mu + \alpha_2 + \beta_2 + (\alpha\beta)_{22} + \varepsilon_{222} \\
\hline
\end{array} \tag{7.6}$$

There are four means and four adjusted means, corresponding to the two levels of each of the two factors. We will contrast the interpretation of these two sets of means in terms of their expected values. For both types of means, we make use of the expected value of the mean of the response in the ijth group: $E(\bar{Y}_{ij.}) = \mu_{ij} = \mu + \alpha_i + \beta_j + (\alpha\beta)_{ij}$.

From Equation 7.4, $E(\bar{Y}_{1..})$ can be determined as

$$\begin{aligned}
E(\bar{Y}_{1..}) &= \frac{2\mu_{11} + \mu_{12}}{3} \\
&= \frac{2[\mu + \alpha_1 + \beta_1 + (\alpha\beta)_{11}] + [\mu + \alpha_1 + \beta_2 + (\alpha\beta)_{12}]}{3} \\
&= \mu + \alpha_1 + \frac{2\beta_1 + \beta_2}{3} + \frac{2(\alpha\beta)_{11} + (\alpha\beta)_{12}}{3}.
\end{aligned}$$

The same procedure can be applied to get all four of the means:

$$E(\bar{Y}_{1..}) = \mu + \alpha_1 + \frac{2\beta_1 + \beta_2}{3} + \frac{2(\alpha\beta)_{11} + (\alpha\beta)_{12}}{3},$$

$$E(\bar{Y}_{2..}) = \mu + \alpha_2 + \frac{\beta_1 + 2\beta_2}{3} + \frac{(\alpha\beta)_{21} + 2(\alpha\beta)_{22}}{3},$$

$$E(\bar{Y}_{.1.}) = \mu + \frac{2\alpha_1 + \alpha_2}{3} + \beta_1 + \frac{2(\alpha\beta)_{11} + (\alpha\beta)_{12}}{3},$$

$$E(\bar{Y}_{.2.}) = \mu + \frac{\alpha_1 + 2\alpha_2}{3} + \beta_2 + \frac{(\alpha\beta)_{12} + 2(\alpha\beta)_{22}}{3}.$$

Each mean reflects not only a factor's main effect, but main effects of the other factor and the interaction terms. Similarly, the difference in means, $E(\bar{Y}_{1..}) - E(\bar{Y}_{2..})$, reflects not only the differences across levels of the factor but differences across the second factor and interaction terms. If interest is on determining the difference in the effects of a single factor, the means are biased.

In contrast, Equation 7.5 and the constraints placed on model terms (see Equation 7.1) can be used to determine the expected value of each of the adjusted means. For example,

$$\begin{aligned} \bar{\mu}_{1.} &= \frac{\mu_{11} + \mu_{12}}{2} \\ &= \frac{\mu + \alpha_1 + \beta_1 + (\alpha\beta)_{11} + \mu + \alpha_1 + \beta_2 + (\alpha\beta)_{12}}{2} \\ &= \mu + \alpha_1. \end{aligned}$$

The same procedure can be applied to get all four of the least square means:

$$\begin{aligned} \bar{\mu}_{1.} &= \mu + \alpha_1, \\ \bar{\mu}_{2.} &= \mu + \alpha_2, \\ \bar{\mu}_{.1} &= \mu + \beta_1, \\ \bar{\mu}_{.2} &= \mu + \beta_2. \end{aligned}$$

Each least square mean is a function of only one level of one factor. Differences in least square means, such as $\bar{\mu}_{1.} - \bar{\mu}_{2.} = \alpha_1 - \alpha_2$, involve effects of only one factor.

As with balanced studies, another way to control for the effect of the second factor in unbalanced studies is restriction, for example, to focus on μ_{ij} — the mean for the ith level of the first factor when restriction is made to the jth level of the second factor.

Which type of mean investigators wish to estimate depends on how they wish to summarize their data. In most experiments, the use of the adjusted means is preferred, since sample sizes aren't proportional to population sizes. Reporting of means can be of use in observational studies, when sample sizes in each group are proportional to corresponding population counts (and if the investigator only wishes to draw inferences on the populations that were sampled). These means estimate the mean for each factor separately; any effect that a second factor may have on the means is ignored. Even in this situation, it can be argued that the adjusted means are preferable to the means because the adjusted means are not contaminated by bias from the second factor. In observational studies, if the sample size n_{ij} for each level of the cross-classification is not proportional to counts in the underlying population, we might prefer to use the adjusted means. Of course, if large interactions exist between the two factors, it might only make sense to consider the restricted means which are computed for restricted values of both factors.

Example. Because of the way that the sampling was done in the cardiac rehabilitation example, we are probably more interested in the means than the adjusted means. This is based on the assumption that the 151 persons in the observational study are representative of persons who complete cardiac rehabilitation. Estimates of both types of means, and their corresponding estimated standard errors, are given in Table 7.3. Regardless of which means are used to summarize the data, the impression is that (1) younger persons and (2) men report higher levels of physical functioning.

When we look at the *means*, we note that persons younger than age 60 report a mean score of 72.2, which is almost 10 points higher than the older persons. But could some of the difference be due to gender? Forty-five of the 58 subjects younger than age 60 are men (78%), while 63 of the 93 subjects age 60 or older are men (67%). Similarly, men had a mean score of 69.3, compared with 59.6 for women — a difference of almost 10 points. Could some of this difference be explained by age group? Sixty-three of the 108 males are age 60 or older (58%), while 30 of 43 women are age 60 or older (70%). To adjust or control for the effects of the second factor, we must examine the adjusted means.

The difference in the adjusted means for the two age groups $(69.5 - 61.5 = 8.0)$ is less than the difference in the means. Similarly, when men and women are compared, the difference in the adjusted means $(70.0 - 61.0 = 9.0)$ is smaller than the difference of the means. The difference between the two types of means can be explained by noting that the majority of persons in the study are older men. The adjusted means for the two age groupings are slightly lower than the means. The adjusted means are computed using equal weight for men and women but there are fewer women than men in each age group. Similarly, the adjusted means for men and women are slightly higher than the means. For each gender, there are more persons aged 60 or older;

when younger and older persons are given equal weight, the average physical functioning appears slightly better.

7.4.2   Standard Errors and Confidence Intervals

Regardless of how the investigators choose to summarize their data, the estimation of the standard errors should be consistent with that of the means. Since both means and adjusted means are linear combinations of means, it is straightforward to obtain the estimates of the standard errors. Most of the larger software packages provide analysts with a choice of which means are estimated and their corresponding estimated standard errors. Point estimates and estimated variances for means, adjusted means, and restricted means are provided in Table 7.4. The table includes information on individual means, differences of means (for levels i and i' for the first factor, or j and j' for the second factor), and linear combinations of means.

Confidence intervals (without any adjustments for multiple comparisons) are obtained in the same way as they were in Equation 5.5. That is, the $100(1 - \alpha)\%$ confidence interval is computed as

$$(\text{point estimate}) \pm t_{1-\alpha/2;\nu} \times \text{standard error},$$

where ν is the number of degrees of freedom used in the estimation of σ^2, here given by $\sum_{i=1}^{a} \sum_{j=1}^{b} (n_{ij} - 1)$, and the standard error is the estimated standard error of the corresponding point estimate.

Example. Now, let's compute confidence intervals for the differences in means for gender and for age group. We must decide which difference of population means we want to consider. Do we want to determine a confidence interval $E(\bar{Y}_{1..}) - E(\bar{Y}_{2..})$ or for $\bar{\mu}_{1.} - \bar{\mu}_{2.}$. For the first interval, calculations based on the means and their estimated standard errors are appropriate because we believe the sample sizes in the four groups reflect the distribution of age group and gender among persons who complete cardiac rehabilitation. The second interval requires the adjusted means and their estimated standard errors. These intervals allow us to assess the magnitude of the effect of age group without any contamination due to gender. For illustration, we will use the first type of interval to illustrate the difference in mean physical functioning for the two age groups, and the second type of interval to illustrate the difference in mean physical functioning by gender.

For the difference in mean physical functioning between persons < 60 years of age and persons ≥ 60 years of age, $E(\bar{Y}_{1..}) - E(\bar{Y}_{2..})$, the appropriate point estimate is $\bar{Y}_{1..} - \bar{Y}_{2..} = 9.2$ (see Table 7.3.) The estimated variance of the difference in means is $s^2(1/n_{1.} + 1/n_{2.}) = 438.96(1/58 + 1/93) = 12.29$, and the estimated standard error is the square root of 12.29 or 3.5 (see Table 7.3). Multiplying the estimated standard error by $t_{[.975,\nu=147]} = 1.976$ and adding

Table 7.3 Means and Adjusted Means, and the Estimated Standard Errors for the Physical Functioning, by Age Group and Gender

	n	Means		Adjusted Means	
		Estimated Mean	Estimated Standard Error	Estimated Mean	Estimated Standard Error
Age:					
< 60	58	72.2	2.8	69.5	3.3
≥ 60	93	63.0	2.2	61.5	2.3
Gender:					
Male	108	69.3	2.0	70.0	2.0
Female	43	59.6	3.2	61.0	3.5

and subtracting the result from 9.2 yields the confidence limits for the difference in mean physical functioning

$$2.3 \leq E(\bar{Y}_{1..}) - E(\bar{Y}_{2..}) \leq 16.1.$$

Thus, there is 95% confidence that the difference in means between younger and older persons is at least 2.3 or at most 16.1. This confidence interval does not cover 0, indicating that the means are unequal. However, some of this difference could be attributed to the differing proportion of males (or females) in the two age groups.

For the difference in the means for physical functioning between men and women, when equal weight is given to the two age groups, we wish to construct a confidence interval for $\bar{\mu}_{.1} - \bar{\mu}_{.2}$. The point estimate is the difference of the least square means, 8.9 (see Table 7.3). The estimated variance of the least square mean for men is $s^2[1/(4n_{11}) + 1/(4n_{21})] = 438.96[1/(4 \times 45) + 1/(4 \times 63)] = 4.18$. Similarly, the estimated variance of the least square mean for women is $s^2[1/(4n_{12}) + 1/(4n_{22})] = 438.96[1/(4 \times 13) + 1/(4 \times 30)] = 12.10$. The estimated variance of the difference in least square means is the sum of the two variances, $4.18 + 12.10$, or 16.28. The estimated standard error of the difference is the square root of 16.28, or 4.0 (see Table 7.3). Multiplying the estimated standard error by 1.976 and adding and subtracting the result from 8.9 yields the confidence limits for the difference in mean physical functioning:

$$1.0 \leq \bar{\mu}_{.1} - \bar{\mu}_{.2} \leq 16.8.$$

In this case, the confidence interval does not cover 0, a result consistent with the F test (see Table 7.2). This interval tells us that we are 95% confident that the difference in mean physical functioning between men and women may be as small as 1.0 or as large as 16.8.

Table 7.4 Means, Adjusted Means, and Restricted Means: Parameters, Point   Estimates, and Estimated Variances

Population Parameter	Point Estimate	Estimated Variance
	Means	
$E(\bar{Y}_{i..})$	$\dfrac{\sum_{j=1}^{b} n_{ij}\bar{Y}_{ij.}}{\sum_{j=1}^{b} n_{ij}}$	$s^2 / \sum_{j=1}^{b} n_{ij}$
$E(\bar{Y}_{.j.})$	$\dfrac{\sum_{i=1}^{a} n_{ij}\bar{Y}_{ij.}}{\sum_{i=1}^{a} n_{ij}}$	$s^2 / \sum_{i=1}^{a} n_{ij}$
$E(\bar{Y}_{i..}) - E(\bar{Y}_{i'..})$	$\dfrac{\sum_{j=1}^{b} n_{ij}\bar{Y}_{ij.}}{\sum_{j=1}^{b} n_{ij}} - \dfrac{\sum_{j=1}^{b} n_{i'j}\bar{Y}_{i'j.}}{\sum_{j=1}^{b} n_{i'j}}$	$s^2 \left(\dfrac{1}{\sum_{j=1}^{b} n_{ij}} + \dfrac{1}{\sum_{j=1}^{b} n_{i'j}} \right)$
$E(\bar{Y}_{.j.}) - E(\bar{Y}_{.j'.})$	$\dfrac{\sum_{i=1}^{a} n_{ij}\bar{Y}_{ij.}}{\sum_{i=1}^{a} n_{ij}} - \dfrac{\sum_{i=1}^{a} n_{ij'}\bar{Y}_{ij'.}}{\sum_{i=1}^{a} n_{ij'}}$	$s^2 \left(\dfrac{1}{\sum_{i=1}^{a} n_{ij'}} + \dfrac{1}{\sum_{i=1}^{a} n_{ij'}} \right)$
$\sum_{i=1}^{a} c_i E(\bar{Y}_{i..})$	$\sum_{i=1}^{a} \dfrac{c_i \sum_{j=1}^{b} \bar{Y}_{ij.}}{\sum_{j=1}^{b} n_{ij}}$	$s^2 \sum_{i=1}^{a} (c_i^2 / \sum_{j=1}^{b} n_{ij})$
$\sum_{j=1}^{b} c_j E(\bar{Y}_{.j.})$	$\sum_{j=1}^{b} \dfrac{c_j \sum_{i=1}^{a} n_{ij}\bar{Y}_{ij.}}{\sum_{i=1}^{a} n_{ij}}$	$s^2 \sum_{j=1}^{b} (c_j^2 / \sum_{i=1}^{a} n_{ij})$
	Adjusted Means	
$\mu + \alpha_i$	$\sum_{j=1}^{b} \bar{Y}_{ij.}/b$	$s^2 (\sum_{j=1}^{b} 1/b^2 n_{ij})$
$\mu + \beta_j$	$\sum_{i=1}^{a} \bar{Y}_{ij.}/a$	$s^2 (\sum_{i=1}^{a} 1/a^2 n_{ij})$
$\alpha_i - \alpha_{i'}$	$\sum_{j=1}^{b} \bar{Y}_{ij.}/b - \sum_{j=1}^{b} \bar{Y}_{i'j.}/b$	$s^2 (\sum_{j=1}^{b} 1/b^2 n_{ij})$
$\beta_j - \beta_{j'}$	$\sum_{i=1}^{a} \bar{Y}_{ij.}/a - \sum_{i=1}^{a} \bar{Y}_{ij'.}/a$	$s^2 (\sum_{i=1}^{a} 1/a^2 n_{ij})$
$\sum_{i=1}^{a} c_i (\mu + \alpha_i)$	$\sum_{i=1}^{a} c_i \sum_{j=1}^{b} \bar{Y}_{ij.}/b$	$s^2 (\sum_{i=1}^{a} c_i^2 \sum_{j=1}^{b} 1/b^2 n_{ij})$
$\sum_{j=1}^{b} c_j (\mu + \beta_j)$	$\sum_{j=1}^{b} c_j \sum_{i=1}^{a} \bar{Y}_{ij.}/a$	$s^2 (\sum_{j=1}^{b} c_j^2 \sum_{i=1}^{a} 1/a^2 n_{ij})$
	Restricted Means	
μ_{ij}	$\bar{Y}_{ij.}$	s^2 / n_{ij}

7.5 CHECKING IF THE DATA FIT THE TWO-WAY MODEL

Many of the procedures which are used to check the appropriateness of the assumptions of two-way ANOVA were discussed in Chapter 2 for one-way ANOVA. Since this material concerning the assumptions of normality, equality of variances, and independence was covered in detail there, it will be only summarized here. Assumptions can also be made about the presence or absence of an interaction. A large, unexpected interaction may indicate a failure of some of the assumptions. Interactions will be discussed following the summary of other model checking procedures.

Plots of the sample variances versus the sample means and of the sample standard deviations versus the sample means for the four groups are shown in Figure 7.2. As there is no clear trend between either the sample variance or the sample standard deviation and the sample mean, there is no indication that a transformation of the data is in order. (See Chapter 2.)

As always, the data should initially be checked for gross outliers.

The assumption of normality can be investigated by normal quantile plots. If sample sizes are large enough, the samples from each population can be checked; otherwise, the normality of the residuals can always be examined.

Example. We should have concern about using the physical functioning score as an outcome variable in an ANOVA because it is an ordinal variable. Thus, strictly speaking, it would probably be preferable to use a nonparametric alternative to the usual two-way ANOVA (see below).

After computing the 151 residuals from the fitting of the two-way ANOVA model to the physical functioning data, the Shapiro-Wilk test for normality yielded a test statistic of $W = 0.97$, suggesting that the residuals are not normally distributed. However, Figure 7.3 provides a normal quantile plot of the 151 residuals. The plot displays some departures from linearity, although nothing serious enough to recommend against using this method.

The assumption of equal variances can also be examined graphically; plots of residuals by group can be made. The variability of the residuals will be comparable when the variances are similar. Hypothesis tests, such as Levene's test, can also be performed. In order to perform tests such as Levene's, the two-way cross-classification must be recast as a one-way classification. Suppose that there are a rows and b columns, then there are ab possible combinations for the two-way ANOVA. The one-way ANOVA would have ab different samples $(i = 1, \ldots, ab)$.

As discussed in Chapter 2, tests for equality of variances tend to be quite sensitive to violations of the assumption of normality. Thus, if there are concerns about normality, the recommendation is usually made to focus on finding a transformation of the data which will produce normality or stabilize the variance.

Example. For the physical functioning data, both gender and age group had two levels, so a single factor is defined with four levels: age < 60 and male, age < 60 and female, age ≥ 60 and male, and age ≥ 60 and female. The ANOVA table for Levene's test, based on the absolute values of the residual deviations, is given in Table 7.5. With a p value of 0.31, there is no evidence that the variances of physical functioning are unequal in the four groups of patients.

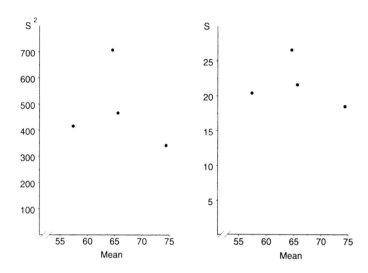

Fig. 7.2 Sample means versus sample variances and sample standard deviations for the four age-group – gender combinations.

Knowledge about the design of the study is generally taken into account when judgments are made concerning the assumption of independence. If the ordering of observations in time or space is available, serial correlations can be computed, as discussed in Chapter 1.

Now, we consider the presence of large interactions. When the data obtained indicate that large interactions exist, it is important to consider if large interactions actually are present in the population means or whether there may be some other explanation for the occurrence of the interactions in the data. Perhaps the two levels of the factors have a catalytic (either synergistic or antagonistic) effect on each other with the result that the mean

Table 7.5 Analysis of Variance Table for Levene's Test for Homogeneity of Variances, Using the Physical Functioning Data

Source of Variation	SS	df	MS	F	p Value
Group	500.9	3	167.0	1.21	0.31
Residual	20208.1	147	137.5		
Total	20709.0	150			

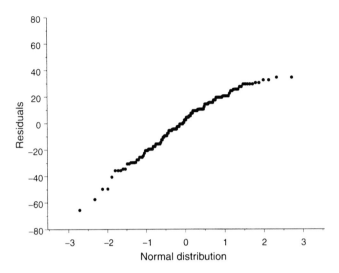

Fig. 7.3 Normal quantile plot of residuals from two-way ANOVA model for the physical functioning data.

response for a combination cannot be expressed in terms of the overall mean plus the main effects. The question of whether interactions exist can often be decided by considering the factors themselves.

Sometimes, when the investigator believes that no interactions exist, the data obtained point to sizable interactions. This could occur, of course, by chance alone. On the other hand, such unexpected interactions may be caused by a problem in the data — there may be an outlier, or the data may be highly skewed. If the observations were not made in a random order, an appreciable time effect may be included in the response. In such a case, the ε_{ijk} can no longer be said to be independent random observations. Some other uncontrolled variable may be affecting the observations. In an experiment involving animals, for example, the position of the cage may have an effect on the outcome variable. Failure of the investigator either to place the animals randomly in the room or somehow to take account of cage position in the design might cause an apparent interaction when none exists. Good test procedure consists in randomizing on every factor that is not controlled in some other way [6]. Random assignment of the experimental units to the treatment combinations is especially important. Thus an unexpected interaction may be a clue to failure in meeting the assumptions of the model being used in the ANOVA. Further discussion on the effects of various failures in assumptions can be found elsewhere [11].

It has been noticed, too, that interactions often occur when the main effects are very large. Interactions frequently disappear if the investigator lessens the differences among the factor levels, making the main effects less pronounced.

Of course, a very small F value obtained from an ANOVA table can also alert analysts to problems in the data set. The value could be explained by chance alone. However, it is possible that the mean square interaction is too small or the mean square residual is too large. The possibilities of unequal variances, lack of independence, or outliers should be explored in the search for an explanation for an unusually small F value [2].

7.6   WHAT TO DO IF THE DATA DON'T FIT THE MODEL

If there are concerns that the violations of the assumptions of the two-way ANOVA are severe, transformations can be considered, or alternative testing strategies can be applied.

Transformations were addressed in detail in Chapters 1 and 2, and will not be covered in much detail here. In addition to using transformations to achieve normality, emphasis is sometimes placed on finding transformations which reduce or eliminate interaction between the factors. If there is little interaction, the results of an ANOVA are simpler to interpret.

If the data are ordinal, or a suitable transformation cannot be found, then nonparametric alternatives may be a reasonable option. In this case, it is appropriate to summarize the data numerically in terms of medians and ranges rather than means and standard deviations.

A variety of methods have been proposed for nonparametric analyses for two-way ANOVA and more complicated designs. One approach for hypothesis testing is to apply the rank transform method [4]. To perform this test, the observations are first ranked from 1 up to the total sample size N. Mean ranks are computed for tied observations (observations which have the same observed value). Then, the ranks are used for the analysis so that sums of squares, mean squares, test statistics (F's) and p values are computed, just as they would be if the actual observations had been used.

This technique has the advantage that it is easy and straightforward to apply. However, the use of rank transformations for two-way and other more complex models has been questioned [8, 10]. Simulation studies have shown that significance levels for the tests can be inflated (e.g. a level of significance of $\alpha = 0.05$ can really be 0.20) and power can be low. Thus, it may be difficult to reject a hypothesis of equal medians when in fact the population medians are unequal. Other drawbacks are that it can only be used for hypothesis testing, so that no confidence intervals can be constructed and that the procedure is not based on any underlying theory. Investigators who question the use of the rank transform method recommend use of the rank-based robust general linear model [8, 10]. These methods can also be applied using standard statistical software but are not discussed here.

Conover gives the following advice in his book [3]. "The recommended procedure in experimental designs for which no nonparametric test exists is to use the usual analysis of variance on the data and then to use the same procedure on the rank transformed data. If the two procedures give nearly identical results the assumptions underlying the usual analysis of variance are likely to be reasonable and the regular parametric analysis valid. When the two procedures give substantially different results, the experimenter may want to take a closer look at the data and to look especially for outliers (observations that are unusually large compared with the bulk of the data) or very nonsymmetric distributions."

Velleman and Wilkinson advocate choosing the analysis based on what will be most useful in answering the question that the investigator has [15]. They argue against strict adherence to basing the choice of analysis on Stevens's proposal for classifying variables [14] since this often results in having to substitute a method that is not designed to answer the questions that the investigator asked. There are a lot more statistical analyses available for interval data than nominal data. But if methods are used that do not meet the assumption of an equal interval scale, the analyst should keep this lack of meeting the assumption in mind, consider possible results of not meeting the assumption, and warn the readers that this assumption was not met.

Alternatively, the two-way classification can always be recast as a one-way classification, with ab levels of the single factor. The advantage of this is that standard nonparametric procedures such as the Kruskal-Wallis test are available; the disadvantage is the analysis is not set up to answer the questions of most interest (viz., the significance of main effects and interaction).

A final alternative is to perform a two-way analysis using the ab sample means, rather than the individual observations. In this case, there is $n = 1$ observation at each combination of factor levels. The analysis would be performed just as if a randomized complete block design were used, with $n = 1$ observation at each combination of factor levels. The assumption of no interaction between the two factors is made. Furthermore, the sample sizes should be approximately the same for each sample. We are making use of the central limit theorem: If a population is distributed with mean μ and variance σ^2, the distribution of the sample mean approaches that of a normal distribution with mean μ and variance σ^2/n, where n is the sample size. If the sample sizes are markedly unequal, there should be concern about the assumption of equality of variances being satisfied.

In the analysis of the physical function data described in Section 7.1, a two-way ANOVA was performed on data that are from a scale that ranges from 0 to 100. Some statisticians would use two-way ANOVA to analyze this data but others would analyze ranks or use some other form of analysis. The use of ordinal data in analyses such as ANOVA is not uncommon in practice but nominal data should not be used.

7.7   SUMMARY

In this chapter, the two-way classification introduced in Chapter 5 was gener-alized to unequal sample sizes. Differences in analyses and in interpretation of the two- way cross-classifications between the simpler case of equal sample sizes and the more complex but frequently occurring case of unequal sample sizes was also reviewed. We indicated that the Type III or adjusted sum of squares is appropriate for hypothesis testing. We illustrated that means and adjusted means are measuring different quantities in unbalanced two-way ANOVA, and we contrasted the interpretation of adjusted means, means, and restricted means. We also went over determining whether the two-way ANOVA is an appropriate procedure, and if not, what some alternatives are. In this chapter, all factors have fixed effects, that is, conclusions were reached only about the populations that were sampled. In the next chapter, we will consider the mixed model, in which one factor is fixed and the other is random.

Problems

7.1   Remove the last observation in Problem 5.2 for men aged 50–80. Sub-stitute the mean for the missing data, and perform a two-way ANOVA on those data. What should the number of degrees of freedom for residuals be? Do any of the mean values change?

7.2   In addition to removing the last observation for men aged 50–80, also remove the last three values for women aged 50–80. Repeat the ANOVA tests using the Type III (or adjusted) sum of squares option and least square (or adjusted) means. Compare the results with those that you obtained from Problem 5.2 when all observations were present. Which means are changed? Obtain 95% confidence limits for the difference between the adjusted means for men and women. Interpret these intervals.

7.3   If you removed all seven observations for men aged 50–80 from Problem 5.2, what type of sums of squares would you use? Perform the ANOVA tests, and compare the results with those in Problem 5.2.

7.4   The following results were obtained from a preliminary study examin-ing whether one of two types of diet combined with aerobic exercise would reduce cholesterol levels. Subjects who participated in the study had elevated cholesterol levels. The cholesterol levels of the 16 subjects at completion of the pretrial were as follows. Perform an ANOVA, and test if these preliminary results indicate that a larger and longer experiment should be done with these diets and exercise program.

Physical Activity	Control	Diet 1	Diet 2
Control	243	236	219
	229	248	228
	252		213
Aerobic	221	212	206
	237	227	199
		209	211

REFERENCES

1. Bennett, C.A. and Franklin, N.L. [1954]. *Statistical Analysis in Chemistry and the Chemical Industry*, New York: John Wiley & Sons, 382.

2. Christensen, R. [2003]. Significantly Insignificant F Tests, *The American Statistician*, 57, 27–32.

3. Conover, W.J. [1999]. *Practical Nonparametric Statistics*, New York: John Wiley & Sons, 417–420.

4. Conover, W.J. and Iman, R. L. [1981]. Rank Transformations as a Bridge between Parametric and Nonparametric Statistics, *The American Statistician*, 35, 124–129.

5. Dean, A. and Voss, D. [1999]. *Design and Analysis of Experiments*, New York: Springer-Verlag, 175–181.

6. Fisher, R.A. [1966.] *The Design of Experiments*, 6th ed., Edinburgh: Oliver and Boyd, 17–21, 40–43.

7. Freund, R.J. and Littell, R.C. [1981]. *SAS for Linear Models*, Cary, NC: SAS Institute, 100–113.

8. Hettmansperger, T.P. and McKean, J.W. [1998]. *Robust Nonparametric Statistical Methods*, London: Arnold, 233–273.

9. Little, R.A. and Rubin, D.B. [1987]. *Statistical Analysis with Missing Data*, New York: John Wiley & Sons, 21–38.

10. McKean, J.W. and Vidmar, T.J. [1994]. A Comparison of Two Rank-Based Methods for the Analysis of Linear Models. *The American Statistician*, 48, 220–229.

11. Miller, R.J. [1986]. *Beyond ANOVA: Basics of Applied Statistics*, New York: John Wiley & Sons, 117-143.

12. Milliken, G.A. and Johnson, D.E. [1984]. *Analysis of Messy Data, Volume 1: Designed Experiments*, Belmont, CA: Wadsworth, Inc., 173–200.

13. Searle, S.R., Speed, F.M., and Milliken, G.A. [1980]. Population Marginal Means in the Linear Model: An Alternative to Least Square Means, *The American Statistician*, 34, 216–221.

14. Stevens, S.S. [1951]. Mathematics, Measurement and Psychophysics, in Stevens, S.S., editor, *Handbook of Experimental Psychology*, New York: John Wiley & Sons, 1–49.

15. Velleman, P. and Wilkinson, L. [1993]. Nominal, Ordinal, Interval, and Ratio Typologies Are Misleading, *The American Statistician*, 47, 65–72.

8

Crossed Factors: Mixed Models

In Chapters 5 and 7 we discussed two-way crossed classifications and limited consideration to situations in which both factors are regarded as fixed. The concept of fixed and random effects was introduced in Chapter 2. A factor has fixed effects if we want to make inferences only about the levels of the factor that are studied. A factor has random effects if the levels of the factor are a sample from a large number of levels that could be selected, and we wish to make inferences about that larger number of levels.

Unlike fixed effects, random effects have variability associated with them, so that the variance of an individual observation reflects not only the residual variance, σ^2, but also the variance of the random effects. The variances which make up the variance of an individual observation are frequently referred to as *components of variance*. When at least some of the effects are considered random, not all observations are independent.

Models for which some factors are fixed and others are random are examples of *mixed* models. The nested, or hierarchical, model presented in Chapter 4 is one example. Mixed models are a very general class of models. The outcome can be expressed as a function of classification variables (factors) and/or continuous variables. (So far in this book, only factors have been addressed; continuous variables are included in the chapters on regression.) When random effects are included in the model, there are multiple ways to describe the lack of independence among the observations.

In this chapter, we focus on a special case of the mixed model, that of a factor with fixed effects being cross-classified with a factor with random effects. Furthermore, we assume that all random effects are independent. Even with these restrictions, the mixed model is more difficult to interpret than the fixed effects. As in Chapter 5, we focus on the special case of equal sample sizes from each of the sampled populations. Random factors can be crossed or nested, and the sample sizes may be equal or unequal.

In Section 8.1 an example is introduced in which one factor is random and the other is fixed. This is followed by a description of the mixed model in Section 8.2. Estimation of fixed effects is addressed in Section 8.3. The breaking apart of the total sum of squares and the ANOVA table is presented in Section 8.4, prior to consideration of estimation of variation components in Section 8.5. Hypothesis testing is presented in Section 8.6. Confidence intervals for population means and variance components are covered in Section 8.7. Some comments on the use of available software are made in Section 8.8, and some extensions of the mixed model are briefly covered in Section 8.9. The chapter is summarized in Section 8.10.

8.1 EXAMPLE

Suppose a manufacturing company is interested in examining factors that affect output. They have $a = 2$ types of machines and want to investigate whether mean output is the same for both machines. They have a large number of persons potentially available to operate the machinery. They select $b = 4$ operators and wish to draw conclusions not just about these operators but about operators in general. Does operator have an effect on mean output? For this study, each operator produces $n = 3$ output measurements using the first machine and $n = 3$ output measurements using the second machine. The data can be summarized in a two-way table, as in Table 8.1. The mean outputs are plotted in Figure 8.1, where the circles indicate machine 1 and the triangles machine 2.

This is an example of a study involving mixed effects, because it has a fixed effect (machine) and a random effect (operator). Machine is considered fixed because the investigators are interested in drawing conclusions about the two machines. Operator is considered random because they wish to draw conclusions about a large population of operators, not just the four who happened to be selected for study.

What are some of the objectives of the study? First, the investigators are likely interested in whether there is an effect of machine on mean output. Second, they are interested in the variability in the output among the operators.

8.2 THE MIXED MODEL

The same expression used for the fixed effects model for an individual observation serves for the mixed model. For example, in the two-way classification with a levels of the first factor and b levels of the second factor, we still use

Table 8.1   Output Data for Two Machines and Four Operators

Machine, i	Operator, j				
	1	2	3	4	
1	16.0	29.5	19.2	23.0	
	12.9	23.6	25.2	23.2	
	15.5	23.2	26.4	29.1	
$\bar{Y}_{1j.}$	14.80	25.43	23.60	25.10	$\bar{Y}_{1..} = 22.23$
2	19.6	24.5	19.1	14.3	
	19.4	15.8	21.6	20.1	
	20.0	17.1	16.9	21.8	
$\bar{Y}_{2j.}$	19.67	19.13	19.20	18.73	$\bar{Y}_{2..} = 19.18$
$\bar{Y}_{.j.}$	17.23	22.28	21.40	21.92	$\bar{Y}_{...} = 20.71$

$$Y_{ijk} = \mu + \alpha_i + \beta_j + (\alpha\beta)_{ij} + \varepsilon_{ijk} \tag{8.1}$$

with

$$i = 1, \ldots, a, \qquad j = 1, \ldots, b, \qquad k = 1, \ldots n.$$

Here a is the number of levels of the first factor, assumed fixed, b is the number of levels of the second factor, assumed random, and n is the number of observations on each factor combination.

The fixed and mixed effects models differ, however, in their statements concerning μ, α_i, β_j, and $(\alpha\beta)_{ij}$. For the mixed effects model we assume

$$\sum_{i=1}^{a} \alpha_i = 0, \qquad \beta_j \sim \text{IND}(0, \sigma_b^2), \qquad (\alpha\beta)_{ij} \sim \text{IND}(0, \sigma_{ab}^2), \qquad \varepsilon_{ijk} \sim \text{IND}(0, \sigma^2)$$

and that the β_j, $(\alpha\beta)_{ij}$, and ε_{ijk} are all mutually independent random effects.

We speak now of a fixed number of levels of the fixed factor and an infinite number of levels of the random factor. For each combination of the levels of the two factors, there exists an infinite population of output measurements. The mean of each of these populations can be broken into four parts: the mean for all possible fixed-random factor combinations (μ), the effect of the level of the fixed factor (α_i), the effect of the level of the random factor (β_j), and the interaction ($(\alpha\beta)_{ij}$).

Example. The investigators are interested in studying exactly $a = 2$ machines but consider the $b = 4$ operators to be a random sample from a large population of operators.

This example of a mixed model might be appropriate in a specific manufacturing plant, where there are two available machines but there are a large number of persons who could operate them.

Let's consider some implications of the assumptions about the random effects and attempt to determine if they are reasonable. Specifying operator as a random effect indicates that the investigators aren't interested in drawing conclusions about the four operators who were selected for study; they want to draw conclusions about operators in general. The population from which the four operators was drawn could be a large number of persons that actually do or could work at the plant. Furthermore, having operator be random allows for correlation in the output produced by a worker. So if operators have an effect on output, it seems reasonable that each of their outputs will be more like each other than those obtained from other operators.

The idea of interaction between operator and machine also seems reasonable. We might anticipate that if one machine is "better" than the other and is used by a "better" operator, then the mean output of this operator-machine combination will be "better" than expected. However, this is *not* implied by the model. The assumption that $(\alpha\beta)_{ij}$ is independent of β_j implies that knowing that one has a "good" machine and a "good" operator tells us nothing about the size of the interaction term.

McLean et al. [2] discussed the reasonableness of this assumption of the mixed model in the context of a similar example, involving a fixed number of

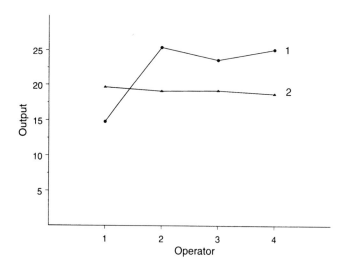

Fig. 8.1 Mean output versus operator, by machine.

machines and randomly selected operators. "This illustration was selected as it easily presents the possibility of the interaction effects being precisely determined when the operator is selected, as would be the case if the interaction is dependent on certain physical characteristics of the operator. It is just as easy to visualize a situation in which the outcome of the interaction is highly dependent on the mental state of the operator at the time of the experiment." Their latter situation corresponds to the mixed model as we have defined it: the interaction term is describing the effect of current mental state of the operator who happens to be working with a particular machine, and it may be reasonable to assume that the effect of the operator, β_j, is independent of the interaction, $\alpha\beta_{ij}$. Assuming dependence between the effect of an operator and the interaction between operator and machine could be reasonable in the former situation.

Correlation between the main effect for operator and the operator-machine interaction is introduced by the specification of an additional assumption, that $\sum_{i=1}^{a}(\alpha\beta)_{ij} = 0$. (Correlation is defined in Appendix A and is addressed in Chapter 11.) The terms of the model have different interpretations than those given in Equation 8.1. There are also differences in how inferences are made from the two alternatives.

We are stressing the model as specified in Equation 8.1 largely because this is the default for most of the software packages. Details regarding how to perform inferences for the mixed model with the constraint that $\sum_{i=1}^{a}(\alpha\beta)_{ij} = 0$ can be found in [2, 6]. Further consideration of using the constrained form of the mixed model is discussed in Voss [8].

Another consequence of the model is that not all observations are independent. We can discuss the variability of an individual observation in terms of its variance and the covariability (a measure of their linear relationship) for two observations in terms of their covariance. When we assume that observations come from normally distributed populations, a covariance of 0 between observations means that they are independent, and a nonzero covariance means lack of independence. Making use of the properties of variances and covariances of linear combinations, we can obtain

$$\text{Var}(Y_{ijk}) = \sigma_b^2 + \sigma_{ab}^2 + \sigma^2, \tag{8.2}$$

$$\text{Cov}(Y_{ijk}, Y_{i'jk'}) = \sigma_b^2, \tag{8.3}$$

$$\text{Cov}(Y_{ijk}, Y_{ijk'}) = \sigma_b^2 + \sigma_{ab}^2. \tag{8.4}$$

That is, the variance of an individual observation is a function of the three variance components, σ_b^2, σ_{ab}^2, and σ^2. The covariance between any two observations that are sampled from the jth level of the random factor but different levels of the fixed factor depends on the variance component for the random factor, σ_b^2. When the component is > 0, the covariance is > 0. This means that observations associated with a particular random effect tend to be more alike than observations in general. Also, observations that are sampled from the ith level of the fixed factor and the jth level of the random factor depend on both σ_b^2 and σ_{ab}^2. If both variance components are 0, all observations are independent. See Appendix A for derivation of these measures of variability and covariability for the mixed model.

Example. In terms of our example, σ_b^2 is the variance of the operator effects, σ_{ab} is the variance component for the interaction between operators and machines, and σ^2 is the residual variation. The variance for an individual output, $\text{Var}(Y_{ijk})$ is the sum of the variance components for operator, for the interaction between operator and machine, and for the residual. The outputs produced from machine 1 and machine 2 when the same person is operating the equipment are not independent; their covariance is σ_b^2, the variance of the operator effects. The outputs produced from one of the machines by a particular operator are also not independent; their covariance is the sum of σ_b^2 and σ_{ab}^2, the variance components for the operators and the operator-by-machine interaction.

8.3 ESTIMATION OF FIXED EFFECTS

For our mixed model, we are generally interested in estimating means associated with fixed effects and in estimating the variance components, σ_b^2, σ_{ab}^2, and σ^2. In this section, we focus on the fixed effects.

As we have done earlier in the book, we can begin with the expression for the mean of the ith level of the fixed factor,

$$\bar{Y}_{i..} = \frac{Y_{i11} + \cdots Y_{i12} + Y_{i21} + \cdots + Y_{i2n} + \cdots + Y_{ib1} + \cdots + Y_{ibn}}{bn}.$$

Since $E(Y_{ijk}) = \mu + \alpha_i$, we can also determine that $E(\bar{Y}_{i..}) = \mu + \alpha_i$. Thus, using properties of expectation, we can verify that $\bar{Y}_{i..}$ is an unbiased estimator for $\mu + \alpha_i$, $\bar{Y}_{...}$ is an unbiased estimator for μ, and $\bar{Y}_{i..} - \bar{Y}_{i'..}$ is an unbiased estimator for $\alpha_i - \alpha_{i'}$, $i \neq i'$. In this chapter, we are using the notation μ_i to denote the mean of the ith population, so μ_i is a shorthand notation for $\mu + \alpha_i$ or $E(\bar{Y}_{i..})$. Note that $\mu_i - \mu_{i'}$ is another way to express $\alpha_i - \alpha_{i'}$.

In order to construct confidence intervals for functions of the fixed effects, we shall need to estimate their standard errors; this will be discussed in Section 8.7.1

8.4 ANALYSIS OF VARIANCE

Before discussing estimation of random effects, we first introduce an ANOVA table. This table can be used for a couple of different purposes. It suggests a method of estimating the variance components σ_b^2, σ_{ab}^2, and σ^2 and this will be our first application of it. Second, as in earlier chapters, it will be used for hypothesis testing.

When sample sizes are equal, the total sums of squares, SS_t, can be separated into the same four parts that were defined in Chapter 5: the sum of squares due to factor A (SS_a), sum of squares due to factor B (SS_b), interaction between factors A and B (SS_{ab}), and residual sum of squares due to error (SS_r). The expressions are equivalent to those given in Chapter 5 and are not repeated in this chapter. The ANOVA table for a general two-way mixed model is given Table 8.2.

Note that the table is equivalent to that given in Table 5.2 except for the EMS and F columns. We are assuming that factor A is fixed and factor B is random. As in earlier chapters, we are using the notation $\phi(\alpha)$ to denote $\sum_{i=1}^{a} \alpha_i^2/(a-1)$ and σ_b^2 to denote the variance component. The EMSs for factors A and B are different from those obtained in the fixed effects model; each includes the interaction variance component, σ_{ab}^2. The EMS for the factor A is a function of two variance components $(\sigma^2, \sigma_{ab}^2)$, and the effects of the levels of factor A. For factor B, it is a function of three variance components: σ^2, σ_{ab}^2, and σ_b^2. These are derived in [6].

It should be noted that some texts (for example, [4]) omit the term $n\sigma_{ab}^2$ in the factor B EMS column. By dropping that term, they assume that a random main effect β_j is correlated with its interaction effect $(\alpha\beta)_{ij}$. Here, we make the assumption that the random main effects are independent of the interaction effects (as described in Section 8.2).

8.5   ESTIMATION OF VARIANCE COMPONENTS

There are several reasons why analysts would be interested in estimating the variance components. For example:

(1) They quantify the amount of variability associated with different sources of variation in the study.

(2) Variances of estimated means are functions of the variance components.

(3) They can be used in the calculation of confidence intervals for population variance components.

(4) They may be useful for the planning of subsequent studies.

With the restrictions that we have made for the model in this chapter, (i.e. two-way cross-classification with one fixed and one random factor, equal sample size from each population), it is straightforward to estimate the variance components.

Referring to the EMS column in Table 8.2, we can solve directly for the variance components σ^2, σ_{ab}^2, σ_b^2 by equating the EMS and the mean squares and expressing the estimates of the variance components as functions of the

Table 8.2   Analysis of Variance, Two-Way Cross Classification, Mixed Effects Model with Equal Sample Sizes

Source of Variation	SS	df	MS	EMS	F
Factor A	SS_a	$a - 1$	MS_a	$\sigma^2 + n\sigma_{ab}^2 + bn\phi(\alpha)$	MS_a/MS_{ab}
Factor B	SS_b	$b - 1$	MS_b	$\sigma^2 + n\sigma_{ab}^2 + an\sigma_b^2$	MS_b/MS_{ab}
Interaction of A and B	SS_{ab}	$(a-1)(b-1)$	MS_{ab}	$\sigma^2 + n\sigma_{ab}^2$	MS_{ab}/s^2
Residual	SS_r	$ab(n-1)$	MS_r	σ^2	
Total	SS_t	$abn - 1$			

Table 8.3   Analysis of Variance Table for Machine-Operator Example, Two-Way Classification, Mixed Effects Model

Source of Variation	SS	df	MS	EMS	F	p
Machines	55.82	1	55.82	$\sigma^2 + 3\sigma_{ab}^2 + 12\phi(\alpha)$	1.30	0.34
Operators	98.97	3	32.99	$\sigma^2 + 3\sigma_{ab}^2 + 6\sigma_b^2$	0.77	0.58
Machine-operator Interaction	129.10	3	43.03	$\sigma^2 + 3\sigma_{ab}^2$	4.04	0.026
Residual	170.43	16	10.65	σ^2		
Total	454.26	23				

mean squares. We don't want to estimate σ_a^2, since factor A represents a fixed effect. The estimates can be obtained directly from an ANOVA table. This estimation procedure is frequently referred to as the *sum of squares* or the *ANOVA* procedure. The population variance components and estimators are given in Table 8.4.

Alternative procedures are also available for estimating variance components. In addition to the sum of squares (ANOVA) method, as described above, three commonly available methods are *minimum variance quadratic estimation* (mivque0), *maximum likelihood* (ML), and *restricted maximum likelihood* (REML). These four methods produce the same values when all estimates are (> 0) and when sample sizes are equal.

As we have seen, estimating variance components by equating the expected mean squares with computed mean squares, as in the sum of squares method, has the advantage that estimates can be obtained directly from an ANOVA table. Thus, if analysts wish to verify a value by hand, it is feasible to do so by this method. However, this method is considered least desirable because the estimates tend to be biased and can yield negative variance components (as we shall see in our example). Of the four methods, the one that is considered preferable is REML [1]. Comparisons among these methods can also be found in [9].

Example. The estimates of the variance components for our example, obtained using the four estimation methods, are summarized in Table 8.5. For example, using the sums of squares in Table 8.3, the estimate for the variance component for interaction is $(43.03 - 10.65)/3 = 10.79$). A couple of things stand out when examining this table. First, the residual variance σ^2 has the same estimated value, regardless of the estimation procedure used; this is always the case. Second, the estimates obtained from the sum of squares and mivque0 procedures are identical; this occurred because the sample sizes in this example were equal, and this is not always true. Note that there is a definite problem with the estimated variance component for operator for both the sum of squares and mivque0 procedures — it is negative. Since variances must be ≥ 0, it is common practice to substitute 0 for the negative values.

As described in Section 8.2, the variance of an individual observation is the sum of the variance components. We can estimate the variance for an individual output by summing the estimated components. For example, using the sum of squares or mivque method (and substituting 0 for the negative estimate -1.67 for operator), the estimated variance for an individual output is $10.79 + 10.65 = 21.44$. Using the REML procedure, the estimated variance for an individual output is $0 + 9.12 + 10.65 = 19.77$.

It can be informative to summarize the data in terms of the percentage of the total variation that is explained by the different sources of variation. For example, using REML estimates, we can say that 0% of the variation is due to the operator, $9.12/19.77 = 46\%$ of the variation is due to the machine by operator interaction, and $10.65/19.77 = 54\%$ of the variation is due to residual variation.

All four methods suggest that there is no variation in the manufacturing output that is due to the operator. All also suggest that both the interaction

Table 8.4 Variance Components: Parameters, Their Interpretation, and Sum of Squares Estimators

Parameter	Interpretation	Sum of Squares Estimator
σ_b^2	Variance component for random effect	$\dfrac{MS_b - MS_{ab}}{an}$
σ_{ab}^2	Variance component for interaction between random and fixed effect	$\dfrac{MS_{ab} - s^2}{n}$
σ^2	Residual variance	s^2

between operator and machine and the residual are large sources of variation in the data. There was no effect of machine in this example; since machine was fixed, a variance component for it was not estimated.

8.6 HYPOTHESIS TESTING

The EMS column of Table 8.2 is particularly important, as it indicates what hypothesis tests can be performed and how they are calculated. These tests are based on the assumptions specified in the mixed model.

The first hypothesis that we are interested in is the hypothesis of no interaction between the two factors:

$$H_0 : \sigma^2_{ab} = 0.$$

The F statistic is the ratio MS_{ab}/MS_r, which follows an F distribution with $\nu_1 = (a-1)(b-1)$ and $\nu_2 = ab(n-1)$ degrees of freedom when the interaction variance component is 0.

Another null hypothesis concerns the variance component σ^2_b:

$$H_0 : \sigma^2_b = 0.$$

The EMSs for the random factor B and the interaction between factors A and B differ with respect to the presence or absence of σ^2_b. This suggests that the F statistic is the ratio MS_b/MS_{ab}. It can be shown that when the H_0 is true, the F statistic follows an F distribution with $\nu_1 = b-1$ and $\nu_2 = (a-1)(b-1)$.

Another null hypothesis concerns the effects of the fixed factor A, which can be expressed in various ways:

$$H_0 : \alpha_1 = \cdots = \alpha_a = 0$$

Table 8.5 Variance Components Estimated Using Four Different Methods

Component	Sum of Squares	Mivque0	ML	REML
Operator	−1.67	−1.67	0	0
Interaction	10.79	10.79	5.95	9.12
(Machine by operator)				
Residual	10.65	10.65	10.65	10.65
Total	21.44	21.44	16.60	19.77
% Operator	0	0	0	0
% Interaction	50	50	36	46
% Residual	50	50	64	54

(Estimation Procedure spans Sum of Squares, Mivque0, ML, REML)

or as

$$H_0 : \mu_1 = \cdots = \mu_a.$$

The F statistic is the ratio MS_a/MS_{ab}, which follows an F distribution with $\nu_1 = a - 1$ and $\nu_2 = (a-1)(b-1)$ when there is no effect of factor A on mean outcome.

Example. The ANOVA table for the machine-operator example is given in Table 8.3. We conclude that there is a significant interaction between machine and operator (i.e. $\sigma_{ab}^2 > 0$), as $F = 4.04$ and $p = 0.024$. But we don't have evidence to conclude that there is a main effect of machine or of operator; that is, the effects of the two machines, α_1 and α_2, may be 0 and the variance component for operator, σ_b^2, may be 0.

The conclusion of the presence of interaction between machine and operator is consistent with what was observed in Figure 8.1. For machine 1, the mean outcome was quite variable across the four operators, while there was essentially no variation in mean output for machine 2.

In general, it is difficult to interpret a model when there appears to be a significant interaction but no significant main effects. Frequently, if an interaction effect is detected, then the main effects of the factors are also included in the model.

Another explanation for our findings is related to our sample size; we may not have had sufficient power to detect effects. Note that the calculated F statistic for testing the main effect of machine, 55.82, is compared with an F distribution with $\nu_1 = 1$ and $\nu_2 = 3$. The $F_{0.95,1,3}$ is equal to 216. If operator is considered fixed rather than random, so that MS_r is used in the denominator, then the calculated F is equal to 5.24; the $F_{0.95,1,16}$ is 3.04. The F distributions with one degree of freedom for the numerator become more spread out as the denominator degrees of freedom are reduced, so that a larger F value is needed to reject the null hypothesis.

8.7 CONFIDENCE INTERVALS FOR MEANS AND VARIANCE COMPONENTS

8.7.1 Confidence Intervals for Population Means

The confidence intervals for fixed effects that are of most interest are those which correspond to particular levels of the fixed effects. Recall that when a factor is considered fixed, investigators want to make inferences about the a fixed levels. It is appropriate to refer to these inferences as concerning a population means even though the samples were drawn from ab populations, since inferences are made by averaging over *all* possible levels of the random factor.

These inferences concern individual means (μ_i), differences of means ($\mu_i - \mu_{i'}$), or general linear combinations of means ($\sum_{i=1}^{a} c_i \mu_i$). Since there is no interest in the particular levels of the random factor that are included in a study, inferences about the ab populations which happened to be selected for study are not made.

We compute confidence intervals for the population means in the usual way, by basing them on t distributions. In Section 8.3 we discussed estimation of the population mean associated with the ith level of the fixed factor, μ_i, by $\bar{Y}_{i..}$.

Next, we need to obtain the variance of $\bar{Y}_{i..}$. This is straightforward, as it only involves taking the variance of a linear combination. As shown in Appendix A, when sample sizes are equal, the variance of $\bar{Y}_{i..}$ is equal to

$$\text{Var} \bar{Y}_{i..} = \frac{\sigma_b^2}{b} + \frac{\sigma_{ab}^2}{b} + \frac{\sigma^2}{bn}. \tag{8.5}$$

This variance reflects variation associated with the random factors, interaction between the fixed and random factor, and the residual variation. We must take into account that the levels of the random factor were selected from a large number of possible levels; we want the variance in the means to reflect this variability. The same is true for the interaction terms. (Recall that in the cross-classifications involving only fixed effects, as in Chapters 5 and 7, there was nothing unknown or uncertain about the levels of the factors included in the investigation.) The covariance between the two means is σ_b^2/b.

Population means and expressions for estimates and their variances that are particularly relevant for inferences in the mixed model are given in Table 8.6.

Estimates of variances can be verified by replacing the unknown variance components with their estimates. Estimated standard errors can be found by taking the square root of the estimated variances. The number of degrees of freedom is that associated with the interaction mean square in the ANOVA table, $(a-1)(b-1)$. Referring back to the EMS column in Table 8.2, it is apparent that the mean square interaction plays an important part in making inferences about the fixed effects.

Example. We wish to construct confidence intervals for the mean output using machine 1, the mean output using machine 2, and the difference in mean output between machines 1 and 2. For some operators, there were large differences in their mean values, and for others the mean values were essentially equal (Figure 8.1). The population parameters, point estimates, estimated standard errors, and confidence intervals are given in Table 8.7.

Each sample mean is calculated over the $bn = 12$ values associated with each level of machine. To estimate the standard error, we need to decide which method to use for estimating the variance components. For this example, we are using the restricted maximum likelihood (REML) estimates, as given in

Table 8.6 Population Parameters, Point Estimates, and Variances of Point Estimates

Population Parameter	Point Estimate	Variance of Estimate
μ_i	$\bar{Y}_{i..}$	$\sigma_b^2/b + \sigma_{ab}^2/b + \sigma^2/bn$
$\mu_i - \mu_{i'}$	$\bar{Y}_{i..} - \bar{Y}_{i'..}$	$2(\sigma_{ab}^2/b + \sigma^2/bn)$
$\sum_{i=1}^{a} c_i \mu_i$	$\sum_{i=1}^{a} c_i \bar{Y}_{i..}$	$\sum_{i=1}^{a} c_i^2 (\sigma_{ab}^2/b + \sigma^2/bn)$

Table 8.5. For each machine, the estimated variance of the sample mean is calculated as

$$\frac{\widehat{\sigma_b^2}}{b} + \frac{\widehat{\sigma_{ab}^2}}{b} + \frac{\widehat{\sigma^2}}{bn} = \frac{0}{4} + \frac{9.12}{4} + \frac{10.65}{12} = 0 + 2.28 + 0.89 = 3.17.$$

The estimated standard error for each sample mean is $\sqrt{3.17} = 1.78$. (The estimated standard errors are the same because the sample sizes are the same for both machines.) The estimated difference of the mean output for the two machines is $22.23 - 19.18 = 3.05$; the estimated variance of the difference is $3.17 + 3.17 = 6.33$, and the estimated standard error is $\sqrt{6.33} = 2.52$.

The final piece of information that we need to determine the confidence interval is the t value, which depends on the desired level of confidence (here, 95%) and on the number of degrees of freedom associated with the interaction mean square [here, $(2 - 1)(4 - 1) = 3$]. The 97.5 percentile of a t distribution with 3 degrees of freedom is 3.182. So the upper and lower limits for the 95% confidence interval for each population mean is its point estimate plus or minus $3.18(1.78) = 5.66$. Similarly, for the difference in means, the upper and lower limits are calculated as the difference in sample means plus or minus $3.18(2.52) = 8.01$.

We are 95% confident that the difference in mean output between machine 1 and machine 2 is between -4.96 and 11.06. Based on this confidence interval, we don't have evidence that mean output is different for the two machines.

Table 8.7 Population Parameters, Point Estimates, Estimated Standard Errors, and 95% Confidence Intervals for the Population Parameters

Population Parameter	Point Estimate	Estimated Standard Error	95% Confidence Interval
μ_1	22.23	1.78	$16.57 < \mu_1 < 27.90$
μ_2	19.18	1.78	$13.51 < \mu_2 < 24.85$
$\mu_1 - \mu_2$	3.05	2.52	$-4.96 < \mu_1 - \mu_2 < 11.06$

Let's go back and take another look at the calculation of the estimated variance of the sample mean. It is not unusual for the contribution to the variance from the residual variability to be smaller than the contribution to the variance from the random effects; the residual variance component is divided by a much larger number ($bn = 12$ versus $b = 4$ in this example). This illustrates the importance of incorporating the different sources of random variation into the variance computations. Note how much smaller the estimated variances, standard errors, and confidence interval lengths would have been if the analyst had considered only the residual variation. The estimated variance for each mean would be less than one-third what it should be (0.89 versus 3.17), and, like the lengths of the confidence intervals, the estimated standard errors would be about one-half what they should be ($\sqrt{0.89} = 0.94$ versus 1.78).

Note that when one factor is fixed and the other is random, the confidence intervals for contrasts in means for the fixed factor are relevant, regardless of the presence or absence of interaction between the two factors. When the interval is determined, we are averaging over all possible random effects and interaction effects. This interpretation of averaging is comparable to that made when all effects are fixed. However, due to a significant interaction, investigators may wish to construct intervals for the difference of means for one factor at specific levels of the second and not only averaged over all levels of the second in the fixed effects setting.

8.7.2 Confidence Intervals for Variance Components

With the exception of the residual variance, it is difficult to determine confidence intervals for individual variance components. In general, estimates of the variance components are highly variable. From one perspective, confidence intervals can be so wide as to be uninformative, and so it is not worthwhile to spend much effort in obtaining them. On the other hand, wide intervals are of value in keeping investigators from having too much faith in the point estimates.

A variety of methods have been proposed for calculating confidence intervals for variance components; these are not presented here. For interested readers, we suggest references where more details can be found [3, 6, 7].

Example. Although we have chosen not to include expressions for variance components, we are including 95% confidence intervals for the variance components for machine-by-operator interaction:

$$2.93 < \sigma_{ab}^2 < 125.09$$

and for the residual variance:

$$5.91 < \sigma^2 < 24.67.$$

The main point of showing these confidence intervals is to demonstrate how wide they are, particularly for σ_{ab}^2. This is not unexpected, particularly in view of the small sample sizes that were used in this illustration.

8.8   COMMENTS ON AVAILABLE SOFTWARE

Before we discuss some extensions or generalizations of the mixed model introduced in this chapter, we feel it is important to emphasize to data analysts the limitations of available software. As of this writing, many software packages have programs appropriate for the fitting of mixed models, but not all do. Traditionally, most of the inferences for mixed models have been made using programs for *general linear models*. (See Chapter 16 for a summary of broad categories of models.) For these models, it is assumed that all factors are fixed, so analysts need to be aware of the limitations of the software. They typically specify appropriate expected mean squares — provided that the assumption of variance components is appropriate — so it is possible that hypothesis tests can be performed correctly. Analysts must be cautious to make sure that other statistical procedures, such as estimating standard errors or confidence intervals, are correct. See [5] for a discussion of some of these issues.

Newer mixed model programs, such as SAS proc mixed, allow analysts to fit a much broader range of models. However, caution must be used in the application of these programs, because it is easy to misunderstand the model that is specified. Analysts can think they are fitting one model when in fact they are fitting a different one. Hypothesis tests for fixed effects are generally available (although ANOVA tables are generally not presented), and standard errors can be estimated correctly to reflect variation other than the residual. Conventional hypothesis tests based on an ANOVA table are not appropriate for many inferences concerning the variances and covariances of random effects.

We recommend using example data sets to fit models using a variety of programs. Seeing what is the same and what isn't the same from the different programs can assist analysts in clarifying what models are fitted and how the computer output is interpreted.

8.9   EXTENSIONS OF THE MIXED MODEL

In this chapter, quite a specific case of the mixed model was introduced: two crossed factors (one fixed and the other random), equal sample sizes, all random effects independent, and variances and covariances expressed as variance components. Here, we consider some extensions or variations on that model.

8.9.1   Unequal Sample Sizes

A couple of things should be kept in mind when sample sizes are unequal. Investigators have to decide which statistics will be used to summarize the data obtained for different levels of a fixed factor. As discussed in Chapter 7, either means (each calculated as the mean of all observations obtained from the specific level of the fixed factor and across all levels of the other factors) or least square (adjusted) means (each calculated as the mean of the means for the specific level of the fixed factor and all levels of the other factors) can be selected, depending on the investigators' interests. Typically, the least square means are preferred in most situations. (Recall that when sample sizes are equal, means and least square means are equal.)

Having unequal sample sizes does not pose a major difficulty for computer-based data analyses, as adjustments can be made to reflect them. If an analyst wants to calculate something by hand (an approach which we find helpful for furthering understanding of concepts), calculations tend to be messier.

8.9.2   Fixed, Random, or Mixed Effects

There are three possible specifications of effects in a two-way classification. Both factors can have fixed effects, both can be random, or there can be one fixed and one random factor. In this chapter, we have focused on the mixed model. In Chapters 5 and 7, both factors had fixed effects.

The possibility that we have not considered so far is that of both factors having random effects. For the variance components models discussed in this chapter, the only modification that we would need to make to the model is to allow $\alpha_i \sim N(0, \sigma_a^2)$. This modification would not change the hypothesis tests, but it would alter the estimation. There is now only one nonrandom term in the model, μ, and inferences for that one parameter — the mean response over all possible levels of the two random factors — could be made. Otherwise, interest would center on estimating the variance components, determining the percentage of variability associated with each one, and possibly determining confidence intervals.

Regardless of the software package that is used, analysts need to specify the model they wish to fit. One piece of this specification includes identifying which factors are fixed and which are random; the details of how to do this vary across the packages.

8.9.3   Crossed versus Nested Factors

Earlier in this book, we considered the possibility of factors being crossed or nested. We mentioned in the introduction to this chapter that the nested or hierarchical model, as we defined it in Chapter 4, is an example of a mixed model. Usually, a factor that is nested in another is random rather than fixed. Mixed models can include models with factors that are crossed and/or nested.

We will illustrate a mixed model with crossed and nested effects in Chapter 9 when we discuss repeated measures.

To fully specify a model, analysts may need to identify which factors are nested in other factors and which are crossed. The details of how to do this can differ across software packages.

8.9.4   Dependence of Random Effects

For the model emphasized in this chapter, the effects of the random factor, (the β_j), the interactions between the fixed and random factors [the $(\alpha\beta)_{ij}$] and the residuals (the ε_{ijk}) were all assumed to be independent. It is possible to assume that there is dependence among the random effects. The form of that dependence is often referred to as their *covariance structure*. We will illustrate an alternative to the assumption of independence in the chapter on repeated measures (Chapter 9).

8.10   SUMMARY

In this chapter, we defined a mixed model as a model which has both fixed and random effects. Our objective was to introduce the concept in the context of a special case: one random factor crossed with one fixed factor, equal sample sizes, and simple covariance structure. We defined the model and addressed its interpretation. We discussed estimation of population means and emphasized the importance of estimating standard errors which reflect the multiple sources of random variation of the estimated means. For random effects, we emphasized estimation of variance components. Inferences in terms of both confidence intervals and hypothesis tests were described for population means and for variance components. More general models than the one used in this chapter were mentioned. Some cautionary notes in using available statistical software were made.

Problems

8.1   A study to compare two teaching methods involved three teachers. Each teacher taught four students by each of the two methods. The data are scores from a final examination. The three teachers were picked at random from a large group of teachers.

Score by Teaching Method
by Student

Teacher	1				2			
	1	2	3	4	1	2	3	4
1	67	73	59	84	75	61	67	58
2	92	84	94	83	54	78	61	70
3	74	72	76	64	42	44	80	83

a)   Plot the sample means. Interpret the data on the basis of this plot.
b)   State an appropriate model and assumptions for the problem.
c)   Obtain an ANOVA table, including the EMS column.
d)   Test $H_0 : \sigma_{ab}^2 = 0$, $H_0 : \sigma_b^2 = 0$, and $H_0 : \mu_1 = \mu_2$.
e)   Estimate by point estimates and confidence intervals μ, μ_1, μ_2, and $\mu_1 - \mu_2$.

8.2   For the Liberty apple study discussed in Chapter 6, measurements were reported only for a single year. In fact, measurements were made for three successive years. If all the data are used, there are three crossed factors: treatment (fungicide versus no fungicide), block, and year. Treatment and year are fixed, and block is random. (Note that with no replication, we must assume no three-way interaction among the three factors.) The data are available on the Wiley ftp site.

a)   State the appropriate three-way ANOVA model.

b)   Perform a three way ANOVA with fruit diameter as the outcome variable. Summarize your findings about the effects of treatment, block and year on mean outcome.

c)   Perform a three-way ANOVA with tree height as the outcome variable. Summarize your findings about the effects of treatment, block, and year on mean outcome.

d)   Perform a three-way ANOVA with yield as the outcome variable. Summarize your findings about the effects of treatment, block, and year on mean outcome.

e)   Perform a three-way ANOVA with percentage of apples with a packout rating of US No. 1 as the outcome variable. Summarize your findings about the effects of treatment, block, and year on mean outcome.

REFERENCES

1. Corbeil, R.R. and Searle, S.R. [1976]. Restricted Maximum Likelihood (REML) Estimation of Variance Components in the Mixed Model, *Technometrics*, 18, 31–38.

2. McLean R.A., Sanders W.L., and Stroup, WW. [1991]. A Unified Approach to Mixed Linear Models, *The American Statistician*, 45, 54–63.

3. Rao, P.S.R.S. [1997]. *Variance Components Estimation*, New York: Chapman and Hall.

4. Scheffé, H. [1958]. *Analysis of Variance*, New York: John Wiley & Sons, 261–274.

5. Schwartz, C.J. [1993]. The Mixed-Model ANOVA: The Truth, the Computer Packages, the Books Part I: Balanced Data, *The American Statistician*, 47, 48–59.

6. Searle, SR. [1971]. *Linear Models*, New York: John Wiley & Sons.

7. Searle S.R., Casella, G. and McCulloch, C.E. [1992]. *Variance Components*, New York: John Wiley & Sons.

8. Voss, D.T. [1999]. Resolving the Mixed Models Controversy, *The American Statistician*, 53, 352–356.

9. Wu, C-T, Gumpertz, M.L., and Boos, D.D. [2001]. Comparison of GEE, MINQUE, ML, and REML Estimating Equations for Normally Distributed Data, *The American Statistician*, 55, 125–130.

9

Repeated Measures Designs

Repeated measures designs are applicable to studies in which more than one measurement of the same response variable is made on each subject. Such designs can be used when treatments are randomly assigned to individuals as well as in surveys in which repeated measurements are made on one or more groups of subjects. A common variable on which measurements are repeatedly taken is time. In this case, the data are frequently referred to as *longitudinal data*, and a repeated measures analysis may be called an analysis of longitudinal data. A defining feature of this type of study is that the repeated measurements are not independent. Analyses need to reflect the correlations among the measurements.

There are many different models which fall under the general category of repeated measures. It is the objective of this chapter to introduce the concept of repeated measures in the context of longitudinal data. The simplest models are considered: when all units belong to a single population and when all units belong to multiple populations, identified by different levels of a single factor. Repeated measurements are made from each unit at the same time points, so that the designs are balanced — sample sizes are equal.

Even the simplest models for longitudinal data are not easy to analyze. Since multiple measurements are made on the same subject, the measurements cannot be assumed to be independent. Recall that independence of units sampled is assumed in many models. When we lose that independence, the models become more complicated.

In Section 9.1, we discuss the situation in which all the individuals belong to a single population. An example introduces the subject, followed by a discussion of the model. The concept of compound symmetry, which defines how the measurements from a single individual are correlated, is described. These subsections are followed by discussions of statistical inference for this particular model. In Section 9.2 we discuss the case in which a populations are to be compared and repeated measures have been taken on all the individuals in each of a samples. Models with effects that are crossed are contrasted with nested effects. In Section 9.3 we discuss how to tell if the data fit the model, and in Section 9.4 we describe what to do if they don't. The chapter is summarized in Section 9.6.

Because of the complexity of this topic, this chapter is meant to be only an introduction to repeated measures ANOVA. For further information see [3] or [9].

9.1   REPEATED MEASURES FOR A SINGLE POPULATION

In some studies, the number of observations made on each individual is just two. For example, a measurement at a first time period can be followed by a measurement at a second time period. The cardiac rehabilitation data illustrated this: self-reported physical functioning was assessed prior to a program of cardiac rehabilitation and after completion of the program. The data could be analyzed using a paired t test or through analysis of a randomized complete block design to investigate whether or not there was a change in mean self-assessment.

The more general one-sample case consists of studies in which each subject is measured on a occasions; a may be greater than as well as equal to two. The subjects are a random sample from a single population. Some examples of such studies are the following:

(1) Each of 10 students took a spelling test four times, once in each of the third, fourth, fifth, and sixth grades.

(2) Systolic blood pressure measurements were made once a week for five weeks on a single sample of individuals attending a clinic.

(3) Lung function measurements were taken once a month for six months on former smokers.

(4) Test animals were injected with three different drugs in the same order. Each animal was injected with the same drug, on successive months, one at a time, and measurements were made after each injection.

9.1.1   Example

As a numerical example, we use the data in Table 9.1, which are scores of 10 students who took a spelling test in each of four grades: grades three, four, five, and six. The grades are the rows, and the students are the columns. In this example, we have $n = 10$ students, who are considered a random sample from a single population of students. We expect that students' scores should be correlated over grade, so that students who scored high in grade three will also score high in grades four, five, and six.

With repeated measures on a single sample, the first step is usually to plot the responses for each subject (here, the student) versus time (here, grade) with straight lines joining the successive observations on a given subject. Such plots are helpful in screening the data for possible outliers and in gaining a general impression of the consistency of the data. For an impression of the overall changes over time for a typical subject, the means at each time, $\bar{Y}_{.j}$, can be plotted for the a time periods. Some investigators like to add to these graphs some information concerning the variability. One method for doing this is to indicate one standard deviation below and above each mean. The resulting *error bar chart* is illustrated for our example in Figure 9.1.

Based on both the table and the figures, it appears that there are no gross outliers to be concerned about. Scores tend to increase from grade to grade. It appears that the increase in score is not linear with grade.

What we are particularly interested in is investigating the effects of grade on mean spelling score. (We are less interested in investigating whether there is an effect of subjects). We shall want to determine whether there is an effect of grade and to describe that effect. The technique of repeated measures analysis will be used for this purpose.

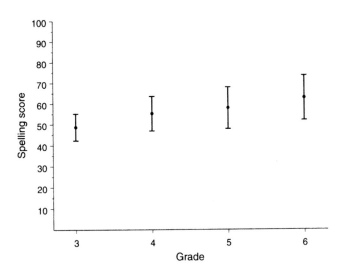

Fig. 9.1 Mean spelling score by grade. Error bars represent one standard deviation.

Table 9.1 Spelling Scores for Ten Students by Grade, i

					Student, j						
i	1	2	3	4	5	6	7	8	9	10	$\bar{Y}_{i.}$
3	48	47	38	48	54	49	52	43	62	46	48.7
4	50	47	50	58	66	58	66	40	60	57	55.2
5	55	50	44	57	70	61	68	42	68	64	57.9
6	70	53	48	72	74	56	69	46	68	72	62.8
$\bar{Y}_{.j}$	55.8	49.3	45.0	58.8	66.0	56.0	63.8	42.8	64.5	59.8	56.2

9.1.2 The Model

For examples such as the one described in Section 9.1.1, each observation can be expressed as

$$Y_{ij} = \mu + \alpha_i + \beta_j + \varepsilon_{ij}, \qquad i = 1,\ldots,a, \quad j = 1,\ldots,b, \qquad (9.1)$$

with $\sum_{i=1}^{a} \alpha_i = 0$, $\beta_j \sim \text{IND}(0,\sigma_b^2)$, $\varepsilon_{ij} \sim \text{IND}(0,\sigma^2)$, and the β_j and the ε_{ij} mutually independent. The parameter μ denotes the overall mean. Here α_i denotes the ith level of the factor which identifies the repeated measurements; this factor is considered fixed and is often represented as "time". The term β_j is the effect of the jth *subject* (unit on which the repeated measurements are determined). Subjects are considered random. In summary, this is a two-way classification with factors of time, which is fixed, and subject, which is random. The two factors are crossed, and because there is no replication, we must assume that there is no interaction between them. This model is equivalent to that given for a complete blocks design with $n = 1$, described in Chapter 6, or as a special case of the mixed model, with $n = 1$ described in Chapter 8.

Example. For the spelling score example, the model is

$$Y_{ij} = \mu + \alpha_i + \beta_j + \varepsilon_{ij}, \qquad i = 1,\ldots,4, \quad j = 1,\ldots,10,$$

and

$$\sum_{i=1}^{4} \alpha_i = 0, \quad \beta_j \sim \text{IND}(0,\sigma_b^2), \quad \varepsilon_{ij} \sim \text{IND}(0,\sigma_e^2).$$

That is, we assume we have a sample of $b = 10$ students from a large population of students. The students are the subjects. Since there is no particular interest in the ten students that were sampled, subject is considered a random effect. Spelling score is determined at $a = 4$ grades in school. Grade corresponds to time, and since we are interested in just these four grades, grade is fixed.

Student and grade are crossed; a spelling score is determined for each student at each of the four grades.

With the usual rule for finding the variance of a linear combination (see Appendix A), the variance of Y_{ij} is $\sigma_y^2 = \sigma_b^2 + \sigma^2$ (i.e., the variance of the effects of the subjects plus the error variance), so that the variability of the Y's is the same in each time period as well as for each subject. The model in Equation 9.1 also implies that the covariances between Y's for the same subject at two different time points are equal, regardless of which two time points are considered. This is another straightforward application of the rule for obtaining covariances of linear combinations of variables; derivations in terms of a mixed model are given in Appendix A. From $Y_{ij} = \mu + \alpha_i + \beta_j + \varepsilon_{ij}$ and $Y_{i'j} = \mu + \alpha_{i'} + \beta_j + \varepsilon_{i'j}$, we can say that for subject j, the covariance between their observation at time i and time i' is equal to

$$\mathrm{Cov}(Y_{ij}, Y_{i'j}) = \sigma_b^2.$$

The model also implies that there is no correlation between responses for different subjects.

The correlation $\mathrm{Corr}(Y_{ij}, Y_{i'j})$ between responses for two time points (i and i') on the same subject (j) is

$$\rho = \mathrm{Corr}(Y_{ij}, Y_{i'j}) = \frac{\mathrm{Cov}(Y_{ij}, Y_{i'j})}{\sqrt{\mathrm{Var}(Y_{ij})\, \mathrm{Var}(Y_{i'j})}} = \frac{\sigma_b^2}{\sigma^2 + \sigma_b^2}. \tag{9.2}$$

We see, then, that the assumptions made in the model in Equation 9.1 imply that response measures for a given subject have equal intercorrelations. This condition is referred to as *compound symmetry*.

For $a = 4$ time points, the covariance matrix Σ can be written as

$$\begin{pmatrix} \sigma^2 + \sigma_b^2 & \sigma_b^2 & \sigma_b^2 & \sigma_b^2 \\ \sigma_b^2 & \sigma^2 + \sigma_b^2 & \sigma_b^2 & \sigma_b^2 \\ \sigma_b^2 & \sigma_b^2 & \sigma^2 + \sigma_b^2 & \sigma_b^2 \\ \sigma_b^2 & \sigma_b^2 & \sigma_b^2 & \sigma^2 + \sigma_b^2 \end{pmatrix},$$

and the correlation matrix R as

$$\begin{pmatrix} 1 & \rho & \rho & \rho \\ \rho & 1 & \rho & \rho \\ \rho & \rho & 1 & \rho \\ \rho & \rho & \rho & 1 \end{pmatrix}.$$

Note that we are assuming that the observations taken over time are dependent (correlated) and we have assumed a simple form for the correlation matrix. We shall return to the assumption of compound symmetry and discuss it, and its alternatives, in Sections 9.3 and 9.4.

9.1.3   Hypothesis Testing: No Time Effect

The null hypothesis usually of most interest is that no differences exist among time periods, that is,

$$H_0 : \mu_1 = \cdots = \mu_a,$$

where μ_i equals $\mu + \alpha_i$, or, in terms of the model,

$$H_0 : Y_{ij} = \mu + \beta_j + \varepsilon_{ij}.$$

The usual ANOVA table for a two-way mixed model with no interaction and with $n = 1$ is given in Table 9.2, and the ANOVA table for the repeated measures model is given in Table 9.3. The total sum of squares, SS_t is separated into three parts: subjects (SS_b), time (SS_a), and residual (SS_r), where, $SS_a = b \sum_{i=1}^{a} (\bar{Y}_{i.} - \bar{Y}_{..})^2$, $SS_b = a \sum_{j=1}^{b} (\bar{Y}_{.j} - \bar{Y}_{..})^2$, and $SS_r = \sum_{i=1}^{a} \sum_{j=1}^{b} (Y_{ij} - \bar{Y}_{i.} - \bar{Y}_{.j} + \bar{Y}_{..})^2$. These sums of squares are the same for Tables 9.2 and 9.3. As before, we are using $\phi(\alpha)$ to indicate $\sum_{i=1}^{a} \alpha_i^2 / (a - 1)$.

The only difference between these two tables is that the EMS column of Table 9.3 has been rewritten in terms of $\rho = \sigma_b^2 / (\sigma^2 + \sigma_b^2)$, the correlation between responses at two different times, and $\sigma_y^2 = \sigma^2 + \sigma_b^2$, the variance of a subject's response. Then σ^2 can be shown to be equal to $\sigma_y^2 (1 - \rho)$.

Under the assumption that no interaction exists between time and subject, we can determine from examining the EMSs in either Table 9.2 or Table 9.3 how to make the test of no effect of time. From the latter, we note that the EMS time and the EMS residual differ by the term $b\phi(\alpha)$. When there is no effect of time, $\phi(\alpha) = 0$, and both mean squares are estimating the same thing. Thus, to test the hypothesis, the appropriate test statistic is $F = MS_a / s^2$. When H_0 is true, this statistic follows an F distribution with $a - 1$ and $(a - 1)(b - 1)$ degrees of freedom.

Usually, no test is made to determine whether there is variability among subjects, although such a test can be made. As with the block designs, we expect there to be an effect of subject. How to perform the test can be seen most easily from the EMS column of either Table 9.2 or 9.3. The appropriate test statistic, $F = MS_b / s^2$, follows an F distribution with $b - 1$ and $(a - 1)(b - 1)$ degrees of freedom when there is no subject effect.

Example. For the spelling example, the ANOVA table is given in Table 9.4. To test the hypothesis of no grade effect, the ratio of the MS grade and the MS residual is calculated as $345.63/21.8 = 15.85$. The p value is < 0.0001. The null hypothesis is rejected, and we conclude that grade does have an effect on mean spelling score. There is also a significant effect of student.

When a significant effect related to time (here, grade) is found, we generally want to describe how time affects the response. We will consider how to do this in Section 9.1.4.

Table 9.2 Analysis of Variance Table for Mixed Model Design

Source of Variation	Sum of Squares	df	Mean Square	EMS
Subjects	SS_b	$b-1$	MS_b	$\sigma^2 + a\sigma_b^2$
Time	SS_a	$a-1$	MS_a	$\sigma^2 + b\phi(\alpha)$
Residual	SS_r	$(a-1)(b-1)$	s^2	σ^2
Total	SS_t	$ab-1$		

9.1.4 Simultaneous Inference

In this subsection, we review linear contrasts and describe specific ones that are useful for identifying how the mean outcome changes over time. The changes we are focusing on here are linear, quadratic, cubic,... trends over time. We discuss inferences in terms of confidence intervals for these contrasts, t tests, and F tests. To apply the F tests, we describe how the sum of squares due to time in an ANOVA table can be subdivided into distinct sums of squares, each with one degree of freedom, which can be used to test for trends over time. (These techniques are not restricted to longitudinal data but they are particularly useful for describing these types of trends. Some of this material was presented in Chapter 3 in the context of multiple comparisons.) This material is written in terms of the special case of a single population, but it is easily generalized to more general cases. Many software programs will produce estimates of these contrasts and sums of squares, as well as hypothesis tests if requested.

Review of Linear Contrasts. As is often the case, investigators aren't interested in merely reporting that means are different on the basis of the F test. They want to describe the differences among the means more completely.

Table 9.3 Analysis of Variance Table for Repeated Measures Design

Source of Variation	Sum of Squares	df	Mean Square	EMS
Subjects	SS_b	$b-1$	MS_b	$\sigma_y^2[1 + (a-1)\rho]$
Time	SS_a	$a-1$	MS_a	$\sigma_y^2(1-\rho) + b\phi(\alpha)$
Residual	SS_r	$(a-1)(b-1)$	s^2	$\sigma_y^2(1-\rho)$
Total	SS_t	$ab-1$		

Table 9.4   Analysis of Variance Table for Spelling Example

Source of Variation	Sum of Squares	df	Mean Square	Computed F	p Value
Students	2383.6	9	264.84	12.15	< 0.0001
Grade	1036.9	3	345.63	15.85	< 0.0001
Residual	588.6	27	21.8		
Total	4009.1	39			

They then consider linear contrasts of the form $\sum_{i=1}^{a} c_i \mu_i$ with the constraint that $\sum_{i=1}^{a} c_i = 0$; these are estimated by

$$\sum_{i=1}^{a} c_i \bar{Y}_{i.} \tag{9.3}$$

When *compound symmetry* holds and the sample size is constant across the a groups, the estimated variance of the linear contrast $\sum_{i=1}^{a} c_i \bar{Y}_{i.}$ is

$$\sum_{i=1}^{a} c_i^2 s^2 / b, \tag{9.4}$$

where b is the common sample size. (This variance reflects *only* the residual variation; the effects of subject cancel out in the contrast, so no variance component associated with subject enters the expression.)

A $100(1 - \alpha)\%$ confidence interval for $\sum_{i=1}^{a} c_i \mu_i$ (where c_i is the ith coefficient and α_i is the effect of the ith level of the factor time, is calculated as:

$$\sum_{i=1}^{a} c_i \bar{Y}_{i.} \pm t_{1-\alpha/2;\nu} \ \text{se} \left(\sum_{i=1}^{a} c_i \bar{Y}_{i.} \right). \tag{9.5}$$

In the context of repeated measures with a single sample, $\nu = (a - 1)(b - 1)$, the number of degrees of freedom used in calculating the residual variance, and the estimated standard error for the linear contrast is $s\sqrt{c_i^2/b}$.

Alternatively, a t test can be made of $H_0 : \sum_{i=1}^{a} c_i \alpha_i = 0$, using the statistic

$$t = \frac{\sum_{i=1}^{a} c_i \bar{Y}_{i.}}{\text{se}(\sum_{i=1}^{a} c_i \bar{Y}_{i.})},$$

to be compared with $t_{1-\alpha/2;\nu}$. Or, by squaring this t statistic, we can obtain the F statistic, to be compared with an F distribution with 1 and $\nu = (a - 1)(b - 1)$ degrees of freedom.

9.1.5 Orthogonal Contrasts

So far, we have only looked at one contrast. But when there are a levels of time, it is possible to construct $a - 1$ *orthogonal* contrasts that can be used to assess trends in the data. A contrast $c_1 \bar{Y}_{1.} + \cdots + c_a \bar{Y}_{a.}$ is said to be orthogonal to another contrast $d_1 \bar{Y}_{1.} + \cdots + d_a \bar{Y}_{a.}$ if $\sum_{i=1}^{a} c_i d_i = 0$.

When $a = 4$, there are three orthogonal contrasts that can be used to investigate the presence of a linear, quadratic, or cubic trend. When the time periods are equally spaced, the coefficients for a linear trend are $c_1 = -3$, $c_2 = -1$, $c_3 = 1$, and $c_4 = 3$. If there is only a linear trend, then a plot of the $\bar{Y}_{i.}$ versus c_i looks like a straight line. (See Table 9.5 for orthogonal coefficients for selected values of a.) For a more complete table of orthogonal contrasts see [2].

When the time periods are equally spaced, the coefficients for a quadratic trend are $c_1 = 1$, $c_2 = -1$, $c_3 = -1$, and $c_4 = 1$. This contrast is orthogonal to the linear trend contrast since $(-3)(1) + (-1)(-1) + (1)(-1) + (3)(1) = 0$. If there is only a quadratic trend, then a plot of $\bar{Y}_{i.}$ versus c_i appears as a parabola. More generally, this is interpreted as a quadratic trend after effects of linear trend have been removed. A quadratic trend has a single inflection point (saucer-shaped), and a cubic trend has two inflection points (S-shaped). This is discussed further in [9].

Similarly, the coefficients for a cubic trend are $c_1 = -1$, $c_2 = 3$, $c_3 = -3$, and $c_4 = 1$. This contrast is orthogonal to those for the linear and quadratic trends, and it is interpreted as the cubic trend after adjustment has been made for linear and quadratic trends.

Estimates of contrasts and their estimated standard errors are used to make t tests or construct confidence intervals for the different trends. Each contrast $\sum_{i=1}^{1} c_i \mu_i$ is a weighted average of the population means. A common application of t tests and confidence intervals is to investigate whether $\sum_{i=1}^{a} c_i \mu_i = 0$, consistent with no trend. These are all applications of the general expression given in Equation 9.5.

Example. Using the orthogonal contrasts, the point estimate for the linear trend in mean spelling scores across grades is calculated by applying Equation 9.3:

$$(-3)\bar{Y}_{1.} + (-1)\bar{Y}_{2.} + (1)\bar{Y}_{3.} + (3)\bar{Y}_{4.},$$

which for this example is calculated as $(-3)(48.7) + (-1)(55.2) + (1)(57.9) + (3)(62.8)$, which is equal to 45.0. Note that if there is no linear trend, we would expect the point estimate to be close to zero. We can't interpret the value 45.0, however, without some estimate of its variability. Its estimated variance is calculated by applying Equation 9.4, with $s^2 = 21.8$ and $b = 10$:

$$(-3)^2 \frac{21.8}{10} + (-1)^2 \frac{21.8}{10} + (1)^2 \frac{21.8}{10} + (3)^2 \frac{21.8}{10} = 43.6.$$

The estimated standard error of this linear contrast is the square root of 43.6, or 6.603. With this information regarding variability, the estimate 45.0 seems high when compared with zero.

To test the hypothesis of no linear trend (i.e., $H_0 : -3\mu_1 - \mu_2 + \mu_3 + 3\mu_4 = 0$), the test statistic is the ratio of the estimated contrast to its estimated standard error. If there were no linear trend, the t statistic would follow a t distribution with $\nu = 27$ degrees of freedom, the number of degrees of freedom associated with the mean square residual. In this case, the calculated test statistic $t = 45.0/6.603 = 6.82$. Since $p < 0.0001$, we reject this hypothesis and conclude that there is a linear trend in mean spelling score across grades.

To obtain a 95% confidence interval for this linear trend, we need the 97.5 percentile of a t distribution with 27 degrees of freedom, or 2.052. The confidence interval for $-3\mu_1 - \mu_2 + \mu_3 + 3\mu_4$ is $45.0 \pm 0.052(6.603)$ or 45 ± 13.5, or $31.5 \leq -3\mu_1 - \mu_2 + \mu_3 + 3\mu_4 \leq 58.5$. We are 95% confident that the population mean of this contrast is between 31.5 and 58.5. We could also use this confidence interval to conclude that there is a linear trend, because the interval does not cover 0.

Similarly, the 95% confidence interval for the quadratic trend, after adjustment for the linear trend, is $-1.6 \pm 2.052(2.953)$, or -1.6 ± 6.1, or $-7.7 \leq \mu_1 - \mu_2 - \mu_3 + \mu_4 \leq 4.5$. This interval does cover 0, so a quadratic trend doesn't seem appropriate. In practice, we would make an adjustment for the number of multiple comparisons made (here, two) using the Bonferroni adjustment, as described in Chapter 3.

Table 9.5 Coefficients of Orthogonal Contrasts, $a = 2, 3, 4$, and 5 Equally Spaced Levels

a	Effect	c_1	c_2	c_3	c_4	c_5
2	Linear	−1	1			
3	Linear	−1	0	1		
	Quadratic	1	−2	1		
4	Linear	−3	−1	1	3	
	Quadratic	1	−1	−1	1	
	Cubic	−1	3	−3	1	
5	Linear	−2	−1	0	1	2
	Quadratic	2	−1	−2	−1	2
	Cubic	−1	2	0	−2	1
	Quartic	1	−4	6	−4	1

9.1.6 F Tests for Trends over Time

Just as orthogonal contrasts can be used to make t tests for investigating trends over time, they can also be used in F tests. We have seen before that the square of a t statistic with ν degrees of freedom is equal to an F statistics with 1 and ν degrees of freedom. This is equally true for testing $H_0 : \sum_{i=1}^{a} c_i \mu_i = 0$. That is, t^2 is equal to

$$F = \frac{b(\sum_{i=1}^{a} c_i \bar{Y}_{i.})^2}{\sum_{i=1}^{a} c_i^2 s^2}. \tag{9.6}$$

It can be shown that $b(\sum_{i=1}^{a} c_i \bar{Y}_{i.})^2 / \sum_{i=1}^{a} c_i^2 s^2$ has an F distribution with 1 and $(a-1)(b-1)$ degrees of freedom. Here s^2 is a χ^2 variable divided by its number of degrees of freedom, and when H_0 is true, $b(\sum_{i=1}^{a} c_i \bar{Y}_{i.})^2 / \sum_{i=1}^{a} c_i^2$ is an independent χ^2 variable divided by its number of degrees of freedom, 1.

When the factor time has a levels, the sum of squares due to time can be divided into $a - 1$ sums of squares, each one due to a particular contrast.

Our objective now is to divide the due time sum of squares into parts that will enable us to make tests to determine the trend in mean response across time. It can be shown that the sum of squares associated with a particular contrast is of the form

$$\frac{b(\sum_{i=1}^{a} c_i \bar{Y}_{i.})^2}{\sum_{i=1}^{a} c_i^2}. \tag{9.7}$$

An ANOVA table can now be written, in which the due time sum of squares has been divided into $a - 1$ parts, one due to each contrast. It can be shown that the expected mean square for any contrast $\sum_{i=1}^{a} c_i \bar{Y}_{i.}$ equals

$$\sigma^2 + \frac{b(\sum_{i=1}^{a} c_i \mu_i)^2}{\sum_{i=1}^{a} c_i^2},$$

which under $H_0 : \sum_{i=1}^{a} c_i \mu_i = 0$ reduces to σ^2. Separate F tests for each contrast can be made. The F statistic is calculated as the ratio of the mean square associated with each contrast to the mean square residual.

Example. In our example, there are $a = 4$ grades, and the number of degrees of freedom associated with the sum of squares due to grade is $a - 1$, or 3. Therefore, this sum of squares can be broken down into three parts: linear trend, quadratic trend, and cubic.

The sum of squares for the linear trend, denoted SS_L is

$$\begin{aligned} SS_L &= \frac{10[-3(48.7) - 1(55.2) + 1(57.9) + 3(62.8)]^2}{(-3)^2 + (-1)^2 + (1)^2 + (3)^2} \\ &= 1012.5. \end{aligned}$$

Similarly, the sum of squares due to a quadratic trend after adjustment has been made for the linear trend, denoted SS_Q is

$$SS_Q = \frac{10[1(48.7) - 1(55.2) - 1(57.9) + 1(62.8)]^2}{(1)^2 + (-1)^2 + (-1)^2 + (1)^2}$$
$$= 6.4.$$

The due time after-quadratic sum of squares can be considered (when $a = 4$) as a due cubic after-quadratic-and-linear sum of squares and calculated in a similar manner. The cubic sum of squares in $SS_C = 18.0$. Note that the three sums of squares, $SS_L + SS_Q + SS_C = 1012.5 + 6.4 + 18.0$, sum to the grade sum of squares, 1036.9.

An ANOVA table is presented with the sum of squares due to grade separated into these three parts in Table 9.6. The sums of squares associated with quadratic and cubic trends are small compared to the residual sum of squares, so that we lack evidence that additional quadratic or cubic trends in mean spelling scores across grades are needed. A formal test of the null hypothesis that there is no quadratic trend is made using $F = 6.4/21.8 = 0.29$, with $p = 0.59$. The test for no cubic trend is made using $F = 18/21.8 = 0.81$, with $p = 0.38$. The linear sum of squares is extremely large; to test the null hypothesis that the $\mu + \alpha_i$ lie on a horizontal line, we compute $F = 1012.5/21.8 = 46.4$ and $p < 0.0001$. These statistical tests strengthen our impressions from Figure 9.1 that the means $\mu + \alpha_i$ change with time in a linear fashion and contain no additional quadratic or cubic trends.

Note that $t^2 = F = 46.44$, so we can see that the test for linear trend can be made using the t test or the F test, based on breaking apart the grade sum of squares into sums of squares for linear, quadratic, and cubic trends.

We note that in some repeated measures studies it is inappropriate to divide the due time sum of squares as was done here. For instance, in the study of the test animals injected with three different drugs, the researchers would not be interested in whether the three $\mu + \alpha_i$ lie on a straight line, but rather in whether certain contrasts, such as $\alpha_1 - \alpha_2$ or $\alpha_1 - \alpha_3$, for example, differ from zero.

In our example with the four grades, the testing times were equally spaced and so orthogonal polynomials could be used directly. However, most software packages handle unequally spaced intervals with ease when the analyst specifies the time points.

9.2   REPEATED MEASURES WITH SEVERAL POPULATIONS

We now consider problems involving a sample of individuals from each of several populations rather than from just one population, again with repeated

Table 9.6   Analysis of Variance Table for Spelling Example

Source of Variation	Sum of Squares	df	Mean Square	Computed F	p Value
Students	2383.6	9	264.84		
Grade:	1036.9	3	345.63	15.85	
Linear trend on grade	1012.5	1	1012.5	46.44	< 0.0001
Quadratic trend after linear trend	6.4	1	6.4	0.29	0.59
Cubic trend after quadratic and linear trends	18.0	1	18.0	0.81	0.38
Residual	588.6	27	21.8		
Total	4009.1	39			

measures on each subject. The different populations could represent different treatment groups (for example, experimental or control) or comparative groups (such as males and females).

9.2.1   Example

The following example is a simple modification of the data on spelling scores that illustrated the one-sample case. Now the ten students have been divided into two groups of five each. Four units have been added to the scores of the five subjects in the second group to determine if the analysis can detect this slight difference between the two treatment effects. Here the two populations might be simply boys and girls. Or they could be children randomly assigned to two methods of teaching spelling. The data are given in Table 9.7, and a graph of mean spelling score versus grade for each treatment group is given in Figure 9.2.

The sorts of questions we wish to study include: Is there an effect of treatment on mean spelling score? Is there an effect of grade on mean spelling score? Is there an interaction between grade and treatment on mean spelling score? If there are differences, we want to describe those differences. As before, we are less interested in investigating the effect of student, as we expect that spelling scores differ from student to student.

Table 9.7 Spelling Scores for Two Groups of Students by Grade

Treatment	Student	Third	Fourth	Fifth	Sixth	
1	1	48	50	55	70	
	2	47	47	50	53	
	3	38	50	44	48	
	4	48	58	57	72	
	5	54	66	70	74	
	$\bar{Y}_{1j.}$	47.0	54.2	55.2	63.4	$\bar{Y}_{1..} = 54.95$
2	1	53	62	65	60	
	2	56	70	72	73	
	3	47	44	46	50	
	4	66	64	72	72	
	5	50	61	68	76	
	$\bar{Y}_{2j.}$	54.4	60.2	64.6	66.2	$\bar{Y}_{2..} = 61.35$
	$\bar{Y}_{.j.}$	50.7	57.2	59.9	64.8	$\bar{Y}_{...} = 58.15$

(Grade spans Third, Fourth, Fifth, Sixth columns.)

9.2.2 Model

To get an idea of an appropriate model, let's first take a closer look at the data in Table 9.7. In this example, there are three factors: treatment, grade, and student. Grade is the variable that contains the repeated measures, and the subjects, on whom the repeated measures are taken, are the students. Note that each of the two levels of treatment appears with each of the four grades; these two factors are *crossed*. Test scores are obtained from each student at each grade, so grade and student are crossed. But a student is only exposed to one of the two treatments. Thus, students are *nested* within treatment. Both treatment and year are considered fixed. Since we aren't interested in the particular students that were selected for study — they represent a random sample of students that could have been chosen, this effect of students nested within treatment is considered random. Grade and treatment are considered fixed; we want to make inferences about these two factors and their interaction.

The model can be expressed (generally) as

$$Y_{ijk} = \mu + \alpha_i + \beta_j + (\alpha\beta)_{ij} + \gamma_{(i)k} + \varepsilon_{ijk},$$

$$i = 1, \ldots, a, \quad j = 1, \ldots, b \quad k = 1, \ldots, c,$$

with

$$\sum_{i=1}^{a} \alpha_i = \sum_{j=1}^{b} \beta_j = \sum_{i=1}^{a} (\alpha\beta)_{ij} = \sum_{j=1}^{b} (\alpha\beta)_{ij} = 0$$

and

$$\gamma_{(i)k} \sim \mathrm{IND}(0, \sigma_c^2), \qquad \varepsilon_{ijk} \sim \mathrm{IND}(0, \sigma^2);$$

the $\gamma_{(i)k}$'s and ε_{ijk}'s are independent. The model for $a = 2$ treatments, $b = 4$ grades, and $c = 5$ students per treatment is

$$Y_{ijk} = \mu + \alpha_i + \beta_j + (\alpha\beta)_{ij} + \gamma_{(i)k} + \varepsilon_{ijk},$$
$$i = 1, 2, \quad j = 1, \ldots, 4, \quad k = 1, \ldots, 5.$$

In the context of our example, Y_{ijk} represents the spelling score for the kth student in treatment i and grade j. The term α_i represents the effect of the ith level of treatment, β_j represents the effect of the jth level of year, $(\alpha\beta)_{ij}$ represents the interaction between the ith treatment and jth grade, $\gamma(i)k$ is the effect of the kth student within treatment i, and ε_{ijk} is the residual.

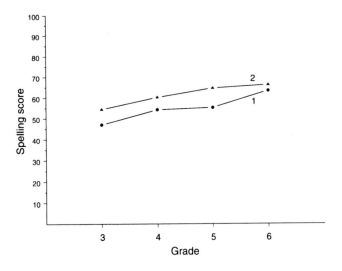

Fig. 9.2 Mean spelling score versus grade for each treatment group separately.

The effects of students within treatment $\gamma_{(i)k}$ are assumed to be independent of one another and follow a normal distribution with mean 0 and variance σ_c^2. The effects of residuals ε_{ijk} are also assumed to be independent of one another and follow a normal distribution with mean 0 and variance σ^2. The $\gamma_{i(k)}$ and ε_{ijk} are assumed to be mutually independent.

The model again implies compound symmetry, for just as in the case of a single sample, Var $(Y_{ijk}) = \sigma^2 + \sigma_c^2$, $\mathrm{Cov}(Y_{ijk}, Y_{ij'k}) = \sigma_c^2$, and $\mathrm{Corr}(Y_{ijk}, Y_{ij'k}) = \sigma_c^2/(\sigma^2 + \sigma_c^2)$. For each student, the correlation matrix for the scores in grades three, four, five, and six is

$$
\begin{pmatrix}
1 & \rho & \rho & \rho \\
\rho & 1 & \rho & \rho \\
\rho & \rho & 1 & \rho \\
\rho & \rho & \rho & 1
\end{pmatrix}.
$$

9.2.3 Analysis of Variance Table and F Tests

Since this is the first time in this book that crossed and nested factors appear together, we illustrate in detail how each deviation $Y_{ijk} - \bar{Y}_{...}$ can be divided into parts that estimate parameters of the model. We have

$$
\begin{aligned}
Y_{ijk} - \bar{Y}_{...} &= (\bar{Y}_{i..} - \bar{Y}_{...}) + (\bar{Y}_{.j.} - \bar{Y}_{...}) + (\bar{Y}_{ij.} - \bar{Y}_{i..} - \bar{Y}_{.j.} + \bar{Y}_{...}) \\
&\quad + (\bar{Y}_{i.k} - \bar{Y}_{i..}) + (Y_{ijk} - \bar{Y}_{ij.} - \bar{Y}_{i.k} + \bar{Y}_{i..}). \qquad (9.8)
\end{aligned}
$$

Here α_i is estimated by $\bar{Y}_{i..} - \bar{Y}_{...}$, β_j by $\bar{Y}_{.j.} - \bar{Y}_{...}$, the interaction $(\alpha\beta)_{ij}$ by $\bar{Y}_{ij.} - \bar{Y}_{i..} - \bar{Y}_{.j.} + \bar{Y}_{...}$, and $\gamma_{i(k)}$ by $\bar{Y}_{i.k} - \bar{Y}_{i..}$; the final term in Equation 9.8 is an estimate of ε_{ijk}. If we square both sides of the equation and sum over all observations, all cross product terms sum to zero and we are left with five sums of squares: SS_a for treatment, SS_b for time, SS_{ab} for the interaction between treatment and time, SS_c for the sum of squares due to subjects within treatments, and SS_r for the residual sum of squares. The ANOVA table is given in Table 9.8. The sources of variation have been put in an order that suggests how inferences are made in repeated measures models such as the one described here. As before, we can get an idea of how to make hypothesis tests by examining the expected mean squares, which are expressed in terms of the correlation ρ and σ_y^2.

There are three tests that are of particular interest. First, we want to test for no interaction between treatment and time,

$$
H_0 : \alpha\beta_{ij} = 0, \qquad i = 1, \ldots, a, \quad j = 1, \ldots, b,
$$

which can be expressed as

$$
H_0 : \mu_{ij} = \mu + \alpha_i + \beta_j
$$

Table 9.8 Analysis of Variance Table for Repeated Measures Design with Several Populations

Source of Variation	Sum of Squares	df	Mean Square	EMS
Treat.	SS_a	$a-1$	MS_a	$\sigma_y^2[1 + (b-1)\rho] + bc\phi(\alpha)$
Subjects(Treat.)	SS_c	$a(c-1)$	MS_c	$\sigma_y^2[1 + (b-1)\rho]$
Time	SS_b	$b-1$	MS_b	$\sigma_y^2(1-\rho) + ac\phi(\beta)$
Treat. by Time Interaction	SS_{ab}	$(a-1)(b-1)$	MS_{ab}	$\sigma_y^2(1-\rho) + c\phi(\alpha\beta)$
Residual	SS_r	$a(b-1)(c-1)$	s^2	$\sigma_y^2(1-\rho)$
Total	SS_t	$abc-1$		

and tested using $F = MS_{ab}/s^2$. As in testing for no effect of time, the corresponding EMSs are both equal to $\sigma_y^2(1-\rho)$ when there is interaction between these two factors. When H_0 is true, the test statistic F follows an F distribution with $\nu_1 = (a-1)(b-1)$ and $\nu_2 = a(b-1)(c-1)$. If a significant result is found, plots of means, as in Figure 9.2, are useful to help identify the interaction. Further suggestions are found in [6].

The test of no effect of treatment,

$$H_0 : \mu_{1.} = \cdots = \mu_{a.},$$

where $\mu_{i.} = \mu + \alpha_i$, is made using $F = MS_a/MS_c$. The expected mean squares are both equal to $\sigma_y^2[1 + (b-1)\rho]$ when there is no effect of treatment. When H_0 is true, the test statistic F follows an F distribution with $\nu_1 = a - 1$ degrees of freedom and $\nu_2 = a(c-1)$ degrees of freedom.

The test of no effect of time,

$$H_0 : \mu_{.1} = \cdots = \mu_{.b},$$

where $\mu_{.j} = \mu + \beta_j$, is made using $F = MS_b/s^2$. The corresponding expected mean squares are both equal to $\sigma_y^2(1-\rho)$ when there is no effect of time. When H_0 is true, the test statistic F follows an F distribution with $\nu_1 = b-1$ degrees of freedom and $\nu_2 = a(b-1)(c-1)$ degrees of freedom.

Note that any terms involving time (for this model, its main effect and its interaction with treatment) are computed using the residual mean square in the denominator of the F statistic. All terms not involving time (here, the main effect of treatment) are computed using the subjects within-treatments mean square.

Sometimes, the sources of variation for the fixed effects are grouped into two groups, called *between subjects* and *within subjects*; these categories reflect the different comparison mean squares used in the F statistics. For this model, treatment is the only source of between-subjects variation. Time and the treatment-by-time interaction reflect the subjects nested within treatment variation.

Example. Table 9.9 is the ANOVA table for the example in which two treatments are compared over four time periods (grades). Since the test of no interaction between treatment and grade is not rejected ($F = 19.7/22.12 = 0.87$ and $p = 0.47$), we proceed to the test of no effect of treatment on mean spelling score. The F statistic for this test is calculated as $409.6/290.75$, or 1.41; note that the mean square for students within treatments is used in the denominator. The test for no effect of grade is computed as $345.63/22.12 = 15.63$. Note that the test for no effect of grade, like the test for no interaction between treatment and grade, uses the mean square residual (22.12) in the denominator.

In this case, only grade was a significant source of variation. To describe how grade is related to mean spelling score, we are interested in determining whether linear or quadratic trends exist. The procedure is identical to what was illustrated earlier in Section 9.1.6, and the results are summarized in Table 9.10. Note that for these confidence intervals, the 97.5 percentile of a t distribution with $\nu = 24$ degrees of freedom (2.064) (Table B.2) is used in the computation of the interval. There is evidence of an increasing linear trend in mean spelling score as grade in school becomes higher.

9.3   CHECKING IF THE DATA FIT THE REPEATED MEASURES MODEL

As we've indicated before, graphing the data is one of the best and easiest ways to get an idea whether or not the data fit the model. The assumptions underlying the foregoing tests and confidence intervals are implicit in the model in Equation 9.1. Here, the β_j and the ε_{ij} are assumed to be independently normally distributed.

Checking for outliers and evaluation of residuals — through normal quantile plots, and through plots of residuals versus levels of the fixed factors to assess normality and equality of variances — is also recommended.

In order to assess normality of random effects besides the residuals, it is necessary to use a computer program which will actually estimate these effects. Typically, these are general programs that can fit mixed models. To assess normality on the basis of a normality quantile plot, there need to be an adequate number of subjects.

As discussed in Section 9.1.2, the model implies that the correlation coefficient between the observations at two time periods is the same regardless of which two time periods are considered. This characteristic of the model is known as *compound symmetry*. In the context of our examples, compound symmetry implies that the correlation between third and fourth grade scores

Table 9.9 Analysis of Variance for Two Groups of Repeated Test Scores

Source of Variation	SS	df	MS	Calculated F	p Value
Treatment	409.6	1	409.60	1.41	0.27
Students(treatment)	2326.0	8	290.75		
Grade	1036.9	3	345.63	15.63	< 0.0001
Treatment by Grade Interaction	57.8	3	19.27	0.87	0.47
Residual	530.8	24	22.12		
Total	4361.1	39			

equals that between third and sixth grade scores. For the first example, the calculated correlation coefficient between the scores for the third and fourth grades is 0.64, and between those for the third and sixth grades is 0.61, so that in this example, the two population correlations may well be equal. Frequently, however, one expects correlations between responses one year apart to be higher than those between responses several years apart. Thus the assumption of compound symmetry is often unrealistic.

If the assumption of compound symmetry is not met, then the F tests given earlier (which involve effects related to time, or use the mean square residual in the denominator) have a true significance that differs from the selected level. The tests are not likely to be conservative, and so analysts cannot trust a rejection decision unless the calculated F is extremely large.

We recommend that simple correlation matrices of the Y's across the repeated measurements be estimated for each treatment group separately to see if gross departures from compound symmetry are apparent.

Graphical methods for checking the assumption of compound symmetry are available [1]. Methods for testing for compound symmetry, such as Mauchly's test [7], are given in [8]; these tests are not described in this book.

Table 9.10 Point Estimates, Estimated Standard Errors (se), and Confidence Intervals for Contrasts

Trend	Point Estimate	Estimated se	95% Confidence Interval
Linear	45.0	6.65	$31.3 \leq -3\mu_{.1} - \mu_{.2} + \mu_{.3} + 3\mu_{.4} \leq 58.7$
Quadratic	−1.6	2.97	$-7.7 \leq \mu_{.1} - \mu_{.2} - \mu_{.3} + \mu_{.4} \leq 5.4$
Cubic	6.0	6.65	$-7.7 \leq -\mu_{.1} + 3\mu_{.2} - 3\mu_{.3} + \mu_{.4} \leq 19.7$

9.4   WHAT TO DO IF THE DATA DON'T FIT THE MODEL

In this section, we focus on the violation of the assumption of compound symmetry. There are two main options, and which way to go depends on the software program that is used. One procedure involves calculating the same F statistic but reducing the number of degrees of freedom. A second option is to assume a correlation structure other than compound symmetry.

If an analyst is using a program in which compound symmetry is assumed, but correlations among responses at different time periods are unequal, the test F statistic has approximately an F distribution [4], but not necessarily with the assumed number of degrees of freedom. The assumed numbers of numerator and denominator degrees of freedom of the F distribution are modified by multiplying each one by an estimate of a function of the variances and covariances of the responses (called *epsilon*). Common ways to estimate epsilon are based on the Greenhouse-Geisser criterion [4] or the Huynh-Feldt criterion [5]. Typically programs present estimates of epsilon and provide p values for the hypothesis tests, based on modification of the degrees of freedom. These are described in greater detail elsewhere (for example, [8]).

The second option involves using a program which fits mixed models. In this case, it is possible to consider alternative correlation matrices. Knowledge of the subject matter should certainly be used in deciding on an appropriate correlation matrix and graphical techniques have been suggested [1]. Examination of the fit of the models should also be considered. One possibility is to use the Akaike information criterion (AIC); the use of this criterion and others is taken up in Chapter 14.

9.5   GENERAL COMMENTS ON REPEATED MEASURES ANALYSES

Since there is a large variety of repeated measures models, analyses of repeated measures data can be difficult to apply and interpret. Furthermore, there are a variety of software programs available, which differ greatly in their sophistication. We have barely scratched the surface in this chapter.

Probably the most important thing to do is to specify the model carefully. Creating a table of the data can be helpful in clarifying which factors are crossed and which are nested. Furthermore, it helps to clarify which factors are fixed and which are random.

Programs that perform general linear modeling can be used to perform repeated measures analyses. One way to use these programs is to specify the model, making sure that factors are specified as crossed or nested and as random or fixed. If an analyst is uncertain how to perform the hypothesis tests, examination of EMS can serve as a guide. Alternatively, some general linear modeling programs have a set of options specifically for performing repeated measures. In this case, it is necessary to specify which variable identifies the repeated measures. If the model is specified correctly, the appropriate analyses are performed. An important point to keep in mind is that these programs typically omit cases with missing data for the variables included in the analysis. Analysts should be careful to check that standard error estimates are calculated as they intended.

Other software fits mixed models with repeated measures as a special case. These programs use different methods for performing the calculations and will handle missing data. As with all programs, it is vital that the model be specified correctly. As with general linear model programs, there are alternative ways of specifying the model to perform repeated measures.

In summary, we feel that a little knowledge of this topic is a dangerous thing. Software programs will generate a set of results, but there is no guarantee that the program was set up correctly. We recommend taking small examples and verifying computer output, if possible, as a way of understanding how the computations are performed. And it is always advisable to consult a statistician who is familiar with the topic and the available software.

Repeated measures designs have been widely used in drug trials, particularly for chronic diseases, where the patients are randomized to treatment groups and their status determined at multiple time points.

Repeated measurements can be determined on factors other than time. For example, five speech therapists might judge the intelligibility of four computer programs written to mimic human speech. Suppose each therapist judges the same four programs in the same order. The judgments from a single therapist are not likely to be independent. For example, a therapist who tends to judge intelligibility highly will tend to assign higher intelligibility values for the four programs.

9.6 SUMMARY

In this chapter, we introduced repeated measures analysis as a technique for analyzing data that include measurements that have been taken multiple times from each subject. Since the measurements obtained from a single subject cannot be assumed to be independent, we need to apply methods to allow for their correlation.

We considered two models in detail. The first dealt with repeated measures on subjects that were drawn from a single population. We described the model and showed how it could be written in terms of a mixed model or as a repeated measures model. For the repeated measures model, we focused on the correlation of observations from a subject over time. We assumed that the correlation matrix of the repeated measurements had a particular structure, referred to as compound symmetry — namely, the correlations between each pair of measurements from an individual subject are equal.

We indicated that the primary inference concerned the mean outcome across time. We described hypothesis tests for investigating whether the mean response is equal across the time points. We discussed linear combinations of the means which can be used for describing trends over time. We focused on orthogonal contrasts for identifying linear and quadratic trends. These contrasts could be used for both hypothesis tests and confidence intervals.

Our second model concerned repeated measurements taken over time from multiple populations, such as subjects exposed to different treatments. We considered the model in which subjects were nested within a particular treatment. We described hypothesis tests and noted that the test for no effect of treatment was made using the mean square associated with subjects within treatment, but that the tests for no treatment-by-time interaction and no effect of time were determined using the residual mean square.

We described how to tell if the data don't fit the model and focused particularly on the assumption of compound symmetry. References were given to methods of analyzing the data when the assumption of compound symmetry does not hold. Finally, we remarked on generalizations of repeated measures models and the wide variety of software available for analyzing repeated measures data.

Problems

9.1   Three drugs were tested in succession on patients with mild hypertension to see if there are differences among the drugs. Systolic blood pressure was measured on each patient. Sufficient time was allowed on a drug before taking the measurement to ensure that no effect of a previous drug could be present.

	Pressure (mm Hg)		
Patient	Drug 1	Drug 2	Drug 3
1	140	128	144
2	124	118	132
3	134	120	140
4	148	134	154
5	136	128	140

a)   Perform a repeated measures ANOVA. Test to see if there is a drug effect on systolic blood pressure.

b)   If appropriate, compute a contrast that would be useful in reporting the results.

9.2   The following data were obtained from a group of 10 adult male smokers during two years, five years apart. They are a measure of lung function called the forced expiratory volume and denoted by FEV1. Subjects are asked to breathe in deeply and then to expel air as rapidly and as fully as possible;

FEV1 is the volume of air expelled during the first second. In adults FEV1 decreases gradually with age, and numerous studies have shown a greater decrease for smokers than for nonsmokers. The data are:

Subject	FEV1 (liters) Year 1	Year 6
1	4.45	4.15
2	4.06	3.83
3	3.73	3.68
4	4.51	4.24
5	3.31	2.81
6	3.69	3.42
7	4.12	3.65
8	3.97	3.82
9	4.08	3.81
10	3.59	3.13

Analyze the data using a paired t test and a single group repeated measures ANOVA. Compare the results of the two analyses.

9.3   The following data represent FEV1 taken from 10 adult male nonsmokers during 2 years, five years apart.

Subject	FEV1 (liters) Year 1	Year 6
1	4.69	4.55
2	5.26	5.18
3	3.96	3.62
4	4.71	4.54
5	4.53	4.51
6	4.47	4.23
7	4.18	3.80
8	3.91	3.87
9	4.58	4.17
10	5.01	4.86

Analyze the data assuming a single-group repeated measures model.

9.4   Combine the data from Problems 9.2 and 9.3, and perform a repeated measures ANOVA. Analyze the data assuming a two-group repeated measures model (smokers and nonsmokers).

9.5   The following systolic blood pressures are from seven normal adult males taken at six-month intervals:

	Pressure (mm Hg)			
Subject	Time 1	Time 2	Time 3	Time 4
1	136	149	149	153
2	122	128	140	143
3	118	117	128	122
4	134	130	131	142
5	127	136	139	135
6	157	160	168	162
7	131	133	140	148

Test the null hypothesis that the means for the four time periods are equal.

9.6   The following data are FEV1 from three groups of males: smokers, nonsmokers, and former smokers. A sample of size four was drawn from each of the three groups. Three measurements were made on each subject at five year intervals. The data are:

		FEV1 (liters)		
Group	Subject	Time 1	Time 2	Time 3
Smokers	1	4.48	4.45	3.99
	2	4.39	3.94	3.42
	3	3.63	3.38	2.87
	4	4.19	3.51	3.43
Former smokers	1	4.85	4.79	4.68
	2	4.53	4.23	4.20
	3	5.00	4.85	4.67
	4	4.30	4.26	4.08
Nonsmokers	1	5.34	5.25	5.14
	2	4.81	4.83	4.57
	3	5.17	4.72	4.61
	4	4.62	4.51	4.50

a)   Calculate and graph means for the three groups and at each time period.

b)   Obtain an ANOVA table and appropriate F test(s).

c)   Compare the graphical and numerical results.

9.7   For the Liberty apple study discussed in Chapter 6, measurements were reported only for a single year. In fact, measurements were made for three successive years. If all the data are used, there are three crossed factors: treatment (fungicide versus no fungicide), block, and year. Treatment and year are fixed and block is random. The data are available on the Wiley ftp site. (Note that this model was not discussed in this chapter.)

a)   State the appropriate repeated measures model.

b)   Use ANOVA to determine whether or not fruit diameter changes over time. Determine orthogonal contrasts, and use them to investigate whether there are linear or quadratic trends over time.

c)   Perform a three-way ANOVA with tree height as the outcome variable. Summarize your findings about the effects of treatment, block, and year on mean outcome.

d)   Perform a three-way ANOVA with yield as the outcome variable. Summarize your findings about the effects of treatment, block, and year on mean outcome.

e)   Perform a three-way ANOVA with percentage of apples with a pack-out rating of US No. 1 as the outcome variable. Summarize your findings about the effects of treatment, block, and year on mean outcome.

REFERENCES

1. Dawson, K.S., Gennings, C., and Carter, W.H. [1997]. Two Graphical Techniques Useful in Detecting Correlation Structures in Repeated Measures Data, *The American Statistician,* 51, 275–283.

2. Fisher, R.A. and Yates, F. [1953]. *Statistical Tables for Biological, Agricultural and Medical Research,* 4th ed., Edinburgh: Oliver and Boyd.

3. Girden, E.R. [1992]. *ANOVA Repeated Measures,* Sage University Series on Quantitative Applications in the Social Sciences, 07-084, Newbury Park, CA: Sage, 1–30.

4. Greenhouse, S.W. and Geisser, S. [1959]. On Methods in the Analysis of Profile Data, *Psychometrika,* 24, 95–112.

5. Huynh, H. and Feldt, L.S. [1976]. Estimation of the Box Correction for Degrees of Freedom from Sample Data in Randomized Block and Split-Plot Designs, *Journal of Educational Statistics,* 1, 69–82.

6. Looney, S.W. and Stanley, W.B. [1989]. Exploratory Repeated Measures Analysis for Two or More Groups, *The American Statistician,* 43, 220–225.

7. Mauchly, J.W. [1940]. Significance Test for Sphericity of a Normal N-Variate Distribution, *Annals of Mathematical Statistics*, 11, 204–209.

8. Rencher, A.C. [2002]. *Methods of Multivariate Analysis*, 2nd ed., New York: John Wiley & Sons, 204–207.

9. Winer, B.J. [1971]. *Statistical Principles in Experimental Design*, 2nd ed., New York: McGraw Hill Book Company, 177–185, 261–308, 514–539.

10

Linear Regression: Fixed X Model

When many measurements are available on each individual, it is often desirable to study them simultaneously. In this chapter, we introduce one method for studying variables simultaneously: regression analysis.

In regression, we are interested particularly in how one variable is related to a set of other variables. The one variable is typically denoted by Y and may be referred to as the dependent, outcome, or predicted variable. The variables are generally denoted by X's and may be referred to as independent, explanatory, or predictor variables, or covariates.

In this chapter, we focus on the simplest applications of regression: investigations involving two variables, which are linearly related to each other. These applications are sometimes referred to as *simple linear regression*. That is, we have a single dependent variable Y and a single independent variable X. Furthermore, we focus on the situations in which the values of the X variable are fixed, or determined by the investigator, and known without error. Similar analyses can be performed when X is not under the control of the investigator, but here we are devoting a separate chapter to what is called the fixed X model. While this model is not used as much as the random X model, we feel regression is easier to introduce when levels of X are fixed, and by describing the two models in separate chapters, we can illustrate subtle differences between them in interpretation and in assessing their fit. Simple linear regression with random X and simple correlation are described in Chapter 11.

In the context of regression, the investigator often wishes to draw a curve that in some sense fits the data as well as possible. There are at least two objectives in fitting a curve:

(1) *General study.* The investigator may wish to study a general underlying pattern connecting the two variables, X and Y.

(2) *Prediction.* The investigator may wish to determine a curve that shows the relation between X and Y, in order to be able to predict Y for a given value of X.

Of the various types of curves that are sometimes fitted to data, the one most commonly used is the straight line. Frequently the decision to fit a straight line is made simply because the line can be fitted easily. On the other hand, the straight line is often an excellent choice for the data. When a straight line does not fit the data well, it is sometimes possible to transform the data in such a way that a straight line fits reasonably well. For example, within a certain range a straight line fitting the logarithm of weight to the square root of age seems to fit better than one fitting weight to age. Alternatively, curves other than straight lines can be fitted to the data.

In Section 10.1 we introduce a simple linear regression example, with levels of the X variable specified by the investigator: fixed X regression. In Section 10.2 we discuss how to fit a straight line through a set of points. In Section 10.3 we state formally the fixed X regression model. Estimation of model parameters is addressed in Section 10.4, followed by confidence interval estimation in Section 10.5 and hypothesis testing in Section 10.6. Section 10.7 concerns how to determine whether the linear regression model fits the data, and Section 10.8 addresses what to do if they don't. In Section 10.9 we consider some practical issues in designing a regression study, including sample size. Comparisons with one-way ANOVA are given in Section 10.10, and the chapter is summarized in Section 10.11.

The objectives and procedures for simple linear regression can be extended to more than two variables. These extensions will be covered in Chapters 12 and 13.

10.1   EXAMPLE

As part of the water quality monitoring of Dungeness Bay (a bay in Puget Sound, off the Olympic Peninsula in Washington State), Washington Department of Health officials have been measuring fecal coliform levels every other month at specific locations in the bay (see Table 10.1).

One way of identifying the locations is in terms of their distance from the mouth of the Dungeness River. We are interested in studying the relation between log fecal coliform levels and distance from the mouth of the river; simple linear regression will be used to investigate this. The Y or dependent variable is $\log_{10}$ fecal coliform level; fecal coliform is measured as the number of organisms per 100 milliliters of water. (It is standard in this field to transform the data to the $\log_{10}$ scale.) The X, predictor, or independent variable is distance, in miles, from the river mouth. Distance is an example of a ratio

Table 10.1 Log Fecal Coliform Levels at 11 Sampling Times at Three Distances from the Mouth of the Dungeness River

Observation	Distance, X	Fecal Coliform	$\log_{10}$ Fecal Coliform, Y
1	0.30	7.8	0.89
2	0.30	4.5	0.65
3	0.30	49.0	1.69
4	0.30	79.0	1.90
5	0.30	4.5	0.65
6	0.30	2.0	0.30
7	0.30	46.0	1.66
8	0.30	33.0	1.51
9	0.30	23.0	1.36
10	0.30	2.0	0.30
11	0.30	1.7	0.23
12	0.95	1.7	0.23
13	0.95	7.8	0.89
14	0.95	7.8	0.89
15	0.95	7.8	0.89
16	0.95	1.7	0.23
17	0.95	4.5	0.65
18	0.95	46.0	1.66
19	0.95	1.7	0.23
20	0.95	11.0	1.04
21	0.95	1.7	0.23
22	0.95	1.7	0.23
23	1.38	2.0	0.30
24	1.38	2.0	0.30
25	1.38	4.5	0.65
26	1.38	1.7	0.23
27	1.38	23.0	1.36
28	1.38	1.7	0.23
29	1.38	33.0	1.52
30	1.38	1.7	0.23
31	1.38	2.0	0.30
32	1.38	1.7	0.23
33	1.38	1.7	0.23

variable, that is, the ratio of any two distances is the same, regardless of the units of measurement, and a distance of 0 is understood.

Specified distances are identified as 0.30, 0.95, and 1.38 miles from the mouth of the river. The last 11 observations at each of these three locations are given in Table 10.1. Note that Department of Health officials specified these distances, or locations, in advance of conducting the sampling. In this sense, the levels of X (0.30, 0.95, and 1.38 miles) were fixed in advance by the officials.

A scatter plot of log fecal coliform versus distance is shown in Figure 10.1, and distance-specific summary statistics are provided in Table 10.2. Combining the data from the three distances, we get $\bar{Y} = 0.73$ and $\bar{X} = 0.88$. Note that for each of the distances, the minimum value of $\log_{10}$(fecal coliform per 100 ml) is 0.23, which corresponds to 1.7 fecal coliform per 100 ml of water. There are one 0.23 at 0.30 (observation 11), five 0.23's at 0.95 (observations 12, 16, 19, 21, 22), and five 0.23's at 1.38 miles (observations 26, 28, 30, 32, 33) in Table 10.1. This seems like a lot of 0.23's. Note in Figure 10.1 that the multiple values of 0.23 are plotted as a single point at the two longer distances, so there appear to be less than 11 observations at these fixed distance. 1.8 coliform per 100 ml is the lower limit at which the laboratory can make accurate measurements. All values less than or equal to 1.8 are reported as 1.7. The result is that on days when the fecal coliform level is very low, the measurement is given the value of 1.7. We will see what effect this has on the results when we perform the regression analyses.

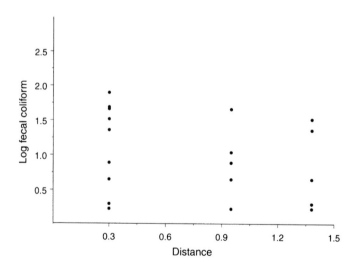

Fig. 10.1 Log fecal coliform levels versus distance from mouth of Dungeness River.

Table 10.2   Summary Statistics for Log Fecal Coliform Levels at Three Distances from the Mouth of the Dungeness River

	Distance		
Summary Statistic	0.30	0.95	1.38
Mean	1.01	0.65	0.51
Standard deviation	0.63	0.49	0.48
Minimum	0.23	0.23	0.23
Maximum	1.90	1.66	1.52
Sample size	11	11	11

We can see from examining the scatter diagram in Figure 10.1 that there are no gross outliers, and that there appears to be a decreasing relation between log fecal coliform concentrations and the distance from the mouth of the river. That is, increased distance from the mouth of the river is associated with decreased $\log_{10}$ coliform levels.

To study the relation between log fecal coliform counts and distance from the mouth of the Dungeness River, we can draw a line through the points to summarize the relation between the two variables or to predict log fecal coliform counts on the basis of distance from the river mouth. In addition, we can determine how these two variables relate to one another. One important question is how distance from the river mouth affects log fecal coliform levels. This will be investigated using confidence intervals and hypothesis tests.

10.2   FITTING A STRAIGHT LINE

Let X and Y denote the measurements on each of n units or individuals. On a scatter diagram, the Y's are measured along the vertical axis, the X's along the horizontal axis. The equation of any straight line except a vertical one can be written in the form

$$\hat{Y} = a + bX.$$

We use $\hat{Y}$ to denote the ordinate of any point on the line, a to denote the Y intercept, and b to denote the slope of the line. Here a is the ordinate or height of the line at the point $X = 0$. The slope, b, is interpreted as follows: when X changes by one unit, the height of the line changes by b units. This does *not* mean that a one unit change in X will *cause* a b unit change in Y.

In order to interpret the slope (the ratio of the change in Y to the change in X) what is meant by "change" must be clear. X and Y should be either interval or a ratio variables. A variable can be classified as interval if equal changes or differences in measurements have the same interpretation, regardless of the initial values. The X variable used in our example, distance, satisfies this requirement, because, for example, the difference between 1 and 2 miles (1 mile) is the same as the difference between 3 and 4 miles (also 1 mile). However, distance can also be classified as a ratio variable because it satisfies a stricter condition: that the ratio of distances is the same regardless of units of measurement (for example, 20 inches / 10 inches = 2; 50.8 centimeters / 25.4 centimeters = 2). Similarly, the Y variable used here is the log transformed fecal coliform concentration, measured as the number of organisms per 100 milliliters of water.

However, many statisticians disagree with a strict adherence to only using interval or ratio data in analyses such as linear regression [13]. These statisticians insist that the analysis used should be chosen based on what will be most useful in answering the questions the investigator has.

The most usual method for fitting a straight line through a set of points is the method of *least squares*. The least squares line has the property that the sum of the squared *vertical* distances from it to points on the scatter diagram is smaller than the corresponding sum for any other line. This is equivalent to saying that a and b are chosen so that the expression

$$Q = \sum_{i=1}^{n}(Y_i - \hat{Y}_i)^2 = \sum_{i=1}^{n}(Y_i - a - bX_i)^2 \tag{10.1}$$

is as small as possible. Here, Y_i denotes the ith observed value of Y, and X_i is the corresponding value of X.

The expression in Equation 10.1 is minimized when

$$a = \bar{Y} - b\bar{X} \tag{10.2}$$

and

$$b = \frac{\sum_{i=1}^{n}(Y_i - \bar{Y})(X_i - \bar{X})}{\sum_{i=1}^{n}(X_i - \bar{X})^2}, \tag{10.3}$$

(See Appendix A for the derivation of the least squares estimates of a and b.) The well-known least squares line then becomes

$$\hat{Y} = (\bar{Y} - b\bar{X}) + bX = a + bX, \tag{10.4}$$

where $(X, \hat{Y})$ denotes any point on the line.

The line can alternatively be written as $\hat{Y} - \bar{Y} = b(X - \bar{X})$. Substituting $X = \bar{X}$ in Equation 10.4, we obtain $\hat{Y} = \bar{Y}$. Thus the least squares line always passes through the point $(\bar{X}, \bar{Y})$; $\bar{Y}$ is the height of the line at the point $\bar{X}$. No assumptions were made in the determination of this least squares line.

Example. For the fecal coliform example, $a = 1.143$ and $b = -0.476$. Thus, the least squares line is $\hat{Y} = 1.143 - 0.476X$. When $X = \bar{X} = 0.877$, $\hat{Y} =$

$\bar{Y} = 0.725$, verifying that the least squares line goes through the point $(\bar{X}, \bar{Y})$. When $X = 0.30$, $\hat{Y} = 1.000$; when $X = 0.95$, $\hat{Y} = 0.690$; and when $X = 1.38$, $\hat{Y} = 0.486$. Note the close correspondence between the observed $\bar{Y}$'s at each distance, as given in Table 10.2, and the values of the $\hat{Y}$'s. They are not exactly the same, however, because different methods of computation were used. The distance-specific sample means in Table 10.2 (1.01, 0.65, 0.51) were computed using only the 11 log fecal coliform values at the specific distance. In contrast, the $\hat{Y}$'s were computed using observations from all three distances, and were based on the assumption that there is a linear relation between log fecal coliform and distance from the mouth of the river. The closeness in the values, however, suggests that the mean log coliform levels may fall on a straight line. The least squares line, on the scatter plot, is shown in Figure 10.2.

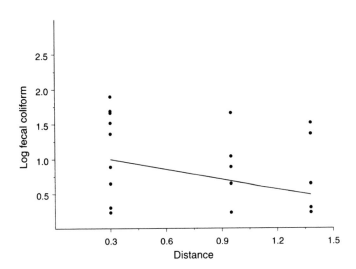

Fig. 10.2 Log fecal coliform versus distance from mouth of Dungeness River, with a regression line.

10.3 THE FIXED X MODEL

A straight line is often fitted to a set of data in the hope of making inferences concerning the underlying populations. When we speak of the populations, we are referring to conditional populations, the populations of Y values for given values of the X variable, frequently denoted $Y|X$. We now state some assumptions about these underlying populations and the sample, in the context of our example:

(1) The log fecal coliform levels at a particular distance from the mouth of the Dungeness River are normally distributed.

(2) Their means all lie on a straight line. In symbols, this assumption is $E(Y|X) = \mu_{Y|X} = \alpha + \beta X$.

(3) Their variances are all equal. This can be expressed as $\mathrm{Var}(Y|X) = \sigma^2$.

(4) All 33 log fecal coliform measurements are independent.

For example, consider a population of log fecal coliform levels at a distance $X = 0.30$ miles from the mouth of the river. This population is assumed to be normally distributed with mean $E(Y|0.30) = \alpha + 0.30\beta$. The population has a variance that is denoted $\mathrm{Var}(Y|0.30)$, or σ^2. For each distance, the assumption is made that a population of log fecal coliform levels exists. The means at the different distances all fall on a straight line, which is called the *population regression line*, $E(Y|X) = \alpha + \beta X$. [We are using the notation $E(Y|X)$ here, but we could just as well use the equivalent notation $\mu_{Y|X}$.] The variances of the log fecal coliform levels are the same, regardless of the distance X.

The model can be summarized more generally by writing

$$Y|X \sim \mathrm{IND}(\alpha + \beta X, \sigma^2), \qquad (10.5)$$

where IND denotes independent and normally distributed.

An alternative way of expressing the model is

$$Y_i = \alpha + \beta X_i + \varepsilon_i, \qquad i = 1, \ldots, n, \qquad (10.6)$$

where $\varepsilon_i \sim \mathrm{IND}(0, \sigma^2)$.

The ε's are assumed to be independent and normally distributed (IND). For example, if we knew that one log fecal coliform level was unusually high for a given distance, this knowledge would tell us nothing about the log fecal coliform levels of any of the other 33 water samples in the data set.

The assumptions that the population means lie on a straight line and that the population variances are equal may be quite unrealistic. Often, however, if X is confined to a moderate range, they are reasonable assumptions. The techniques which were derived to make inferences about the population parameters (both hypothesis testing and confidence intervals) are based on the model assumptions.

10.4   ESTIMATION OF MODEL PARAMETERS AND STANDARD ERRORS

10.4.1   Point Estimates

Let's first consider the estimation of the population regression line, and the two parameters α and β which define it. The regression line computed from a sample is called the *sample regression line*. This is the well-known least squares line, which was given in Equation 10.4.

We estimated α by a, β by b, and the population regression line by $\hat{Y} = a + bX$. The sample intercept a is an unbiased estimator of α, and b is an unbiased estimator of β. That is, if we took repeated random samples of (X, Y) from a large population of (X, Y) and each time computed a and b, the average of the a's would equal α and the average of the b's would equal β.

By estimating the population regression line, Equation 10.4 can also estimate the mean value of Y for a given value of X. Denote this given value of X by X^*. That is,

$$\hat{E}(Y|X^*) = a + bX^*.$$

This would be of particular interest if the focus of an investigation were on prediction of Y for specified values of X.

For a given data set, the estimate e_i of ε_i can be calculated as $Y_i - a - bX_i$, or $Y_i - \hat{Y}_i$. These are usually referred to as residuals, and represent vertical deviations of an individual observation (X_i, Y_i) from $(X_i, \hat{Y}_i)$.

The variance of the Y's for all values of X, that is, σ^2, is estimated by $s^2 = \sum_{i=1}^{n}(Y_i - \hat{Y}_i)^2/(n-2)$. It is natural to use the sum of squared deviations around the sample regression line to estimate the variance of the population. s^2 is computed from the residuals. It is often called the *residual mean square* or *variance of the residuals*. If we had known the true parameters α and β, we could have used $\sum_{i=1}^{n}(Y_i - \alpha - \beta X_i)^2/n$ to estimate σ^2. On the average, the use of $a = \bar{Y} - b\bar{X}$ for α and b for β underestimates σ^2 in repeated sampling, and to take account of this we subtract 2 from n and divide by $n - 2$. We say that 2 degrees of freedom have been used in estimating α and β; $n - 2$ remain.

No assumptions were required to estimate any parameters that define the population regression line. We assumed that the distributions of $Y|X$ exist and each has the same variance, σ^2, when we set out to estimate σ^2. If it turns out the variance is not constant, s^2 may not be of interest, as it will not have a clear interpretation. The parameters, corresponding point estimates, and interpretation of the point estimates are summarized in Table 10.3.

Table 10.3 Parameters of the Simple Linear Regression Model, Their Point Estimates, and Interpretation of the Estimates

Parameter	Estimate	Interpretation of Estimate
α	a	Y intercept of sample regression line
β	b	Slope of sample regression line
$E(Y \vert X) = \alpha + \beta X$	$a + bX$	Sample regression line
$E(Y \vert X^*) = \alpha + \beta X^*$	$a + bX^*$	Estimated mean of $Y \vert X^*$
σ^2	s^2	Estimate of $\mathrm{Var}(Y \vert X)$

10.4.2 Estimates of Standard Errors

We can derive variances for each of the point estimates presented above. They are straightforward to derive, as each estimate (involving a and/or b) is a linear combination of the Y's. Thus, getting the variances only involves taking the variances of linear combinations, which is described in Appendix A; the derivations are based on the assumptions that $Y_1 \vert X_1, Y_2 \vert X_2, \ldots, Y_n \vert X_n$ are independent and that the distributions of $Y \vert X$ all have the same variance, σ^2. Standard errors are obtained by taking the square root of the variances. Estimated standard errors are obtained by replacing the unknown population variance σ^2 by its estimate, s^2. We will rely on statistical software to generate the point estimates and estimated standard errors for us. Expressions for the point estimates and their estimated standard errors are given in Table 10.4.

Looking at the expressions for the estimated standard errors is informative. First, consider the slope, b. The denominator of the slope's estimated standard error is $\sqrt{\sum_{i=1}^{n}(X_i - \bar{X})^2}$. Thus, the variability of the slope is related to the differences between the X_i and $\bar{X}$ values. What would this suggest about how to select values of X if one were interested in minimizing the variability of the slope estimate? We will return to this in Section 10.9, when planning of studies with X fixed is addressed.

Second, consider the estimate Y when X is fixed at X^*, $\hat{Y} \vert X^* = a + bX^*$. One of the terms in the expression for the estimated standard error involves $(X^* - \bar{X})^2$ in the numerator. This tells us that the variability of the $\hat{Y}$'s is not constant, but varies with X^*. At what value of X will the estimated standard error be the smallest?

Example. For the fecal coliform example, selected point estimates and their estimated standard errors are given in Table 10.5. As we saw in Section 10.2, $a = 1.14$ and $b = -0.48$. The sample regression line is $\hat{Y} = 1.14 - 0.48X$.

These estimates can be used to estimate mean log fecal coliform levels at specified distances from the mouth of the river. The $\hat{Y}_i$ are 1.00 at 0.30, 0.69 at 0.95, and 0.49 at 1.38. So far, we have only made estimates at distances

Table 10.4 Population Parameters, Point Estimates, and Estimated Standard Errors in Simple Linear Regression

Parameter	Point Estimate	Estimated Standard Error
$\alpha + \beta \bar{X}$	$\bar{Y}$	$se(\bar{Y}) = s/\sqrt{n}$
α	$a = \bar{Y} - b\bar{X}$	$se(a) = s\sqrt{\dfrac{1}{n} + \dfrac{\bar{X}^2}{\sum_{i=1}^{n}(X_i - \bar{X})^2}}$
β	b	$se(b) = s/\sqrt{\sum_{i=1}^{n}(X_i - \bar{X})^2}$
$E(Y\|X^*)$	$\hat{Y} = a + bX^*$	$se(\hat{E}(Y\|X^*)) = s\sqrt{\dfrac{1}{n} + \dfrac{(X^* - \bar{X})^2}{\sum_{i=1}^{n}(X_i - \bar{X})^2}}$
σ^2	s^2	-

where measurements were actually taken. There is nothing to preclude our estimating mean $\log_{10}$ coliform values at other distances. For example, for the 33 observations, the mean distance $\bar{X}$ was 0.88; the mean $\log_{10}$ fecal coliform level at $\bar{X} = 0.88$ is $\bar{Y} = 0.73$. It is not a good idea to predict Y outside the range of the measured X's, as we don't know if the linear relation holds outside the range.

Next, consider some of the residuals. All 11 determinations of log fecal coliform drawn at $X = 0.30$ from the river mouth had a predicted value of 1.000. Because their actual values ranged from 0.30 to 1.90, their residuals (observed minus predicted values) ranged from -0.70 (for $\log_{10}$ fecal coliform of 0.30) to 0.90 (for $\log_{10}$ fecal coliform of 1.90). Similarly, all 11 determinations taken at $X = 0.95$ had a predicted $\log_{10}$ fecal coliform level of 0.69. Because the actual values ranged from 0.23 to 1.66, their residuals ranged from -0.46 to 0.97. Finally, all 11 determinations taken at $X = 1.38$ had a predicted $\log_{10}$ fecal coliform level of 0.49. Since the actual values ranged from 0.23 to 1.52, their residuals ranged from -0.26 to 1.03.

The sum of the residuals over all 33 determinations is 0. If the residuals were squared, summed over the 33 determinations, then divided by $n - 2 = 31$, the value would be 0.274. This is the estimated variance of each population of log fecal coliform values, the mean square error, or $s^2 = 0.274$; the estimated standard deviation is $s = 0.523$.

In Table 10.5, as expected, the estimated standard errors for $\hat{Y}|X^*$ increase as X^* gets further away from the sample mean $\bar{X}$. The estimated standard error of $\hat{Y}$ is the smallest at $\bar{X} = 0.877$. At this point it is $0.523/\sqrt{33} = 0.091$.

Table 10.5   Point Estimates and Estimated Standard Errors for the Example

Point Estimate	Estimated Standard Error
$\bar{Y} = 0.725$	$se(\bar{Y}) = 0.091$
$a = 1.143$	$se(a) = 0.202$
$b = -0.476$	$se(b) = 0.205$
$\hat{Y}|0.30 = 1.00$	$se(\hat{Y}|0.30) = 0.149$
$\hat{Y}|0.88 = 0.73$	$se(\hat{Y}|0.88) = 0.091$
$\hat{Y}|0.95 = 0.69$	$se(\hat{Y}|0.95) = 0.092$
$\hat{Y}|1.38 = 0.49$	$se(\hat{Y}|1.38) = 0.138$
$s^2 = 0.274$	—

10.5   INFERENCES FOR MODEL PARAMETERS: CONFIDENCE INTERVALS

This section and the next one involve statistical inference for the simple linear regression model. The derivation of the procedures for determining confidence intervals or performing hypothesis tests were based on all of the model assumptions (see Equation 10.5): the distributions of $Y|X$ are normally distributed with mean $\alpha + \beta X$ and variance σ^2, and all observations are independent. To review, no assumptions were made in determining the sample regression line, and the assumptions of equal variance and independence of observations were required for obtaining the estimated standard errors. Now we make use of the additional assumption of normality of the distributions of $Y|X$.

Confidence intervals for α, β, and $E(Y|X^*)$ are given in Table 10.6. In Section 10.4, we discussed point estimates and estimated standard errors. The only other piece of information that is needed to construct the confidence interval is the t value. For a $100(1 - \alpha)\%$ confidence interval, we add and subtract the $100(1 - \alpha/2)$ percentile of a t distribution with number of degrees of freedom equal to that used in the estimation of σ^2, here $n - 2$. As we have seen throughout the book, these interval estimates can be used to give a plausible range of values that the parameter can assume, or they can be used for hypothesis testing.

Most frequently, interest is in obtaining the confidence interval for β. Interval estimates of α may or may not be of interest. They are of interest if the Y intercept is something meaningful (i.e., it makes sense and it is possible for X to assume a value of 0) and sampling has been done near or at $X = 0$.

It is possible to compute a confidence interval for $E(Y|X)$ for all X values. However, it is important to construct these for the X values within the range where data were collected; there isn't any evidence about the relation between Y and X for X values far away from values at which Y was determined.

Table 10.6 Confidence Intervals in Linear Regression

Parameter	$100(1-\alpha)\%$ Confidence Interval
$\alpha + \beta \bar{X}$	$\bar{Y} \pm t_{1-\alpha/2;n-2} \ \text{se}(\bar{Y})$
α	$a \pm t_{1-\alpha/2;n-2} \ \text{se}(a)$
β	$b \pm t_{1-\alpha/2;n-2} \ \text{se}(b)$
$E(Y\vert X^*)$	$(a + bX^*) \pm t_{1-\alpha/2;n-2} \ \text{se}(\hat{E}(Y\vert X^*))$

If we were to construct intervals for $E(Y\vert X^*)$ for a range of values of X and plot the upper and lower limits, then hyperbolic curves, symmetric about the least squares line, would be drawn. The curves would reach a minimum vertical distance from the least squares line at $X = \bar{X}$; this is the point where the estimated standard error of $\hat{E}(Y\vert X^*)$ is minimized. The curves would fan away from the line as the distance of the X values from $\bar{X}$ was increased, reflecting the greater uncertainty in estimating $\hat{Y}$ away from $\bar{X}$. For each X^*, a $100(1-\alpha)\%$ confidence interval is presented.

Example. Selected parameters and their 95% confidence intervals are provided in Table 10.7 for the fecal coliform example. In Section 10.4, we obtained point estimates and estimated standard errors. The only other thing we need is the t value. Since $\nu = n - 2 = 31$, we want the 97.5 percentile of a t distribution with 31 degrees of freedom, $t_{(0.975;31)} = 2.0395$.

The 95% confidence interval for β is $b \pm 2.0395 \cdot \text{se}(b)$, or numerically $-0.476 \pm 2.0395(0.205)$, or $-0.894 < \beta < -0.059$. There is 95% confidence that the population slope lies between -0.894 and -0.059. Besides giving a plausible range of values for β, the interval can be used to test the hypothesis that $\beta = 0$ (or some other number of interest). Because the interval does not include 0, we can conclude that $\beta \neq 0$.

Table 10.7 Confidence Intervals for Fecal Coliform Example

Parameter	Point Estimate	Estimated Standard Error	Confidence Interval
β	-0.48	0.21	$-0.89 < \beta < -0.059$
$E(Y\vert 0.30)$	1.00	0.15	$0.70 < E(Y\vert 0.30) < 1.30$
$E(Y\vert 0.95)$	0.69	0.092	$0.50 < E(Y\vert 0.95) < 0.88$
$E(Y\vert 1.38)$	0.49	0.14	$0.21 < E(Y\vert 1.38) < 0.77$

Now, consider the 95% confidence interval for $E(Y\vert X^*)$. As shown in Table 10.7, the widths of the confidence intervals reflect the estimates of the standard errors. The further away X^* is from $\bar{X}$, the wider the confidence interval is. This can also be seen from the confidence bands, shown in Figure 10.3.

The intervals provide a range of values for *mean* $\log_{10}$ coliform concentrations at a specified distance from the river mouth. Confidence intervals for mean coliform counts and coliform counts at a specified distance could be obtained by computing the antilog of the lower and upper confidence limits. For example, to get the confidence interval for the mean coliform concentrations at $X = 0.3$ miles from the river mouth, the lower and upper limits of this interval would be $10^{0.70} = 4.97$ and $10^{1.30} = 20.14$.

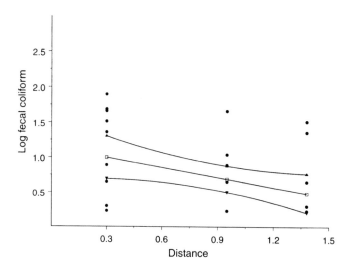

Fig. 10.3 Log_{10} fecal coliform versus distance from river mouth — observed data, sample regression line, 95% confidence bands.

10.6   INFERENCE FOR MODEL PARAMETERS: HYPOTHESIS TESTING

10.6.1 t Tests for Intercept and Slope

One of the key questions that an investigator should want to examine is whether or not the slope of the population regression line is 0. If β does not equal zero, and the model is specified correctly, then the means of the populations of Y's at different levels of X all fall on a straight line, which depends on X. Knowledge of X potentially can give information concerning

Y. If β equals zero, then $E(Y|X) = \alpha$; thus at each value of X, there is a normally distributed population of Y's, all with the same mean and the same variance. Knowledge of X can give us no information concerning Y; our best estimate of Y is simply $\bar{Y}$.

We can state the hypothesis to be tested in words: the population regression line has slope of 0. Alternatively, we can make use of the model to state what the hypothesis of particular interest is, for example:

$$H_0 : Y_i = \alpha + \varepsilon_i$$

or

$$H_0 : E(Y|X) = \alpha$$

or

$$H_0 : \beta = 0.$$

When this hypothesis is rejected, we conclude that $\beta \neq 0$. If it is not rejected, we conclude that the line on which the means of the Y's for the different values of X lie may be horizontal.

There are several equivalent ways to perform the hypothesis test. One way, as seen above, is to use a confidence interval for β. Alternatively, we can use a t test, where the test statistic is

$$t = \frac{b}{se(b)}.$$

When H_0 is true, the test statistic follows a t distribution with $n - 2$ degrees of freedom. Finally, we can use the ANOVA F test, as described in Section 10.6.3.

Sometimes, there may be interest in determining whether or not the slope is equal to some specified value, β_0. For example, we might wish to test that $\log_{10}$ fecal coliform decreases by $\beta_0 = 0.5$ for each mile from the river mouth. Again, the confidence interval for β can be constructed; if the hypothesized value β_0 is not included in the interval, the hypothesis is rejected. Equivalently, to test $H_0 : \beta = \beta_0$, we compare the statistic

$$t = \frac{b - \beta_0}{se(b)}$$

with $t_{1-\alpha/2;n-2}$. This test has a significance level of α.

While the test that $\beta = 0$ is of primary interest in the majority of investigations, tests about the intercept α can be informative as well. Of particular interest is testing that α is 0, that is, that the population regression line goes through the origin. Many statistical packages routinely provide tests of both $\alpha = 0$ and $\beta = 0$.

Example. In the context of the example, we are interested in whether the line for the regression of log fecal coliform counts on distance from river mouth has a slope of 0. The calculated t statistic is $b/se(b) = -0.476/0.205 = -2.32$ ($p = 0.027$). Because the p value is so small, we reject H_0 and conclude that $\beta \neq 0$.

To test that $\beta = -0.5$, the calculated $t = (-0.476 - (-0.5))/0.205 = 0.12$ and $p = 0.91$; β could possibly be 0.5.

We do not make any inferences about α in this example. A test that the regression line goes through the origin is not sensible in this situation. Furthermore, no fecal coliform counts were taken at the mouth of the river (i.e. no sampling was done at $X = 0$); we would not want to assume that the same linear relation between log coliform values and distance that exists between $X = 0.30$ miles and $X = 1.38$ miles from the river mouth holds nearer the mouth.

10.6.2   Division of the Basic Sum of Squares

In the ANOVA models of the earlier chapters, each deviation of an observation from the overall mean of the data was divided into two or more parts. Similarly, in simple linear regression, the ith deviation from $\bar{Y}$, $Y_i - \bar{Y}$, can be divided into two parts and expressed as follows:

$$Y_i - \bar{Y} = (\hat{Y}_i - \bar{Y}) + (Y_i - \hat{Y}_i). \tag{10.7}$$

One part, $\hat{Y}_i - \bar{Y}$, is the distance at $X = X_i$ of the sample regression line from the horizontal line representing $\bar{Y}$. The other, $Y_i - \hat{Y}_i$, is the vertical distance of Y_i from the sample regression line (the residuals).

When all n deviations are broken into two parts in this way, squared, and added, the cross-product terms add to zero, and we have

$$\sum_{i=1}^{n}(Y_i - \bar{Y})^2 = \sum_{i=1}^{n}(\hat{Y}_i - \bar{Y})^2 + \sum_{i=1}^{n}(Y_i - \hat{Y}_i)^2. \tag{10.8}$$

For convenience, we denote the total sum of squares on the left-hand side of the equation as SS_t. On the right-hand side, $\sum_{i=1}^{n}(\hat{Y}_i - \bar{Y})^2$ is called the *regression* on the X sum of squares and is denoted by SS_{reg}; $\sum_{i=1}^{n}(Y_i - \hat{Y}_i)^2$ is the residual sum of squares, SS_r — it is sometimes called the "error" sum of squares or the "deviation from regression on the X sum of squares.

Example. Let's consider the breaking apart of the total sum of squares for the log fecal coliform study. As an example, consider the fourth observation in the data set (see Table 10.1), with $X_4 = 0.30$ and $Y_4 = 1.898$. (This particular observation was chosen simply because it was the largest at $X = 0.30$; any other point would have worked about as well.) The estimate $\hat{Y}_4 = a + bX_4 = 1.143 - 0.476 \times 0.30 = 1.000$. The deviation from the overall mean is $Y_4 - \bar{Y} = 1.898 - 0.725 = 1.173$. This deviation can be broken down into the part explained by the regression of log fecal coliform counts on distance,

$\hat{Y}_4 - \bar{Y} = 1.000 - 0.725 = 0.275$, and the part explained by the deviations from the regression of log fecal coliform on distance, $Y_4 - \hat{Y}_4 = 1.898 - 1.000 = 0.898$. (Note: $0.275 + 0.898 = 1.173$.) Calculating these deviations, squaring them, and summing over all 33 observations gives $SS_t = 9.957$, $SS_{reg} = 1.474$, and $SS_r = 8.483$. Thus, the total variation in the data set has been broken down into two parts — variation due to the regression of log fecal coliform on distance and residual variation — and quantified in terms of sums of squares.

10.6.3   Analysis of Variance Table and F Test

We can use ANOVA to test for zero slope. The two sources of variation in the observations were identified and quantified in terms of sums of squares. As before, mean squares are determined by dividing sums of squares by numbers of degrees of freedom. Note that the residual mean square corresponds to the estimate of $\text{Var}(Y|X)$, or s^2.

Table 10.8 gives the ANOVA table for linear regression in formulas.

Table 10.8   Analysis of Variance Table for Simple Linear Regression

Source of Variation	Sum of Squares	df	Mean Square	EMS	Computed F
Regression	SS_{reg}	1	MS_{reg}	$\sigma^2 + \beta^2 \sum (X_i - \bar{X})^2$	MS_{reg}/s^2
Residual	SS_r	$n - 2$	s^2	σ^2	
Total	SS_t	$n - 1$			

The calculated F is used for testing the hypothesis $H_0 : \beta = 0$. If β is zero, the ANOVA table provides two independent estimates of σ^2: MS_{reg} and s^2; their ratio, $F = MS_{reg}/s^2$, is used as the test statistic. If β is not zero, MS_{reg} estimates something greater than σ^2. In this case, the F statistic follows a non-central F distribution with parameters $\nu_1 = 1$, $\nu_2 = n - 2$ and a noncentrality parameter λ which depends on β.

Example. For our example, the calculated F statistic is $F = MS_{reg}/s^2 = 5.39$ and $p = 0.027$ (Table 10.9). When testing at level of significance $\alpha = 0.05$, this hypothesis is rejected; our conclusion, therefore, is that β is not equal to zero. Note that, as before, $t^2 = F$, that is, $(-2.32)^2 = 5.39$.

10.7   CHECKING IF THE DATA FIT THE REGRESSION MODEL

With the wide availability of statistical software, performing repeated analyses to check and recheck that data fit specified regression models is not difficult to do. As in other chapters, this process should be viewed as something that

Table 10.9 Analysis of Variance Table for the Regression of Log Fecal Coliform on Distance from Mouth of River

Source of Variation	Sum of Squares	df	Mean Square	Computed F	p Value
Regression	1.47	1	1.47	5.39	0.027
Residual	8.48	31	0.27		
Total	9.96	32			

you don't do just once, but repeatedly, to evaluate the effect of transforming variables, deleting observations, and so on.

Before determining if the data fit the fixed X simple linear regression model, we recommend checking for gross outliers by examining a scatter diagram, such as Figure 10.1. Checking of the data then proceeds after obvious errors and outliers are removed.

One common way of assessing the fit of a model is to calculate the *coefficient of determination*, $R^2 = \mathrm{SS}_{reg}/\mathrm{SS}_t$. It is sometimes referred to as "R-square" on output from statistical software. For the fixed X model, R^2 should not be interpreted as the square of a correlation coefficient (see Section 11.2), and its square root has no interpretation. It gives the reduction in variation in Y obtained by fitting the regression line to the data. We have noted previously that R^2 can range from 0 to 1. If all points fall on a straight line with nonzero slope, then $\mathrm{SS}_r = 0$ and $R^2 = 1$; if the sample regression line has slope 0, $\mathrm{SS}_{reg} = 0$ and $R^2 = 0$.

When R^2 is close to 1, most of the variation in Y can be explained by the linear relationship between X and Y. But there could be violations of the regression model: unequal variances, lack of normality, lack of independence, lack of linearity, or outliers. Thus, there could be concerns about making inferences, even in this situation.

There are a couple of ways to interpret an R^2 close to 0. It may be that the variables aren't particularly strongly related, so that a line that is fitted is not much better than a horizontal line drawn at $\bar{Y}$. Or it may be that the variables have some relation other than a linear one (for example, a quadratic one).

Thus, R^2 is good for an overall summary of the fit of a model, but we will want to do something more to identify outliers and to examine the model assumptions of linearity, normality, and equal variances. These assessments will provide us with some idea of the appropriateness of the inferences we wish to make about the underlying populations. To do this, we will focus on the observed data and the residuals obtained from fitting the linear regression model.

The methods of checking the appropriateness of a regression model are sometimes referred to as *regression diagnostics*. With simple linear regression, we can get a fairly good idea of whether or not the model is an appropriate representation of the relationship between the two variables simply by examining a scatter plot. Here, we have introduced more formal methods for checking if the data fit the model; discussion of outliers, linearity, equality of variances, and normality is taken up in the following subsections.

The methods are typically used in more complex settings, say with multiple X variables; here, we can focus on the techniques and avoid the complexity. We rely on statistical software to aid us in evaluating the fit of a model. Further details can be found in other sources [1, 2, 3, 5, 7, 10].

10.7.1   Outliers

With fixed X regression, we are more concerned with detecting outliers — unusual values in Y for given values of X — than with unusual values for Y or X per se. Because the X values are fixed, there shouldn't be any unusual values. If there are, they are likely data entry errors and should have been detected during initial data screening. A value of Y that seems unusual in initial data screening may or may not be an outlier in the context of regression.

Thus, outliers are best identified through simultaneous consideration of Y and X. A simple graphical approach is to examine a scatter diagram of Y versus X. Alternative approaches make use of residuals, $e_i = Y_i - \hat{Y}_i$, which are functions of both Y and X. For any example, the mean of the e_i is 0, and their variance is $s^2 = MS_r$. Most any univariate summarization of the residuals can identify unusually small or large values. Stem and leaf diagrams or histograms make effective graphical summarizations, while listings of extreme values provide good numerical summarizations.

10.7.2   Checking for Linearity

Now, consider the assumption of linearity. When there are multiple Y values determined at each specified value of X, we would like, ideally, to see the scatter diagram shown in Figure 10.4a. The means all fall on a straight line, and it appears that the variances are equal across different X values. Sometimes, boxplots are drawn at each distinct value of X for the same purpose. Another alternative to the plot of Y versus X is a *residual plot*, that is, a plot of $e_i = Y_i - \hat{Y}_i$ versus X, as in Figure 10.4b. When the residuals are computed, the linear effect of Y on X is removed. Thus, if there is a linear relation between Y and X, there should be no apparent relation between the residuals and X; if a least squares line were drawn through the n points (e_i, X_i), the slope of the line drawn through the points should be close to 0. These plots are informative for assessing linearity regardless of how many Y's are measured at each X.

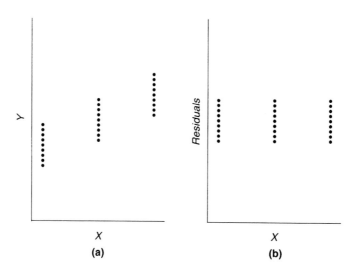

Fig. 10.4 Scatter diagrams showing no violations of assumptions: (a) Y versus X; (b) residuals versus X.

A nonlinear relation between Y and X would be detected from the original scatter diagram or from the residual plot. For example, if there were a quadratic relation between Y and X, the scatter diagrams of the original data and the residual plot would have a quadratic shape, as in Figure 10.5a and Figure 10.5b. With the fixed X model, when there are multiple observations associated with each X value, it is possible to test for linearity, as described, for example, in [1].

10.7.3 Checking for Equality of Variances

Next, consider the assumption of equality of variances. Recall that the distributions of Y (or, equivalently, the residuals ε_i) for given values of X are assumed to have equal variances. Whether or not this assumption is violated can also be assessed from the scatter diagrams and residual plots. If the assumption is correct, there should be no apparent pattern in the range of Y values across values of X in a scatter diagram of Y versus X or in the range of residuals across values of X in a residual plot.

The scatter diagram and residual plot presented in Figure 10.6a and Figure 10.6b suggests a trend of increasing variability of Y with increasing X. Indeed, a common indication of inequality of variances or nonnormality is an

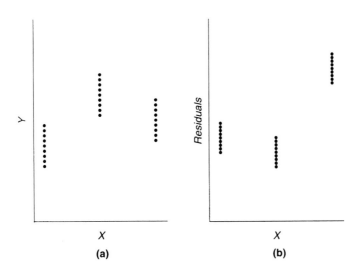

Fig. 10.5 Scatter diagrams showing violation of assumption of linearity: (a) Y versus X; (b) residuals versus X.

increasing range of Y (or residuals) with increasing values of X when the slope of the regression line is positive; the reverse is true when the slope is negative.

Another common indication of inequality of variances is an increasing range of Y (or residuals) with increasing values of Y. This violation can be detected through a plot of residuals versus fitted values $(e_i, \hat{Y})$; an increasing range of residuals as fitted values are increased suggests this.

However, we must be cautious in interpreting these plots, particularly when the number of Y's determined at a fixed X is not constant, as the range depends on sample size; greater spread would be expected with a greater number of observations measured. When there are multiple Y's at each value of X, a hypothesis test for equality of variances, such as Levene's test discussed in Chapter 2, can also be considered. When there are few responses (or even just one) at each value of X, there aren't good alternatives to looking at the plots.

10.7.4 Checking for Normality

To assess the assumption of *normality* of $Y|X$, normal quantile plots are helpful. As discussed in Chapter 2, if the sample size is large enough at each X, normal quantile plots of the observed responses can be made for each of the populations. Otherwise all of the residuals can be considered at the same time

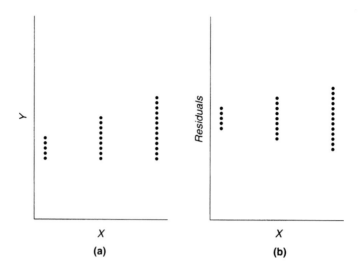

Fig. 10.6 Scatter diagrams showing violation of assumption of equal variances: (a) Y versus X; (b) residuals versus X.

and a single plot constructed. If the populations are normally distributed, a straight line should be observed. If a linear relationship is not obtained, some indication of the nonnormality should be suggested by the shape of the curve. As we've noted before, the residuals are slightly correlated. Stem and leaf plots, boxplots, and histograms of the residuals are also useful for evaluating normality.

Example. For our example, $R^2 = 0.15$. This means that 15% of the variation in log fecal coliform is due to its linear regression on distance, and 85% is due to something else. This suggests that there is not a particularly strong linear relation between the two variables.

   We can assess linearity and equality of variances by examining the plot of log coliform versus distance, in Figure 10.1, and the plot of the residuals versus distance, in Figure 10.7. As at the beginning of the chapter, when we first viewed the data, it appeared that there was some linear tendency toward more coliform bacteria closer to the mouth of the river. We can arrive at the same conclusion from the plot of the residuals versus distance. There is some concern about lack of equality of variances. The range of observed values (and residuals) seems greater at a distance of 0.30 miles than at 1.38 miles. (It is appropriate to make some comparison of the ranges because of the equal sample size of 11 at each distance.) However, Levene's test for equality of variance (described in Chapter 2) did not reject: $p = 0.18$.

Normality can be assessed from the normal quantile plot of the residuals, given in Figure 10.8. The plot shows some mild departures from normality; the shape of the curve is consistent with a distribution that is skewed to the right. (The skewness of the residuals $= 0.61$.) The Shapiro-Wilk statistic is $W = 0.92$ with $p = 0.023$. These results suggest that the log transformation of the coliform concentrations made the distribution of the outcome less skewed, but there was still some skewness remaining. We are reluctant to try alternative transformations, as use of the $\log_{10}$ transformation is standard in this field.

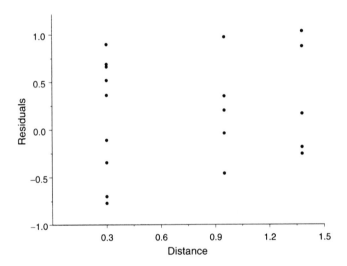

Fig. 10.7   Plot of residual of log coliform concentration versus distance.

Independence of the Y values is often checked by plotting them versus time, or whatever other factor might be association with the lack of independence (see Section 1.3.4 in Chapter 1). In the fecal coliform example, there are several factors that might result in a seasonal trend in the data set. Some of the streams whose water goes eventually to the bay receive water from irrigation ditches that can become contaminated by animal or human wastes. The ditches are used mainly in late summer and early fall when rainfall is low. Also, the bay is enclosed by a spit that is a wildlife refuge, so the bay is used by seals and birds at particular times of the year. Using data from multiple sites and years, investigators have found a small seasonal trend in the fecal coliform levels. In this example, all the measurements for each site

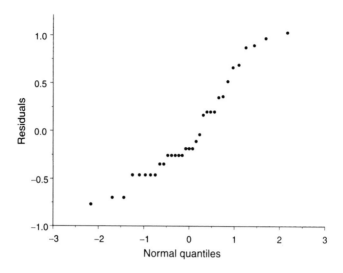

Fig. 10.8 Normal quantile plots of 33 residuals from coliform study.

were taken on the same day, so to that any seasonal effects affect the three sites equally; it is balanced across sites.

There are no gross outliers or unusual points apparent from the graphs or from the listing of residuals, given in Table 10.10. The largest residual, 1.03, is associated with the 29th observation in the data set: $X_{29} = 1.38$, $Y_{29} = 1.52$. Previous data sets have included values of log fecal coliform concentrations as large as 1.52 or larger. The Health Department is concerned about high levels of fecal coliform, so it makes sense to retain the larger values.

One thing to keep in mind when interpreting the data is the presence of 11 values of log coliform concentrations of 0.23, indicating that that the actual count was below the detection range. It isn't known what effect, if any, this has on the slope. We could speculate that if a more sensitive method of testing were devised, so that a lower detection limit could be specified, the slope would be greater in magnitude (i.e., more negative), as more values below the current detection limit were found at greater distance from the river mouth. Having log fecal coliform concentrations below 0.23 would also lower the skewness of its distribution and make it more symmetric.

10.7.5 Summary of Screening Procedures

Table 10.11 contains a summary of procedures that can be applied for checking various assumptions for simple linear regression. For each of the assumptions

Table 10.10 Observed Y, Predicted Y ($\hat{Y}$), and Residual (e_i) for Coliform Study

Observation	Y_i	$\hat{Y}_i$	e_i
1	0.89	1.00	−0.11
2	0.65	1.00	−0.35
3	1.69	1.00	0.69
4	1.90	1.00	0.90
5	0.65	1.00	−0.35
6	0.30	1.00	−0.70
7	1.66	1.00	0.66
8	1.52	1.00	0.52
9	1.36	1.00	0.36
10	0.30	1.00	−0.70
11	0.23	1.00	−0.77
12	0.23	0.69	−0.46
13	0.89	0.69	0.20
14	0.89	0.69	0.20
15	0.89	0.69	0.20
16	0.23	0.69	−0.46
17	0.65	0.69	−0.04
18	1.66	0.69	0.97
19	0.23	0.69	−0.46
20	1.04	0.69	0.35
21	0.23	0.69	−0.46
22	0.23	0.69	−0.46
23	0.30	0.49	−0.19
24	0.30	0.49	−0.19
25	0.65	0.49	0.17
26	0.23	0.49	−0.26
27	1.36	0.49	0.88
28	0.23	0.49	−0.26
29	1.52	0.49	1.03
30	0.23	0.49	−0.26
31	0.30	0.49	−0.19
32	0.23	0.49	−0.26
33	0.23	0.49	−0.26

discussed above, we include what methods should be used and what we would expect to see if they are satisfied.

10.8 WHAT TO DO IF THE DATA DON'T FIT THE MODEL

Research workers may know theoretically or from looking at their data that the three assumptions underlying the linear regression model are not true.

Table 10.11   Summary of Methods for Checking Assumptions of Model

Assumption	How to Check	What Will Be Seen if Assumption Satisfied
No outliers	Scatter diagram	No outlying Y values
	Residuals	No outlying residuals
Linearity	Plots of residuals versus X	No pattern
Equal variances	Plot of residuals versus X	Constant spread
	Plot of residuals versus fitted values	Constant spread
Normality	Stem and leaf plot of residuals	Normal shape
	Histogram of residuals	Normal shape
	Normal quantile plots of residuals	Straight line

For each X, the Y's may not be normally distributed, their variances may be unequal, or their means may lie on a curve rather than on a straight line.

If a scatter diagram of the data shows points lying along a curve rather than a straight line, at least two options can be considered. One option is to fit a curve to the data. For example, if there appears to be a quadratic relation between the X and Y variables, a polynomial in X, such as a quadratic curve, can be fitted to the data. This technique will be covered in Chapter 14.

An alternative method which is widely used when assumptions are not met is that of transforming the data. Recall that transformations were introduced in Chapter 1. However, in that chapter we focused on using transformation only to achieve normality. We are asking more of transformations in the context of regression. Transformations are made with the objective of obtaining new variables that satisfy all three assumptions: normality, equal variances, and means on a straight line. Since nonlinearity tends to be associated with unequal variances, it is frequently the case that one transformation will take care of both violations of these assumptions simultaneously.

The appropriate transformation is sometimes based on graphical analysis and sometimes on professional knowledge of the variables. It can also be chosen by a trial-and-error approach: various transformations are tried, lines are fitted, and the residuals are examined over the range of X. If the transformation is decided upon by examining the scatter diagram, particular transformations to be considered can be selected on the basis of the general shape of the curve along which the data lie.

The objective is to transform the data so that they are approximately linear in the new variable. For example, if the data can be fitted by an equation $Y = \alpha + \beta \log X$, then it is not linear in X, but is linear in $\log X$. The techniques of this chapter can still be used, but with the independent variable $\log X$ instead of X; all statistical statements must then be made in terms of Y and $\log X$.

In regression analysis, the transformation can be made on X, on Y, or on both. Frequently used transformations are those discussed in Chapter 1 — the log transformation, the square root, and other power transformations being common. Effects of transformations on nonlinear curves are shown in Figure 10.9.

Suppose a scatter diagram of Y versus X shows that the data fall approximately on the curve given in Figure 10.9a. This curve suggests that Y varies as the log of X. A straight line could be produced in one of two ways. We could transform X to $\log X$ and plot Y versus $\log X$; as shown in Figure 10.9b the scale on the X axis is compressed. Alternatively, we could transform Y to e^Y and plot e^Y versus X; as shown in Figure 10.9c the scale on the Y axis is stretched.

As another example, suppose the data points fall approximately on the curve given in Figure 10.9d. This suggests that there is an exponential relation between the two variables: Y varies as e^X. To obtain a linear transformation, we could transform X to e^X and plot e^X versus Y, as in Figure 10.9e; note that this has the effect of stretching the X axis. Or we could transform Y to $\log Y$ and plot $\log Y$ versus X, as in Figure 10.9f; here the Y axis is compressed.

It is generally easier for most people to interpret the regression equations if transformations are made on X. In the example discussed in this chapter, however, the dependent variable is transformed; people are used to looking at the logarithm of the fecal coliform level.

10.9 PRACTICAL ISSUES IN DESIGNING A REGRESSION STUDY

When planning a study with X fixed, several important question to ask include: is regression an appropriate technique? what values of X should be selected? what is an appropriate sample size? We address these here.

10.9.1 Is Fixed X Regression an Appropriate Technique?

Let's reiterate some important points about what X's are and are not acceptable as independent variables in simple linear regression.

Nominal variables, which are discrete and have no ordering associated with them, are not good choices for simple linear regression. Examples include

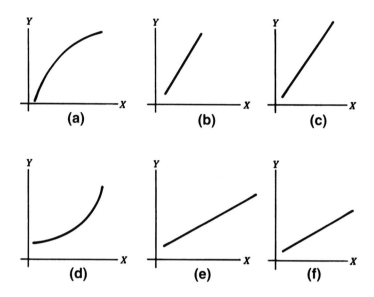

Fig. 10.9 Effects of transformation on nonlinear curves: (a) pretransformed; (b) Y versus log X; (c) e^Y versus X; (d) pretransformed; (e) Y versus e^X; (f) log Y versus X.

race and religion. Because there is no order to these values, it doesn't make sense to try to consider them as single independent variables in simple linear regression. Reasonable alternatives are to use one-way ANOVA or to use regression but transform these nominal variables to a set of dummy variables, as described in Chapter 14.

Ordinal variables (discrete variables that are ordered) have limitations as well. Examples include measures of disease severity (classified as "mild," "moderate," and "severe"). We don't know how to assign numbers to these categories. For example, we could call "mild" a 1, "moderate" a 2, and "severe" a 3. But does the difference between moderate and mild mean the same thing as the difference between severe and moderate? Does the difference between severe and mild mean twice the difference between mild and between moderate or moderate and severe? When the underlying variable being measured is thought to be interval and the scale that approximates it allows for a considerable range of values and is likely highly correlated with the underlying variable, then many investigators would use simple linear regression using ordinal data. Otherwise, if the ordinal can assume only a few values, it is probably better to use ANOVA or to construct a series of dummy variables for use in a regression analysis, as described in Chapter 14.

10.9.2   What Values of X Should Be Selected?

When planning a study, an important task is to choose values of X. Certainly, investigators have in mind the range of values of X, based on preliminary study or knowledge of the field, but there are statistical considerations that should be considered as well. Focusing only on statistics, how should the levels of X be selected? A trade off needs to be made between the number of populations sampled and the number of observations drawn from each one. Usually there is an upper limit in sample size beyond which the investigator cannot afford to go. Determinants can be money, space (for example, available cages or tanks), or time.

Many of the statistics in Table 10.4 have estimated variances with a term which has $\sum(X_i - \bar{X})^2$ in the denominator. This suggests that to obtain a small variance and narrow confidence intervals, it is desirable for the investigator to select X values that are spread out, so that the sum of squared deviations of X is large. Power is maximized by selecting two values of X, the smallest and largest values that are of interest, and taking equal-size samples; this can be a dangerous procedure, however, for it does not provide an opportunity to see whether a straight line fits the data. It is best to sample values of X throughout the range of values of interest. An illustration of the effect that selected X values have on the variability of the slope as well on the generalizability of a study is provided by Kraemer and Thiemann [9].

10.9.3   Sample Size Calculations

Once it is decided how many levels of X will be selected, the size of the sample must be determined. It is generally recommended that equal sample sizes be used. For our calculations, we have assumed that the X values are equally spaced and the sample size is constant across all X values. To perform the sample size calculation, we need to know the following: desired power, one-sided or two-sided test, values of X, slope to be detected (β), and common variance σ^2.

How to perform sample size calculations for simple linear regression with fixed X's can be found in [9]. A variety of software packages, such as SAS and [6], among others, can be used for determining the required sample size.

10.10   COMPARISON WITH ONE-WAY ANOVA

The way in which the data are generated when the fixed X regression model is applied looks a lot like that for one-way ANOVA. Indeed, the example which we considered, the fecal coliform study in Dungeness Bay, Washington, was used for problems at the end of Chapter 2. It is interesting to compare and contrast what we learned from the one-way ANOVA and from the simple linear regression for this example.

First, when we think of a one-way ANOVA, the first thing we tend to think of doing is the one-way ANOVA F test. When we tested for equality of means, the p value associated with the test was $p = 0.087$. If we made the hypothesis test at $\alpha = 0.05$, we might have been inclined to stop there and conclude that we had no evidence that the means were unequal; we could have explained this by saying either that the means are equal and that mean $\log_{10}$ fecal coliform concentration is not associated with distance from the mouth of the Dungeness River, or that we didn't have the power to detect an inequality. We could have looked for linear trends, using the techniques described in Chapter 3, although this would be somewhat complicated by the fact that the distances were not chosen to be equally spaced.

In contrast, we focus on the possibility that distance affects $\log_{10}$ fecal coliform in the context of simple linear regression. Assuming that a linear relation exists, a sample regression line can be determined and predictions can be made easily at other distances at which sampling did not take place. We also have the ability to assess something about the error associated with a predicted value at a distance that either was or was not sampled. Thus, the objective to be achieved determines whether one-way ANOVA or simple linear regression is to be used.

This example illustrates an important point about sample size calculations: they should reflect the investigator's research hypothesis. In our example, a nonzero slope was found, even though a test for equality of means was not rejected. More generally, the results depend on the relative power of the two tests and also on the particular sample that is taken.

10.11   SUMMARY

In this chapter, we introduced simple linear regression, that is, straight line regression with a single X or independent variable. We restricted consideration to the fixed X model, which is appropriate when the values of X are fixed, or selected by the investigator.

We introduced an example for which levels of X were fixed in advance of measuring values of the response variable Y. We first reviewed how to draw a line through a set of points, using the method of least squares. We described the fixed X regression model, with the main assumptions being that for any value of X (within the range of X values that were sampled) there is a normally distributed population of responses; the means of these populations all fall on a straight line, called the population regression line, which is a function of X, and their variances are constant, and so do not depend on X.

We then discussed estimation of the parameters of the model and how the estimates could be used to make inferences about the population regression line, its intercept, and its slope; both confidence intervals and hypothesis tests were described.

Next, we discussed how to assess whether assumptions — linearity, normality, equality of variances, independence — were violated and what to do if they were. We then mentioned some things to keep in mind when planning a study for which simple linear regression with fixed X values was contemplated. Finally, we compared and contrasted the techniques used here with one-way ANOVA, discussed in Chapter 2.

In the next chapter we will consider simple linear regression with X random, or not under control of the investigator, and simple correlation. We shall see that most of the techniques discussed in the chapter are applicable in the next, but more can be done when X is random and further assumptions are made about the distributions of X and Y.

The fixed X regression model will be extended from one X to multiple X variables in Chapter 12. The techniques are a bit more complex, but the objectives are essentially the same.

Problems

10.1   The following data were reported by the National Center for Health Statistics [11]. X is the year of a baby's birth and Y is the percentage of mothers aged 15–44 years who breast-fed their baby. You wish to investigate the relation between the percentage of mothers who breast-feed and the year of the baby's birth.

Year of Baby's Birth	% of Mothers Breast Feeding
1972–74	30.1
1975–77	36.7
1978–80	47.5
1981–83	58.1
1984–86	54.5
1987–89	52.3
1990–92	54.2
1993–94	58.1

a)   Explain why simple linear regression with fixed X is appropriate here.

b)   List the points (X_i, Y_i) that you would use in constructing a scatter diagram. Draw the scatter diagram. Determine the least squares estimates a and b and the sample regression line $\hat{Y} = a + bX$. Draw the sample regression line on the scatter plot. Interpret a and b.

c)   What concerns, if any, would you have in assuming the simple linear regression model with fixed X, as specified in Equation 10.5?

10.2   The following data were reported by the National Center for Health Statistics [12]. X is the year, and Y is the prevalence (percentage) of cigarette smoking by persons 25 years and older in the United States. You wish to investigate the relation between prevalence of smoking and year.

Year	Prevalence
1974	37.1
1979	33.3
1983	31.7
1985	20.2
1987	29.1
1990	25.6
1991	26.0
1992	26.5
1993	24.8
1994	25.1

a)   Explain why simple linear regression with fixed X is appropriate here.

b)   Choose the points (X_i, Y_i) that you would use to construct a scatter diagram. Draw the scatter diagram. Determine the least squares estimates a and b and the sample regression line $\hat{Y} = a + bX$. Draw the sample regression line on the scatter plot. Interpret a and b.

c)   What concerns, if any, would you have in assuming the simple linear regression model with fixed X, as specified in Equation 10.5?

10.3   This problem uses made-up data to illustrate the effects that outliers in Y have on a, b, $se(a)$, $se(b)$, and residuals. For each of the following three subproblems, calculate these estimates.

a)   For this first data set, there are no outliers:

X	Y
1.0	0.25
1.0	1.00
1.0	1.75
2.0	1.25
2.0	2.00
2.0	2.75
3.0	2.25
3.0	3.00
3.0	3.75

b)   For this second data set, there is an outlier at $\bar{X}$:

X	Y
1.0	0.25
1.0	1.00
1.0	1.75
2.0	1.25
2.0	2.00
2.0	4.75
3.0	2.25
3.0	3.00
3.0	3.75

c) For this third data set, there is an outlier at the largest X.

X	Y
1.0	0.25
1.0	1.00
1.0	1.75
2.0	1.25
2.0	2.00
2.0	2.75
3.0	2.25
3.0	3.00
3.0	5.75

d) Comparing the results of the three analyses, what do you conclude about the effects of an outlier near $\bar{X}$? away from $\bar{X}$?

10.4 Blood glucose level was measured on four individuals 1 h after glucose load, on seven individuals at 2 h after load, and on six individuals at 4 h after load. (There were 17 individuals involved altogether.) The data obtained were as follows:

Interval	Observation Number						
	1	2	3	4	5	6	7
1	106.5	124.7	123.5	158.5			
2	86.2	59.8	64.5	106.8	95.8	117.5	59.2
4	72.7	62.5	51.8	58.8	44.0	41.0	

a) Calculate the least squares line fitting blood glucose level to interval after load.
b) Plot a scatter diagram and the least squares line.
c) Assuming that the regression is linear, obtain an ANOVA table.

d)   Test whether $\beta = 0$.

e)   Find a 95% prediction interval for the blood level of an individual 3 hours after glucose load.

10.5   IQ tests were given to children of three different age groups. The scores were as follows:

Age (years)	IQ Scores							
3	105	94	108	101	100			
4	96	119	103	107	110	112	106	
5	120	114	121	116	128	115	118	123

a)   State a possible model.

b)   Write out the least squares regression line for predicting IQ from age.

c)   Plot the data and the regression line.

d)   Obtain an ANOVA table.

e)   Test whether $\beta = 0$.

f)   Give a 95% confidence interval for β.

g)   Give and interpret a 95% confidence interval for the mean IQ for children of age 4.

10.6   The following data represent yields of rye for four preselected levels of fertilizer:

Level of Fertilizer	Yield (bushels per acre)									
50	13.1	28.0	12.2	10.1	13.8	5.2	8.2	38.3	11.1	14.5
60	29.6	25.7	28.6	33.8	29.7	9.0	4.4	27.0	16.1	12.4
70	33.7	42.6	22.1	41.3	23.5	36.4	35.3	26.5	35.4	34.3
	15.3	46.4	20.1	46.0	16.5					
80	26.8	31.4	25.6	24.2	33.8	32.7	22.0	42.1	40.9	30.1

a)   State a possible model.

b)   Obtain the estimated regression line.

c)   Calculate and interpret a 95% confidence interval for β.

d)   Test the hypothesis $H_0 : \beta = 0$ using a t test and an F test. Verify that $t^2 = F$.

e)   Give a 95% confidence interval for the population mean yield for 75 lbs of fertilizer per acre.

f)   Give a 95% confidence interval for the population mean yield with no fertilizer.

g) Do you have as much faith in the confidence interval in part (e) as in the one in part (f)? Why?

10.7 Express the estimated slope b as a linear combination of the Y's. Using the rules for finding the mean and variance of a linear combination, verify that $E(b)$ is equal to β and the variance of b is equal to $\sigma^2 / \sum_{i=1}^{n}(X_i - \bar{X})^2$. (See Appendix A for details on obtaining means and variances of linear combinations.)

10.8 Express the sample regression line at X^* as $\bar{Y} + b(X^* - \bar{X})$. This can be regarded as a linear combination of $\bar{Y}$ and b.

    a) Determine the variance of $\bar{Y}$.

    b) Verify that the covariance of $\bar{Y}$ and b is 0.

    c) Determine the variance of $\bar{Y} + b(X^* - \bar{X})$.

REFERENCES

1. Afifi, A.A. and Azen, S.L. [1972]. *Statistical Analysis: A Computer Oriented Approach*, New York: Academic Press, 98–100.

2. Belsey, D.A., Kuh, E., and Welsch, R.E. [1980]. *Regression Diagnostics: Identifying Influential Data and Sources of Collinearity*, New York: John Wiley & Sons, 6–84.

3. Chatterjee, S. and Hadi, A.S. [1988]. *Sensitivity Analysis in Linear Regression*, New York: John Wiley & Sons, 71–127.

4. Cook, R.D. [1977]. Detection of Influential Observation in Linear Regression, *Technometrics*, 19, 15–18.

5. Cook, R.D. and Weisberg, S. [1982]. *Residuals and Influence in Regression*, New York: Chapman and Hall.

6. Elashoff, J. D. [2002]. *nQuery Advisor Version 5.0 User's Guide*, Saugas, MA: Statistical Solutions.

7. Fox, J. [1991]. *Regression Diagnostics: An Introduction*, Sage University Paper Series on Quantitative Applications in the Social Sciences, 07-079. Newbury Park, CA: Sage, 21–39.

8. Hoaglin, D.C. and Welsch, R.E. [1978]. The Hat Matrix in Regression and ANOVA, *The American Statistician*, 32, 17–22.

9. Kraemer, H.C. and Thiemann, S. [1987]. *How Many Subjects*, Newbury Park, CA: Sage, 60–65.

10. Miller, R.J. [1986]. *Beyond ANOVA: Basics of Applied Statistics*, New York: John Wiley & Sons, 164–220.

11. National Center for Health Statistics. [1997]. *Health, United States, 1996–1997 and Injury Chartbook*, Hyattsville, MD, 97.

12. National Center for Health Statistics. [1997]. *Health, United States, 1996–1997 and Injury Chartbook*, Hyattsville, MD, 183.

13. Velleman, P. and Wilkinson, L. [1993]. Nominal, Ordinal, Interval and Ratio Typologies Are Misleading, *The American Statistician, 47*, 65–72.

11

Linear Regression: Random X Model and Correlation

In Chapter 10 we discussed simple linear regression where the values of X were fixed. In this chapter, we are considering two topics.

The first topic is simple linear regression with random X values. As the name implies, values of X are not chosen in advance (preselected) by an investigator, but are determined by some random process, as the Y values are. As in the previous chapter, we are restricting consideration to the simple case, when there is one X and one Y.

The second topic is correlation between the two variables X and Y. With some additional assumptions, it is possible to interpret a measure of the strength of the linear association between the two variables, the *simple correlation* — something that is not possible when X is fixed.

In Section 11.1 we briefly introduce an example which will be used throughout the chapter, in which both X and Y are random. This is followed in Section 11.2 by a consideration of various ways to numerically summarize the relationship between two variables. In Section 11.3, noting that the model described in Chapter 10 is applicable whether X is random or fixed, we review inferences about the population regression line when the predictor, or independent variable X, is random. In Section 11.4 we introduce the bivariate normal distribution. When we make the additional assumption that the two variables are jointly normally distributed, it is now appropriate to address making inferences (both confidence intervals and hypothesis tests) about the correlation coefficient ρ as well as the population regression line. How to check if the data fit the bivariate normal model is covered in Section 11.5, and what to do if it doesn't in Section 11.6; the latter section introduces the commonly used nonparametric alternative to the correlation coefficient, Spearman's ρ. A summary of the chapter is given in Section 11.7.

11.1 EXAMPLE

As part of a longitudinal study of a 3-month cardiac rehabilitation program [1], subjects with coronary artery disease underwent a variety of assessments at baseline, that is, prior to the start of their program. We consider two variables here: baseline physical functioning and baseline peak exercise capacity. The dependent variable, Y, is self-reported physical functioning. This was assessed using the Medical Outcomes Study–Short-Form Questionnaire (MOS-36); the scale is from 0 to 100, with higher values indicating better functioning [14, 15]. The independent or predictor variable X is peak exercise capacity, defined as the peak exercise intensity attained during a progressive treadmill exercise test. It is measured in METS (metabolic equivalents).

11.1.1 Sampling and Summary Statistics

After the subjects agreed to enter the cardiac rehabilitation study, their self-reported physical functioning (Y), their peak exercise capacity (X), and a variety of other measures related to cardiovascular health were assessed. Most of the analyses presented in this chapter are restricted to a sample of $n = 43$ women who completed the 3-month cardiac rehabilitation program. The data are presented in Table 11.1, in an order corresponding to that in which women entered the study. The sampling units are women with coronary artery disease. We assume that the women were sampled at random. Both variables are considered random because their observed values depend on who was entered into the study. The observed values are drawn from the *joint*, or *bivariate*, distribution of the two variables. In other words, women at pre-selected levels of peak exercise capacity were not identified for inclusion in the study, as they would have been if sampling consistent with the fixed X model had been used.

Univariate summary statistics for these two variables are given in Table 11.2. Exercise capacity ranges from 2 to 10 and assumes discrete values. The mean is higher than the median, and the distribution is skewed to the right. The Shapiro-Wilk W test rejects the hypothesis of normality ($p = 0.012$). Self-reported physical functioning is an ordinal variable, which ranges from 0 to 95, with a distribution which is slightly skewed to the left, all despite the W test being nonsignificant ($p = 0.27$).

In the previous chapter, there was summarization of the Y variable for each value of the X variable. We could consider the conditional distributions of $Y|X$ because this reflected the sampling. It didn't make sense to report summary statistics for both variables separately, because the X's were taken at fixed levels.

EXAMPLE   267

Table 11.1   Peak Exercise Capacity X (in METS) and Self-Reported Physical Functioning Y (MOS-36 Scale)

Obs	Peak Exercise Capacity	Self-Reported Physical Functioning	Obs	Peak Exercise Capacity	Self-Reported Physical Functioning
1	7.0	90	23	5.0	75
2	2.0	30	24	3.5	75
3	6.0	65	25	7.0	60
4	4.0	40	26	2.0	45
5	6.0	75	27	7.0	95
6	8.0	75	28	5.0	40
7	7.0	80	29	7.0	65
8	3.0	40	30	5.0	55
9	3.0	80	31	4.0	35
10	3.0	15	32	4.0	60
11	6.0	60	33	6.0	35
12	4.0	60	34	5.0	50
13	8.0	65	35	4.0	35
14	2.0	65	36	4.0	55
15	2.5	0	37	10.0	95
16	3.0	55	38	9.0	85
17	8.0	35	39	5.0	65
18	5.0	50	40	2.0	75
19	2.0	70	41	7.0	90
20	2.0	45	42	3.0	85
21	3.0	55	43	3.0	30
22	2.0	90			

In contrast, since subjects were sampled and observations for both variables obtained, we can consider alternative distributions: the distribution of peak exercise capacity, the distribution of self-reported physical functioning, and the joint or bivariate distribution of the two variables; the last reflects how the sampling was actually carried out. The statistics in Table 11.2 are summary univariate statistics for the distribution of each variable by itself, sometimes referred to as the *marginal* distributions.

A scatter diagram, or plot, of self-reported physical functioning versus peak exercise capacity, as shown in Figure 11.1, provides an indication of how the two variables are related to each other. This plot suggests that a linear relation exists between physical functioning and peak exercise capacity, with higher (i.e., better) physical functioning scores associated with higher (i.e., better) peak exercise capacity.

Table 11.2 Univariate Summary Statistics for Baseline Characteristics

Statistic	Peak Exercise Capacity	Physical Functioning
n	43	43
Minimum	2	0
Q_1	3	40
Median	4	60
Q_3	7	75
Maximum	10	95
Mean	4.74	59.65
Standard deviation	2.17	22.37
Variance	4.73	500.47
Skewness	0.59	-0.42
Interquartile range	4	35
p value for W test	0.012	0.27

11.2 SUMMARIZING THE RELATIONSHIP BETWEEN X AND Y

While the scatter diagram gives a graphical representation of the relationship
between X and Y, we can also obtain statistics to summarize how the variables
are related. Knowing that we have sampled X and Y from their bivariate
(joint) distribution, it is appropriate to consider the *covariance* and the *simple
correlation* between the variables, as well as determine the least squares, or
sample, regression line.

One measure of the linear association between two variables is the population *covariance* σ_{XY}, which is defined as $E(X - \mu_X)(Y - \mu_Y)$. It is estimated
as

$$s_{XY} = \frac{\sum_{i=1}^{n}(X_i - \bar{X})(Y_i - \bar{Y})}{n - 1}. \tag{11.1}$$

The covariance can assume both negative and positive values (as well as
0). The sign provides an indication of how the X and Y variables are related.
If it is positive, this suggests observed values X_i that are below $\bar{X}$ tend to
appear with observed values of Y_i that are below $\bar{Y}$. This means that small
values of X are associated with small values of Y and that large values of X
are associated with large values of Y. Sometimes we say there is a *positive* or
increasing relation between the two variables. In contrast, if observed values
X_i that are below $\bar{X}$ tend to appear with values of Y_i that are above $\bar{Y}$, the
covariance is negative. Here, we can say there is a *negative* or *inverse* relation
between the two. If the covariance is 0, there is no tendency for smaller values
of X to be observed either with smaller or with larger values of Y.

The covariance is difficult to interpret by itself, because it doesn't have any upper or lower bounds. Thus, in practice, it isn't used as a measure of the magnitude or strength of a linear association between two variables.

Frequently, the sample variances and covariances are summarized together in a *sample covariance matrix*. The covariance between a variable and itself is its variance. The sample covariance matrix is expressed with the variances on the diagonal of the matrix and the covariance off the diagonal, as follows:

$$\begin{pmatrix} s_X^2 & s_{XY} \\ s_{YX} & s_Y^2 \end{pmatrix}.$$

This is a symmetric matrix: $s_{XY} = s_{YX}$.

Another indicator of the linear association between the two variables is the population *correlation coefficient*, ρ, which is defined as

$$\rho = \frac{\sigma_{XY}}{\sigma_X \sigma_Y}. \tag{11.2}$$

It is sometimes written as ρ_{XY} to indicate that it is the correlation between X and Y. Since we are concerned with one X and one Y in this chapter, the subscripts X and Y are eliminated. ρ is sometimes referred to as a *simple* correlation because it involves only two variables. This distinguishes it from multiple correlations and partial correlations, which are functions of more

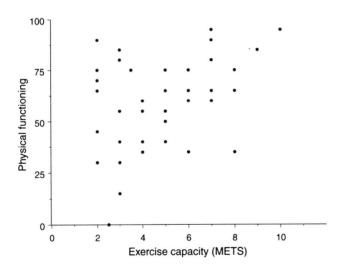

Fig. 11.1 Scatter diagram of self-reported physical functioning versus peak exercise capacity.

than two variables; we discuss these in Chapter 13. The ρ is estimated by the *sample correlation coefficient*,

$$r = \frac{s_{XY}}{s_X \cdot s_Y} = \frac{\sum_{i=1}^{n}(X_i - \bar{X})(Y_i - \bar{Y})}{\sqrt{\sum_{i=1}^{n}(X_i - \bar{X})^2 \sum_{i=1}^{n}(Y_i - \bar{Y})^2}}. \tag{11.3}$$

(The $n - 1$'s in the numerator and denominator cancel out.)

The advantage of the correlation coefficient over the covariance is that it is bounded between -1 and 1. Thus, in addition to its sign, its value can also be informative about the strength of the association between the two variables. From looking at Equation 11.3, we see that the denominator is always positive, so that the sign of the correlation is determined by the sign of the numerator, or the covariance between the two. The correlation is negative or positive for the same reason that the covariance is negative or positive. We can also see that the correlation between a variable and itself is 1. Frequently, the correlations between two variables are summarized in terms of a *sample correlation matrix*, with ones on the diagonal (corresponding to the correlation of X with X and the correlation of Y with Y) and the simple correlation of X with Y off the diagonal:

$$\begin{pmatrix} 1 & r \\ r & 1 \end{pmatrix}$$

Like the covariance matrix, this is a symmetric matrix. We will say much more about the simple correlation in Section 11.4.2.

Finally, the population regression line, $E(Y|X) = \alpha + \beta X$, can be viewed as a summary of the relation between X and Y. As in Chapter 10, we estimate α by

$$a = \bar{Y} - b\bar{X}, \tag{11.4}$$

β by

$$b = \frac{\sum_{i=1}^{n}(Y_i - \bar{Y})(X_i - \bar{X})}{\sum_{i=1}^{n}(X_i - \bar{X})^2}, \tag{11.5}$$

the population regression line $E(Y|X)$ by

$$\hat{Y} = a + bX,$$

and the population variance $\text{Var}(Y|X) = \sigma^2$ by

$$s^2 = \sum_{i=1}^{n}(Y_i - \hat{Y}_i)^2 / (n - 2).$$

For convenience, we repeat Table 10.4, given in Chapter 10 for the point estimates and their estimated standard errors, as Table 11.3. Note that all of these formulas are the same as those for the fixed X model.

Table 11.3   Population Parameters, Point Estimates, and Estimated Standard Errors in Simple Linear Regression

Parameter	Point Estimate	Estimated Standard Error
$\alpha + \beta \bar{X}$	$\bar{Y}$	$se(\bar{Y}) = s\sqrt{\frac{1}{n}}$
α	$a = \bar{Y} - b\bar{X}$	$se(a) = s\sqrt{\frac{1}{n} + \frac{\bar{X}^2}{\sum_{i=1}^{n}(X_i - \bar{X})^2}}$
β	b	$se(b) = s\sqrt{\frac{1}{\sum_{i=1}^{n}(X_i - \bar{X})^2}}$
$E(Y\|X^*)$	$\hat{Y} = a + bX^*$	$se(\hat{E}(Y\|X^*)) = s\sqrt{\frac{1}{n} + \frac{(X^* - \bar{X})^2}{\sum_{i=1}^{n}(X_i - \bar{X})^2}}$
σ^2	s^2	—

No distributional assumptions were made for the computation of the sample covariance, the sample simple correlation, or the estimates that make up the least squares line. As indicated in the previous chapter, the derivation of the standard errors of the Y intercept a, the slope b, and $\hat{Y}$ were made assuming that all observations were independent and the conditional distributions $Y|X$ had constant variance, σ^2.

Example. For the cardiac rehabilitation example, the sample covariance matrix for peak exercise capacity and self-reported physical functioning is

$$\begin{pmatrix} 4.73 & 20.80 \\ 20.80 & 500.47 \end{pmatrix}.$$

The sample covariance is given off the diagonal as $s_{XY} = 20.80$. The sample variances $s_X^2 = 4.73$ and $s_Y^2 = 500.47$ are on the diagonal of the covariance matrix and are also given as univariate summary statistics in Table 11.2.

The sample correlation matrix for the two variables is

$$\begin{pmatrix} 1.00 & 0.43 \\ 0.43 & 1.00 \end{pmatrix}.$$

The sample regression line is $\hat{Y} = 38.79 + 4.40X$. (See Table 11.4 for point estimates and the estimated standard errors.) The Y intercept a is 38.79; this is not of particular interest, other than for constructing the line, as a peak exercise capacity of 0 METS is meaningless. The slope of the line is 4.40, indicating that for every change of one MET, self-reported physical functioning is changed by 4.40 points. We can compute $\hat{Y}$ for selected values of X, say X^*. So, for example, at $X = \bar{X} = 4.7$ METS, $\hat{Y} = \bar{Y} = 59.7$. The estimate of σ^2 for physical functioning scores is $s^2 = 418.98$; the standard deviation, the square root of s^2, is $s = 20.47$.

Like the scatter diagram, the positive sample covariance $s_{XY} = 20.80$, the positive sample correlation $r = 0.43$, and the positive slope $b = 4.40$ all suggest that higher values of peak exercise capacity are associated with higher values of self-reported physical functioning.

Of course, so far, we have only computed estimates; no inferences have been made for this example. We will do this after we have introduced the random X model.

11.3   INFERENCES FOR THE REGRESSION OF Y ON X

Let's go back and take another look at the assumptions that were made for the model assumed in Chapter 10. The assumptions concerning the underlying populations can be summarized by writing

$$Y|X \sim \text{IND}(\alpha + \beta X, \sigma^2) \tag{11.6}$$

or as

$$Y_i = \alpha + \beta X_i + \varepsilon_i, \qquad i = 1, \ldots, n, \tag{11.7}$$

where $\varepsilon_i \sim \text{IND}(0, \sigma^2)$.

For this model, there are no assumptions about the distribution of X or Y; it doesn't matter if the values of X were fixed by the investigator or were selected at random. The assumptions are made only about the conditional distribution of $Y|X$. Thus, all of the inferences that were performed in the previous chapter can be performed with the X variable regarded as fixed or random, provided that the same model and underlying assumptions are made.

The inferences are made in the same way that they were for the fixed X model. For convenience, the confidence intervals presented in Table 10.6 are repeated in Table 11.5. This table could be used for either interval estimation or for hypothesis testing. Similarly, the ANOVA table for testing $H_0 : \beta = 0$ in Table 10.8 is reproduced here as Table 11.6. The only difference in the ANOVA table is the EMS due to regression. Here, the EMS is expressed as a function of σ_X^2 rather than $\sum_{i=1}^{n}(X_i - \bar{X})^2$ and so reflects the different sampling schemes which are assumed in the fixed X and random X models. For the ANOVA test, when H_0 is true, the F statistic follows an F distribution with $\nu_1 = 1$ and $\nu_2 = n - 2$ degrees of freedom. When H_0 is not true, the F statistic follows a noncentral F distribution with $\nu_1 = 1$, $\nu_2 = n - 2$ and noncentrality parameter $\lambda = n\beta^2 \sigma_X^2$.

Table 11.4 Estimates of Model Parameters for the Cardiac Rehabilitation Example

Term	Interpretation	Estimate	Standard Error
a	Y-intercept	38.79	7.56
b	Slope	4.40	1.45
s^2	Variance	418.98	—
s	Standard deviation	20.47	—

Table 11.5 Confidence Intervals in Linear Regression

Parameter	$100(1 - \alpha)\%$ Confidence Interval
α	$a \pm t_{1-\alpha/2;n-2}\,\mathrm{se}(a)$
β	$b \pm t_{1-\alpha/2;n-2}\,\mathrm{se}(b)$
$E(Y\mid X^*)$	$(a + bX^*) \pm t_{1-\alpha/2;n-2}\,\mathrm{se}(\hat{Y}\mid X^*)$
$\alpha + \beta\bar{X}$	$\bar{Y} \pm t_{1-\alpha/2;n-2}\,\mathrm{se}(\bar{Y})$

Example. The question of greatest interest for the cardiac rehabilitation example is whether a positive linear relationship exists between physical functioning and peak exercise capacity. We can use a confidence interval for β, or a t test for $H_0 : \beta = 0$, or the ANOVA F test.

The expression for the 95% confidence interval for β is $b \pm t_{[0.975;41]}\,\mathrm{se}(b)$. Since the sample size is $n = 43$, the degrees of freedom associated with s^2 are $n - 2$, or 41. The 97.5 percentile of a t distribution with 41 degrees of freedom is 2.02. As shown in Table 11.4, the slope $b = 4.40$ and the estimated standard error of b is $\mathrm{se}(b) = 1.45$. Thus, the 95% confidence interval is computed as $4.40 \pm 2.02 \times 1.45 = 4.40 \pm 2.93$, or $1.47 < \beta < 7.33$. There is 95% confidence that the slope lies between 1.47 and 7.33. Because the interval does not include 0, we can conclude that $\beta \neq 0$. The calculated t statistic is $b/\mathrm{se}(b) = 4.40/1.45 = 3.03$ ($p = 0.0042$), and the calculated F statistic is $\mathrm{MS}_{reg}/\mathrm{MS}_r = 3841.67/418.98 = 9.17$ (see Table 11.7). As before, $t^2 = F$ (note that in the text, they aren't exactly the same, due to rounding error).

Table 11.6 Analysis of Variance Table for Simple Linear Regression

Source of Variation	Sum of Squares	df	Mean Square	EMS	F
Regression	SS_{reg}	1	MS_{reg}	$\sigma^2 + n\beta^2\sigma_X^2$	MS_{reg}/s^2
Residual	SS_r	$n-2$	s^2	σ^2	
Total	SS_t	$n-1$			

Thus, using any of the equivalent procedures, we conclude that $\beta \neq 0$; peak exercise capacity and physical functioning are related.

Figure 11.2 provides a plot of the data, along with the sample regression line and 95% confidence bands for the population regression line. The sample regression line and 95% confidence bands were not drawn outside the range of peak exercise capacities included in the study. As in Chapter 10, the confidence bands are narrowest at the point $(\bar{X}, \bar{Y})$ and become wider as values of X move further away from $\bar{X}$.

11.3.1   Comparison of Fixed X and Random X Sampling

We now wish to distinguish between the two methods of obtaining data on X and Y, the fixed X and random X sampling. We will use the cardiac rehabilitation data as an example. The fixed X method is one in which values of peak exercise capacity are specified by the investigator before data on physical functioning are collected. For example, the investigator could have decided to sample six women with peak exercise capacity of 2 METS, six women with peak exercise capacity of 5 METS, and so on. Each observation on physical functioning is from the distribution of Y for a fixed X value. We say that we have sampled from the fixed X distributions or from the conditional distributions.

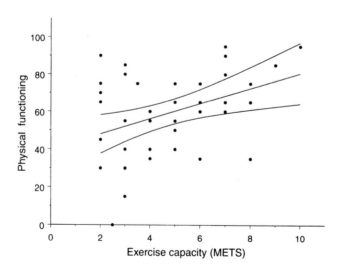

Fig. 11.2 Physical functioning versus peak exercise capacity, with sample regression line and 95% confidence bands.

Table 11.7   Analysis of Variance Table for the Regression of Physical Functioning on Peak Exercise Capacity

Source of Variation	Sum of Squares	df	Mean Square	Computed F	p Value
Regression	3841.67	1	3841.67	9.17	0.0042
Residual	17178	42	418.98		
Total	21020	43			

An alternative method, the one which was actually used, may be termed the random X method. In this case, the X, Y measurement on each woman is an observation from the joint distribution of X and Y. We say we have sampled from the joint distribution of X and Y. That is, the investigator selects the women and measures both their peak exercise capacity and their physical functioning.

The regression analyses as given in this chapter and the previous one can be performed regardless of which of the two sampling methods was employed, provided the investigator is willing to make the assumptions implied in Equations 11.6 and 11.7. Thus in our example, even though the observations were sampled from the joint distribution, we can consider an entire population of physical functioning scores divided into subpopulations, each consisting of physical functioning scores for women with the same peak exercise capacity. If the investigator is willing to assume normality, linearity of means, and equality of variances for the Y's of these fixed X populations, then the regression analysis is appropriate, regardless of which way the sampling is performed.

We stress the two types of sampling procedure because there are important differences between them in what can be estimated. When sampling is done from the fixed X distributions, we are able to estimate the following: (1) the mean of the Y's for any given value of X, (2) the slope of the regression line, and (3) the variance of the Y's for any given X. In the cardiac rehabilitation example, if we had selected women on the basis of their peak exercise capacity, the regression parameters could be estimated, but it is clear that we could not hope to estimate the mean peak exercise capacity, the mean physical functioning, or any of the other parameters which are estimated in Table 11.2. When sampling is done from the joint distribution of X and Y, parameters of the distributions of X and Y (means, variances, quantiles, etc.) can be estimated as well as descriptors of their joint distribution such as the covariance and correlation. Table 11.8 summarizes the parameters and their estimates for the two types of sampling. In order to make inferences about the correlation coefficient ρ, further assumptions about the joint distribution of Y and X must be made.

Table 11.8   Parameters and Estimates for Fixed X and Random X Sampling

Parameter	Type of Sampling	
	Fixed X	Random X
α	a	a
β	b	b
$E(Y\|X)$	$\hat{Y}$	$\hat{Y}$
$\mathrm{Var}(Y\|X)$	s^2	s^2
$E(Y)$	—	$\bar{Y}$
$\mathrm{Var}(Y)$	—	s_Y^2
$E(X)$	—	$\bar{X}$
$\mathrm{Var}(X)$	—	s_X^2
$\mathrm{Cov}(X,Y)$	—	$s_{X,Y}^2$
ρ	—	r

11.4   THE BIVARIATE NORMAL MODEL

As mentioned earlier, when observations are drawn from the joint distribution of Y and X, one can estimate certain parameters and perform a regression analysis provided one assumes the model in Equations 11.6 and 11.7; that is, for particular X values, the Y populations are normally distributed, have means on a straight line, and have equal variances. A second model is frequently appropriate when sampling from the joint distribution, namely the bivariate model, which enables us to make inferences concerning the *correlation* between Y and X. In this model, X and Y are assumed to have a *bivariate normal distribution*.

11.4.1   The Bivariate Normal Distribution

If X and Y denote two measurements on the same individual, and if each of them is normally distributed, then in most cases we can expect them to be jointly normally distributed. The expression for the bivariate normal distribution is

$$f(x,y) = \frac{1}{2\pi\sigma_X\sigma_Y\sqrt{1-\rho^2}}$$

$$\times \exp\left\{-\frac{\left[\frac{(x-\mu_X)^2}{\sigma_X^2} - \frac{2\rho(x-\mu_X)(y-\mu_Y)}{\sigma_X\sigma_Y} + \frac{(y-\mu_Y)^2}{\sigma_Y^2}\right]}{2(1-\rho^2)}\right\}. \quad (11.8)$$

Theoretically, it is possible that two variables, each of which is normally distributed, have some joint distribution other than the bivariate normal distribution. We are not concerned with this possibility; in practical situations of the type we are discussing, it seldom occurs.

For two normally distributed variates X and Y, the bivariate normal distribution is described by five parameters. Four of these are μ_X, σ_X (or σ_X^2), μ_Y, and σ_Y (or σ_Y^2). The fifth is the covariance σ_{XY} of X and Y or their correlation, $\rho = \sigma_{XY}/\sigma_X\sigma_Y$, defined in Section 11.2. For many purposes, it is more convenient to work with ρ.

When X and Y have a joint normal distribution, a plot of Y versus X has an elliptical shape and is referred to as a *concentration ellipse*. The shape of the ellipse depends on the correlation ρ. To demonstrate this effect, we show in Figure 11.3 concentration ellipses for $\rho = -0.5, 0, 0.5, 0.9$ when $\mu_X = \mu_Y = 0$ and $\sigma_X^2 = \sigma_Y^2 = 1$. These plots were generated by randomly selecting $n = 100$ observations from the specified bivariate normal distribution. When $\rho = 0$, the concentration ellipse is a circle; there is no relation between the two variables. When $\rho = 0.5$, there is a positive relationship between the two variables, that is, increasing values of X are associated with increasing values of Y. When $\rho = -0.5$, there is an inverse relationship between the two, that is, increasing values of X are associated with decreasing values of Y. At $\rho = 0.9$, there is a stronger linear relationship than there was at $\rho = 0.5$, as indicated by the narrower concentration ellipse.

When the two variables are jointly normally distributed, all the assumptions of the fixed X model are met. For example, if women's weights (Y) and heights (X) have a bivariate normal distribution, then there is a population of weights of women of any particular height. These populations are normally distributed; their means lie on a straight line, $\mu_{Y|X} = E(Y|X) = \alpha + \beta X$; and their variances are equal (σ^2). In terms of the five parameters characterizing the joint distribution, the population mean weight for any height X is

$$\mu_{Y|X} = E(Y|X) = \left(\mu_Y - \rho\frac{\sigma_Y}{\sigma_X}\mu_X\right) + \rho\frac{\sigma_Y}{\sigma_X}X = \alpha + \beta X, \qquad (11.9)$$

and the variance is

$$\sigma_{Y|X}^2 = \mathrm{Var}(Y|X) = \sigma_Y^2(1-\rho^2) = \sigma^2. \qquad (11.10)$$

Thus the slope of the population regression line of Y on X is $\beta = \rho(\sigma_Y/\sigma_X)$, and its intercept is $\alpha = \mu_Y - \rho(\sigma_Y/\sigma_X)$. The variance of Y for a particular X value is $\sigma^2 = \sigma_Y^2(1-\rho^2)$.

Because the joint normal distribution model implies all the assumptions of the fixed X model, one can sample from the bivariate normal distribution of X and Y and then analyze the data as if they had been drawn from the distributions of Y with X fixed. This includes making the point and confidence interval estimates and tests presented earlier in this chapter. Everything is performed in precisely the same way as when sampling from the fixed X distributions. In addition, one can estimate and test hypotheses concerning μ_X, μ_Y, σ_X^2, σ_Y^2, and ρ.

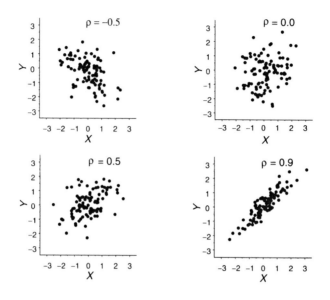

Fig. 11.3   Concentration ellipses for $\rho = -0.5$, 0, 0.5, 0.9 for samples of size $n = 100$.

We need learn very little for the joint model, in addition to what we know for the fixed X model. We already know how to obtain point and confidence interval estimates and make tests for $\mu_X, \mu_Y, \sigma_X^2, \sigma_Y^2, \alpha$, and β. There remains only ρ, whose point estimate r was defined in Equation 11.3. In some texts, r is called the Pearson correlation.

11.4.2   The Correlation Coefficient

We can learn important characteristics of ρ when X and Y are jointly normally distributed simply by examining the equations for β, $\mu_{Y|X}$, and $\sigma_{Y|X}^2$, given above, expressed as functions of ρ.

Consider first $\sigma_{Y|X}^2 = (1 - \rho^2)\sigma_Y^2$. What can we say about ρ from this expression? Since variances must be ≥ 0, we can tell that ρ must range between -1 and $+1$. When $\rho = \pm1$, $\sigma_{Y|X}^2 = 0$; that is, when X is specified, there is no variation in Y. Thus, there is a perfect linear relation between Y and X. When $\rho = 0$, $\sigma_{Y|X}^2 = \sigma_Y^2$. The equality of these two variances indicates that knowing X provides no information about Y. For the bivariate normal model, $\rho = 0$ implies that X and Y are independent. Since the absolute value of ρ varies between 0 and 1, it is considered a measure of the *strength of the linear relation* between between X and Y.

Next, consider the expression for β. When $\rho = 0$, $\beta = 0$, so we can also conclude from this that $\rho = 0$ indicates no linear relationship between X and

Y. Since σ_Y and σ_X are both > 0, the correlation coefficient must have the same sign as the slope. If Y increases with X, both ρ and β are positive. If Y increases with decreasing X, both parameters are negative. This also can be seen graphically in Figure 11.3. Furthermore, we can see that ρ has the advantage of being independent of the units of measurement; both Y and X are in both the numerator and denominator of the expression for ρ, so that any transformations of either one or both will not affect ρ.

In terms of a specific example, if an entire population of weights and ages lies on a straight line with either positive or negative slope, then ρ is ± 1: $+1$ if the slope of the line is positive, -1 if it is negative. If X and Y are statistically independent, and an individual's weight bears no relation to his or her age, ρ equals zero. If weights are measured in kilograms instead of pounds, the covariance and variance are changed, but the correlation coefficient remains the same. It measures the linearity of the relationship between X and Y.

Now, consider an interpretation for r^2 which arises from breaking the total sum of squares, SS_t, into two parts (regression and residual) but expressing these two sums of squares in terms of r rather than b. See Table 11.9 for the ANOVA table expressed in terms of r^2. Using b as defined in Equation 11.5 and r as defined in Equation 11.3, the regression and residual sums of squares are

$$SS_{reg} = \sum_{i=1}^{n}(\hat{Y}_i - \bar{Y})^2$$

$$= b^2 \sum_{i=1}^{n}(X_i - \bar{X})^2$$

$$= r^2 \sum_{i=1}^{n}(Y_i - \bar{Y})^2$$

and

$$SS_r = (1 - r^2) \sum_{i=1}^{n}(Y_i - \bar{Y})^2. \tag{11.11}$$

These sums of squares are presented in Table 11.9. From this table, we see that $1 - r^2$ is the proportion of the original total variation $[SS_t = \sum_{i=1}^{n}(Y_i - \bar{Y})^2]$, that is left after fitting the straight line. The quantity r^2 is the proportion of the original sum of squared deviations that is removed by fitting the straight line ($r^2 = SS_{reg}/SS_t$). Another way to say this is that r^2 is the proportion of the original variation that is explained by the linear relation between X and Y. Thus, if $r = 0.5$, only one-fourth of the total sum of squares is removed by the sample regression line (explained by the linear relation between the two variables). Three-fourths of the variation is left over. The square of the correlation coefficient is calculated in the same

Table 11.9 Analysis of Variance Table in Terms of r^2

Source of Variation	Sums of Squares	df	Mean Square	EMS
Regression	$r^2 \mathrm{SS}_t$	1	$r^2 \mathrm{SS}_t$	$\sigma^2 + n\rho^2\sigma_Y^2$
Residual	$(1 - r^2)\mathrm{SS}_t$	$n - 2$	$\frac{(1-r^2)\mathrm{SS}_t}{n-2}$	σ^2
Total	SS_t	$n - 1$		

way as the coefficient of determination R^2. When two variables have a joint normal distribution, we can talk about the correlation and its square. When two variables do not have a joint normal distribution, we can talk about the coefficient of determination, but it cannot be interpreted as the square of the correlation coefficient and its square root doesn't have an interpretation.

An equivalent way to express r and b is in terms of the sample covariance s_{XY} and the sample variances s_X^2 and s_Y^2. That is, r can be expressed as

$$r = \frac{s_{XY}}{s_X s_Y},\tag{11.12}$$

and b as

$$b = \frac{s_{XY}}{s_X^2}\tag{11.13}$$

The sample variances and covariances all have the same denominator $(n - 1)$, which cancels out in the formulas.

11.4.3   The Correlation Coefficient: Confidence Intervals and Tests

The shape of the distribution of the statistic r depends heavily on the value of the population correlation coefficient ρ, as well as on the sample size. See Figure 11.4 for some distributions of r when $\rho = 0, 0.5$, or 0.9 and $n = 40$. The distribution for $r = 0$ is symmetric; for ρ large in magnitude, it is highly skewed. Only for tests of $H_0 : \rho = 0$ can we make t and F tests. For making confidence intervals for ρ and for testing $H_0 : \rho = \rho_0$, r must be transformed to another variable, whose distribution is known and readily available. We give here first a method for testing $H_0 : \rho = 0$, and then a method for making confidence intervals for ρ and for testing $H_0 : \rho = \rho_0$.

The t test of $H_0 : \rho = 0$. For a test of $H_0 : \rho = 0$, we form the statistic

$$t = \frac{r\sqrt{n - 2}}{\sqrt{1 - r^2}}.\tag{11.14}$$

If ρ is actually zero, this statistic has a t distribution with $n - 2$ degrees of freedom. The null hypothesis is rejected for small or large values of t.

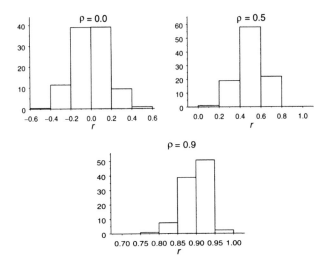

Fig. 11.4   Distribution of r for $\rho = 0$, 0.5, 0.9 and $n = 40$.

The F test of $H_0 : \beta = 0$ is equivalent to this test. From Table 11.9, the test statistic can be written

$$F = \frac{r^2 \sum_{i=1}^{n}(Y_i - \bar{Y})^2}{(1 - r^2) \sum_{i=1}^{n}(Y_i - \bar{Y})^2 / (n - 2)} = \frac{r^2(n - 2)}{1 - r^2}. \qquad (11.15)$$

When H_0 is true, this statistic follows an F distribution with 1 and $n - 2$ degrees of freedom. From Equation 11.14 and Equation 11.15, we see that the calculated F statistic is the square of the calculated t statistic. As mentioned earlier, the square of a t variable with ν degrees of freedom is an F variable with 1 and ν degrees of freedom. It should not be surprising that this test of $H_0 : \rho = 0$ is really the same test as the previous test of $H_0 : \beta = 0$. As discussed above, the relation $\beta = \rho(\sigma_Y / \sigma_X)$ implies that if either β or ρ is zero, both are zero. When ρ is not equal to zero, the statistic follows a noncentral F distribution, $\nu_1 = 1$, and $\nu_2 = n - 2$ degrees of freedom and noncentrality parameter $\lambda = n\rho^2\sigma_Y^2$.

Example. Let's go back to the cardiac rehabilitation example. The sample variances are $s_X^2 = 4.731$ for peak exercise capacity and $s_Y^2 = 500.471$ for self-reported physical functioning, and the standard deviations are $s_X = 2.175$ and $s_Y = 22.371$ (see Table 11.2). The covariance between the two variables is estimated as $s_{X,Y} = 20.80$, as reported in Section 11.2. The correlation between the two variables is $r = 0.43$. The positive correlation indicates that increasing levels of one variable are associated with increasing levels of the other one. The $r = 0.43$ is a measure of the strength of the linear relation between peak exercise capacity and physical function. We can verify that $r = bs_X/s_Y = (4.40 \times 2.175/22.371) = 0.43$.

The square of the correlation coefficient is $r^2 = 0.43^2 = 0.18$. This indicates that 18% of the variation in physical functioning is explained by the linear relation between physical functioning and peak exercise capacity, and 82% is *not* so explained. Thus, there is a lot of variation in physical functioning that is not being accounted for by the relation between the two variables. When physical function was plotted against exercise capacity in Figure 11.1, it didn't look like there was a very strong relation between the two.

The residual sum of squares, $SS_r = 17,178$, as reported in Table 11.7, can be shown to be equal to $SS_t(1 - r^2) = 21,020[1 - (0.43)^2)] = 17,178$.

To test the hypothesis $H_0 : \rho = 0$, we determine

$$t = \frac{0.43\sqrt{41}}{\sqrt{1 - (0.43)^2}} = 3.03,$$

which is identical to the calculated t statistic when we tested $H_0 : \beta = 0$. Similarly, using ANOVA, $F = 9.17$ and $p = 0.0042$. These are the same values that were determined when testing whether the slope β is equal to 0 (see Table 11.7).

Fisher's Z Statistic. A simple way of obtaining confidence intervals for ρ or for testing the null hypothesis that ρ equals any particular value ρ_0 makes use of the statistic

$$Z = \frac{1}{2} \log_e \frac{1 + r}{1 - r}. \tag{11.16}$$

(Note that we are using a capital Z for $[1/2] \log_e[(1 + r)/(1 - r)]$ and a small z for a standard normal variable.) It has been shown that the statistic Z is approximately normally distributed, with mean

$$\mu_Z \approx \frac{1}{2} \log_e \frac{1 + \rho}{1 - \rho}$$

and variance

$$\sigma_Z^2 \approx \frac{1}{n - 3}.$$

In other words, we have

$$Z \sim \text{ND}\left(\mu_Z, \frac{1}{n - 3}\right) \tag{11.17}$$

To obtain a confidence interval for ρ, a $100(1 - \alpha)\%$ confidence interval is first obtained for μ_Z, namely,

$$Z \pm z_{[1-\alpha/2]} \frac{1}{\sqrt{n-3}}.$$ (11.18)

The upper and lower limits of this confidence interval are then used to obtain upper and lower limits of the $100(1-\alpha)\%$ confidence interval for ρ. First, ρ is expressed in terms of μ_Z:

$$\rho = \frac{e^{2\mu_Z} - 1}{e^{2\mu_Z} + 1}.$$ (11.19)

Then, substituting in the upper and lower limits of the confidence interval for μ_Z, the upper and lower limits of the confidence interval for ρ are obtained. This interval can be used to provide a plausible range of values that ρ could have, or it can be used to test the hypothesis $H_0 : \rho = \rho_0$.

The same Z statistic can be used to make a formal test of $H_0 : \rho = \rho_0$, where ρ_0 is any value between -1 and $+1$ (with the foregoing t test in Equation 11.14 we can test only $H_0 : \rho = 0$):

$$z = \frac{Z - \mu_Z}{\sigma_Z}.$$ (11.20)

Here ρ_0 is transformed to μ_Z, r is transformed to Z, and $\sigma_Z = \sqrt{1/(n-3)}$. When H_0 is true, the test statistic follows a standard normal distribution. This test is usually constructed as a two-sided test, so the hypothesis is rejected for large and small values of the statistic.

Example. From the cardiac rehabilitation study, $r = 0.43$ and

$$Z = \frac{1}{2}\log_e \frac{1 + 0.43}{1 - 0.43} = 0.46.$$

A 95% confidence interval for μ_Z is computed using Equation 11.18, namely, $0.46 \pm 1.96/\sqrt{40}$, or $0.15 < \mu_Z < 0.77$.

Because the value of μ_Z increases as ρ increases, if μ_Z lies between 0.15 and 0.77, ρ lies between the numbers corresponding to 0.15 and 0.77. Substituting the lower limit of the interval, 0.15, into Equation 11.19, we find the lower limit of the confidence interval for ρ is 0.15. Similarly substituting the upper limit, 0.77, into Equation 11.19, we find the upper limit of the confidence limit of ρ is 0.65. The 95% confidence interval for ρ is therefore $0.15 < \rho < 0.65$. Note that $r = 0.43$ is not at the midpoint of the interval.

The Z statistic can also serve in testing whether two population correlation coefficients, taken from separate samples, are equal. For example, we might wish to test whether the correlation between physical functioning and exercise capacity is the same in men and in women. If the two population correlations are ρ_1 and ρ_2, the null hypothesis is $H_0 : \rho_1 = \rho_2$. If the sample correlations r_1 and r_2 are based on independent samples of size n_1 and n_2, we have

$$Z_i \sim \text{ND}\left(\mu_{Z_i}, \frac{1}{n_i - 3}\right), \qquad i = 1, 2, \tag{11.21}$$

and

$$Z_1 - Z_2 \sim \text{ND}\left(\mu_{Z_1} - \mu_{Z_2}, \frac{1}{n_1 - 3} + \frac{1}{n_2 - 3}\right). \tag{11.22}$$

Under $H_0 : \rho_1 = \rho_2$, we have $\mu_{Z_1} - \mu_{Z_2} = 0$; therefore, $Z_1 - Z_2$ is normally distributed with mean equal to 0 and variance equal to $1/(n_1 - 3) + 1/(n_2 - 3)$. The test statistic for testing equality of correlation coefficients is

$$z = \frac{Z_1 - Z_2}{\sqrt{\frac{1}{n_1 - 3} + \frac{1}{n_2 - 3}}}. \tag{11.23}$$

The test statistic follows a standard normal distribution when the two correlation coefficients are equal.

Example. We have already seen that for women, $n_1 = 43$, $r_1 = 0.43$, and $Z_1 = 0.46$. A sample of $n_2 = 106$ men was also included in the cardiac rehabilitation study. Repeating the analyses for men, we obtain $r_2 = 0.47$ and $Z_2 = 0.51$. The standard error of $Z_1 - Z_2$ is $\sqrt{(1/40) + (1/103)} = \sqrt{0.0347} = 0.186$. Using Equation 11.23, the calculated test statistic is equal to $(0.46 - 0.51)/0.186 = -0.27$. The corresponding p value is the probability that a standard normal variable is greater than 0.27 or less than -0.27, which is 0.79. Alternatively, a confidence interval for the difference of the two population correlation coefficients can be constructed. Using techniques described above, a 95% confidence interval is $-0.39 < \rho_1 - \rho_2 < 0.30$. Whether the hypothesis test or the confidence interval is used, the null hypothesis is not rejected, and we conclude that the correlation between peak exercise capacity and physical functioning may be the same in men and women.

If ρ_1 is the correlation between physical functioning and peak exercise capacity and ρ_2 is the correlation between physical functioning and age, and if r_1 and r_2 have been calculated from a single sample of women with measurements on the three variables, then r_1 and r_2 are not statistically independent. We no longer have $\text{Var}(Z_1 - Z_2) = 2/(n - 3)$, since Z_1 and Z_2 are undoubtedly correlated, and the foregoing test does not apply. See [8, 9, 13] for a discussion of dependent correlations.

11.5 CHECKING IF THE DATA FIT THE RANDOM X REGRESSION MODEL

Example. Before we consider specific methods for checking if the data fit the regression model, we first make some comments on its applicability in the cardiac rehabilitation example. Based on what we know about the data collection and the variables, we can say that the data do not satisfy the assumptions of the regression model. Clearly, the self-reported physical functioning variable is ordinal, rather than continuous or ratio. Another violation of the assumptions is that the subjects were not selected at random. (As stated earlier in Section 11.1, the investigators enrolled all subjects who had contact with the cardiac rehabilitation center and who were willing and able to participate.) The assumption of a random sample is frequently violated in a longitudinal study. Even though the subjects are not truly selected at random, however, the assumption is made that they represent a hypothetical population of persons with coronary artery disease who would have been willing to participate in the study. To evaluate this, investigators may make comparisons between those who were and were not willing to participate. Ideally, there will be no major differences.

Just as the procedures for making inferences for the fixed X regression model are identical for the random X regression model, so are the techniques for determining whether or not the model fits the data. Thus, the methods discussed in Section 10.7 for identifying outliers and checking for linearity, constant error variances and normally distributed errors are applicable here and are not repeated.

The assumption of bivariate normality should also be checked if the bivariate normal model is assumed. While there are formal tests for bivariate normality, it is simplest to make use of one of the characteristics of a bivariate normal distribution: if X and Y have a bivariate normal distribution, then X is normally distributed and Y is normally distributed. Checking that each variable is normally distributed, as described in Chapter 1, is generally adequate (although X and Y can each be normally distributed but do not follow a bivariate normal distribution). Another informal check is to examine the scatter diagram of X and Y values and see if the points fall within an ellipse.

For studies involving random X's, there may be only one or a few values of Y associated with each measured X. If only one Y_i exists at each X_i, we have simply n samples of size 1. The residuals, $Y_i - \hat{Y}_i$, can be considered to be a single sample of size n. Examination of the residuals through residual plots is a good way to check for linearity and equality of variances. Normal quantile plots of the residuals are useful for assessing normality. Thus, residual plots can always be used, regardless of how sampling was done.

In Chapter 10, we were more concerned about outliers in Y and less concerned about unusual values in X. Here, there is greater concern about unusual X values, as these could signal violations of assumptions of the random X regression model. Thus, methods for evaluating X values are discussed here.

11.5.1   Checking for High-Leverage, Outlying, and Influential Observations

So far, we have devoted a lot of attention to the residuals, the e_i. Residuals can be of interest in and of themselves. Unusually large values should be of concern, as they suggest either that there are outliers in the data set or that a nonlinear relation exists between the two variables.

However, residuals should not be relied upon exclusively for these purposes, especially when looking for outliers. The numerical value of each residual is affected by any outliers used in fitting the regression line. Outlying observations *may* shift the regression line closer to their Y value by changing both the slope and the intercept value. The resulting residual may be small. Thus, residual plots should be viewed along with the scatter diagram in the case of one X and one Y variable.

Another problem with the sample residuals is that they do not have equal variance. In simple linear regression, while we assume that each ε_i has the same variance σ^2, this does not imply that the sample residuals, the $e_i = Y_i - \hat{Y}_i$, all have the same variance. The observations that have their X value far away from $\bar{X}$ tend to have smaller residuals because they have a larger influence on the placement of the sample regression line. Thus, it can be difficult to tell whether a residual is "large" or "small."

Thus, we want to consider modifications to the e_i which have desirable properties such as (1) constant variance and (2) a known distribution. This will enable us to establish some criteria or rules of thumb for deciding what observations are or are not outliers.

But first, we define the term *leverage*: it means how far away an X value is from $\bar{X}$. Observations that have an X value that is located far from $\bar{X}$ are often called high leverage points, and those close to $\bar{X}$ are called low leverage points. The high leverage points have the potential to have a large influence on the regression line if their Y value is an outlier. The usual measure of leverage is called the *hat value*, and for the ith observation it is frequently denoted h_i,. In simple linear regression, it is defined as

$$h_i = \frac{1}{n} + \frac{(X_i - \bar{X})^2}{\sum_{j=1}^{n}(X_j - \bar{X})^2}. \tag{11.24}$$

The values of h_i satisfy $1/n < h_i < 1$; they are functions only of the X and not the Y. Recall that this expression was used in the estimated variance of $\hat{Y}_i | X_i = s^2 h_i$ (see Table 10.4).

The h_i are of interest because (1) a large value might suggest an outlier in X, (2) the point (X_i, Y_i) could be having a large effect on regression estimates if X_i is indeed an outlier, and (3) the variance estimate of the e_i and its modifications can be expressed in terms of them (see below).

The estimated variance of e_i is equal to $s^2(1-h_i)$. (From this expression, we can see that high leverage points, with large values of h_i, have small variances.) Its estimated standard error is the square root, $\text{se}(e_i) = s\sqrt{1 - h_i}$. Taking the ratio of the residual to its standard error seems like a good idea; they have variances of 1. We will refer to the residual divided by its estimated standard error as a *standardized residual* and denote the ith standardized residual as r_i. It is calculated as

$$r_i = \frac{e_i}{s\sqrt{1 - h_i}}. \tag{11.25}$$

This quantity has assumed a variety of other names, such as the Studentized residual, or the internally Studentized residual. We have opted to make use of the notation and definition of this term in *The Cambridge Dictionary of Statistics* [10].

The standardized residual is often adjusted further so that the numerator and denominator are independent and the resulting residual has a t distribution with $\nu = n - p - 1$ degrees of freedom, where p is equal to the number of parameters that define the population regression line (in this chapter $p = 2$ for α and β) [3]. This is accomplished by deleting, say, the ith observation from the regression analysis. Using the remaining $n - 1$ observations [i.e., not including (X_i, Y_i)], the simple linear regression analysis is repeated. The residual for each of the $n - 1$ observations is computed as the difference between the observed value and the fitted value, determined from the sample regression line that does *not* include Y_i. The sample variance of the $n - 1$ residuals is denoted by $s^2_{(-i)}$. The estimated standard error of e_i is obtained as $s_{(-i)}\sqrt{1 - h_i}$. We will refer to the ith residual divided by $s_{(-i)}\sqrt{1 - h_i}$ as a *Studentized residual* and will denote it by t_i:

$$t_i = \frac{e_i}{s_{(-i)}\sqrt{1 - h_i}}. \tag{11.26}$$

By deleting each observation from the regression analysis one at a time, a Studentized residual can be computed for each of the n observations. The t_i have also assumed a variety of other names, such as deleted residual or externally Studentized residual. There is little uniformity in the names for the Studentized and deleted residuals in texts and statistical packages. (Again, we are using the term Studentized residual as defined in [10].) It is safest to see how they are computed.

Another way to think about individual data points in a regression analysis is in terms of their influence on estimates, usually the coefficients that make up the sample regression line. Points that have a large effect on the magnitude and variability of these coefficients are said to be *influential*.

One commonly used measure of influence is *Cook's distance*. There is a value of Cook's distance associated with each observation in the data set. It refers to a distance between sample regression coefficients when an observation is and is not deleted in the computation of the coefficients. Cook's distance D_i can be expressed succinctly as

$$D_i = \frac{r_i^2}{p} \frac{h_i}{1 - h_i}. \tag{11.27}$$

Carefully examining this equation indicates that Cook's distance should be large when the Y_i and/or X_i are influential. As discussed above, outliers in Y should be identified by large values of the standardized residuals, and unusual values of X should be identified by large leverages. Sometimes, the standardized residual r_i and the ratio $h_i/(1 - h_i)$ do not identify an influential point, but in combination they do.

It's best to use good judgment and knowledge of the subject matter in deciding what to do about points that have high leverage, are outliers, and/or are influential. Some recommendations have been given, however, which we briefly mention here. Belsey et al. [3] suggest that observations with hat values which exceed $2p/n$ be given a closer look as high-leverage observations. Fox suggests observations with Studentized residuals that exceed 2 (in absolute value) be given further consideration as potential outliers and that observations with Cook's distance of $D_i > 4/(n - p)$ be examined more closely as influential observations. More detailed information can be found in [3, 5, 11, 12], among others.

Example. We discuss assessing whether the model fits the data for the cardiac rehabilitation example. Note that $r^2 = 0.18$. This means that 18% of the variation in Y is explained by the linear regression of physical functioning on peak exercise capacity. That isn't particularly large, but it is not an atypical value of r^2 for an investigation in this field. We might not expect a great fit. There are lots of reasons self-reported physical functioning may not relate exclusively to peak exercise capacity; for example, patients might have other characteristics, such as arthritis, that would affect their self-reported physical functioning.

For assessing violations of the model assumptions, we focus on Studentized residuals, hat values, and Cook's distance. (The results for residuals e_i, standardized residuals r_i, and Studentized residuals t_i are essentially equivalent and are not repeated.)

Some of the diagnostics introduced in this chapter are summarized in Table 11.10. The Studentized residuals ranged from -2.67 (observation 15) to 2.24 (observation 22). These two women had low peak exercise capacities (2.5 and 2.0, respectively), and both reported their physical functioning (0 and 90, respectively) as quite discrepant from what the model predicted (49.78 and 47.58, respectively).

The largest hat values (0.162 and 0.114) are associated with peak exercise capacities of 9 and 10. This is expected, as these exercise capacities are the

Table 11.10 Peak Exercise Capacity X in METS, Self-Reported Physical Functioning Y, and Diagnostics: Studentized Residuals, Hat Values, and Cook's Distance

Obs	Exercise Capacity	Physical Functioning	Studentized Residual	Hat Value	Cook's Distance
1	7.0	90	1.024	0.049	0.027
2	2.0	30	−0.884	0.061	0.026
3	6.0	65	−0.009	0.031	0.000
4	4.0	40	−0.807	0.026	0.009
5	6.0	75	0.483	0.031	0.004
6	8.0	75	0.052	0.077	0.000
7	7.0	80	0.518	0.049	0.007
8	3.0	40	−0.592	0.039	0.007
9	3.0	80	1.413	0.039	0.039
10	3.0	15	−1.900	0.039	0.068
11	6.0	60	−0.254	0.031	0.001
12	4.0	60	0.177	0.026	0.000
13	8.0	85	0.556	0.077	0.013
14	2.0	65	0.876	0.061	0.025
15	2.5	0	−2.674	0.049	0.159
16	3.0	55	0.149	0.039	0.000
17	8.0	35	−2.058	0.077	0.163
18	5.0	50	−0.528	0.024	0.003
19	2.0	70	1.134	0.061	0.042
20	2.0	45	−0.129	0.061	0.001
21	3.0	55	0.149	0.039	0.000
22	2.0	90	2.241	0.061	0.149
23	5.0	75	0.699	0.024	0.006
24	3.5	75	1.034	0.031	0.017
25	7.0	60	−0.475	0.049	0.006
26	2.0	45	−0.129	0.061	0.001
27	7.0	95	1.284	0.049	0.042
28	5.0	40	−1.028	0.024	0.013
29	7.0	65	−0.226	0.049	0.001
30	5.0	55	−0.282	0.024	0.001
31	4.0	35	−1.060	0.026	0.015
32	4.0	60	0.177	0.026	0.000
33	6.0	35	−1.521	0.031	0.036
34	5.0	50	−0.528	0.024	0.003
35	4.0	35	−1.060	0.026	0.015
36	4.0	55	−0.067	0.026	0.000
37	10.0	95	0.649	0.162	0.041
38	9.0	85	0.341	0.114	0.008
39	5.0	65	0.206	0.024	0.001
40	2.0	75	1.398	0.061	0.062
41	7.0	90	1.024	0.049	0.027
42	3.0	85	1.681	0.039	0.054
43	3.0	30	−1.098	0.039	0.024

farthest away from the mean value of 4.74. Note that the hat values for observations 15 and 22 were 0.049 and 0.061; the peak exercise capacities were not unusual.

There were three values of Cook's distance which were large: 0.159 (observation 15), 0.163 (observation 17) and 0.149 (observation 22). In each case, the Cook's distance is reflecting discrepancies between predicted and observed physical functioning; in none of these cases is peak exercise capacity unusual. For the two highest leverage points, the residuals are quite small and Cook's distance is also small. Sometimes residuals associated with high leverage points are small because the points are *influential* in determining the predicted values. This is likely not the case here, since the Cook's distance, which seeks to combine effects of the leverage and outliers, is not particularly large.

Thus, by examining the individual points, we have detected some discrepancies between observed and predicted physical functioning. Recall that these Studentized residuals are used to identify potential outliers in self-reported physical functioning. The values may be unusual, but they are plausible; the investigators felt they were genuine self-reports which should not be deleted.

This study was conducted with the peak exercise capacity levels random, not fixed by the investigator. However, because of the nature of the data, there are multiple values of self-reported physical functioning for some values of peak exercise capacity.

Whether or not the assumptions of linearity and constant error variances are appropriate can be assessed by examining the plot of the Studentized residuals versus peak exercise capacity as shown in Figure 11.5. We don't see any pattern in the plot that would suggest that the relation between self reported physical functioning and peak exercise capacity is not linear. There may be a suggestion that the variance of the residuals is greater for the lower values of peak exercise capacity. It is difficult to say something definitive here, because of the small sample size at each level. However, it is possible that this is the case.

The normal quantile plot of the Studentized residuals is shown in Figure 11.6. The residuals fall approximately on a straight line; the Shapiro-Wilk statistic is $W = 0.99$, and $p = 0.95$. These two pieces of information suggest that the Studentized residuals are approximately normally distributed.

From our checks of the assumptions, some appear satisfied and some don't. This sort of situation is fairly typical with real data. We recommend that researchers give limitations of their results when not all assumptions are satisfied.

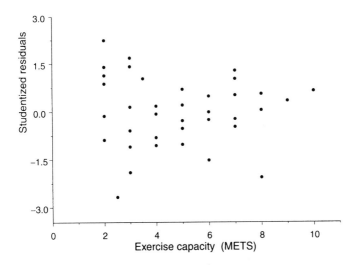

Fig. 11.5 Studentized residuals versus peak exercise capacity.

11.6 WHAT TO DO IF THE DATA DON'T FIT THE RANDOM X MODEL

If a suitable transformation cannot be found, either the reader should be warned or more robust procedures should be used.

11.6.1 Nonparametric Alternatives to Simple Linear Regression

When the relationship between X and Y is not linear, analysts can try fitting different models (for example, through use of transformations). An alternative approach is not to restrict the distribution of the errors (for example, not to require they be normally distributed) or the form of the relation between $E(Y|X)$ and X. This is referred to as *nonparametric regression*. There are a variety of methods which can be used, they are all computer-intensive and at this time are not routinely available in all software packages. A reference for a nonparametric procedure based on ranks is [6]; an introduction to smoothing techniques (kernel and nearest–neighbor approaches) is found in [2] .

11.6.2 Nonparametric Alternatives to the Pearson Correlation

When X and Y have a bivariate normal distribution, we know that there is a linear relation between the two variables. If they do not, there still may be a relation between them; it may or may not be linear. Since r is a measure of the strength of the linear relation between two variables, it may not be the best statistic to summarize the strength of the relation between the two variables.

One alternative to the Pearson correlation is the Spearman, or rank, correlation, r_s. Rather than obtain the correlation using the *measured* values of X and Y, the values of X are ranked from 1 to n and the values of Y are ranked from 1 to n, and the correlation of the *ranks* is calculated. That is, the Spearman correlation is the Pearson correlation using the ranks of the measurements rather than the measurements themselves. The Spearman correlation measures the tendency of X to increase or decrease with Y. If a linear relation does indeed exist between the two variables, then the Pearson and Spearman correlations should be similar. If there is an increasing relation between the two variables, for example, a quadratic relation, the Spearman correlation should be higher than the Pearson correlation. While the Pearson r may be strongly influenced by outliers, the Spearman r_s is insensitive to them. Like the Pearson r, the Spearman r_s can assume values between -1 and $+1$. Values of -1 indicate large values of X are associated with small values of Y and all points lie on a curve. Values of $+1$ indicate large values of X are associated with large values of Y and all points lie on an increasing

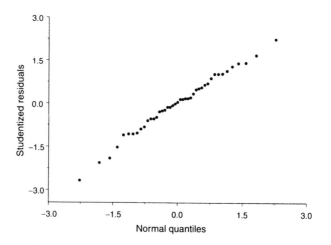

Fig. 11.6 Normal quantile plot of Studentized residuals for women in study.

or decreasing (monotonic) curve. Values of 0 indicate there is no tendency for X to increase or decrease with Y. Another advantage that the Spearman rank correlation has over the Pearson correlation is that it is appropriate for ordinal data; ideally, Pearson correlation is used for interval and ratio types of variables.

Tests of the hypothesis $H_0 : \rho_s = 0$ are made using the same procedures (t or F tests), as described in Section 11.4.3, with the substitution of ranks for the observations (or r_s for r).

Example. For the cardiac rehabilitation example, the Spearman rank correlation between physical functioning and peak exercise capacity is $r_s = 0.38$, which is quite close to the Pearson correlation of $r = 0.43$.

As with the other summary statistics and tests, we rely on the computer to make the appropriate calculations.

11.7 SUMMARY

In this chapter, we expanded our discussion of the regression of a dependent variable Y on an independent variable X to applications in which both X and Y are random. We referred to the underlying model as the random X regression model. In these applications, it is appropriate to summarize the data in terms of the sample means and sample standard deviations of the two variables as well as the sample regression line and sample correlation between the two. Since all of the inferences that were made when X is fixed are applicable when X is random, the procedures for making inferences about the population regression line — for the slope β, the mean $E(Y|X)$ of Y for given value of X, and so forth — are identical.

We further assumed that the two variables X and Y have a bivariate normal distribution. We summarized properties of this distribution and its dependence on the means and standard deviations of X and Y and the population correlation coefficient ρ. We described ρ as a measure of the strength of the linear relation between the two variables. When this model holds, we indicated that it is appropriate to estimate and make inferences about ρ and described procedures for hypothesis testing and confidence intervals for ρ.

Next, we considered how to check whether the assumptions of the random X model were violated. The procedures that were discussed in Chapter 10 are still appropriate here, but we also included looking for unusual X values, introduced the concepts of leverage and influence, and defined other measures — standardized and Studentized residuals and Cook's distance — which are useful for regression diagnostics.

Finally, we discussed what to do if the data don't fit the random X model. Transforming the data, as described in Chapter 10, was mentioned. Nonparametric regression was referenced. Spearman's correlation, the correlation of the ranks of the observed data, was introduced as an example of a nonparametric alternative to the Pearson correlation coefficient.

Problems

11.1   Using the data from Chapter 1, investigate the relation between total biovolume of algae and species richness. (The data are available on the Wiley ftp site.)

  a)   Construct a scatter diagram of total biovolume versus species richness. Are any outliers apparent?

  b)   Regress total biovolume on species richness. Are any outliers apparent? Why?

  c)   Are the residuals normally distributed? Why?

  d)   Plot the residuals versus species richness. Are any violations from the assumptions of the regression apparent? Which ones and why?

  e)   What is the Pearson correlation between the two variables? the Spearman correlation? Which summary statistic would you choose to report? Why?

  f)   Repeat parts (a)–(e) using log biovolume instead of biovolume.

  g)   Repeat parts (a)–(e), deleting outlying observations. Comment on the appropriateness of the deletions.

  h)   What do you conclude about the relation between total biovolume and species richness?

11.2   For the cardiac rehabilitation study, regress physical functioning on sex, coded as 0=male and 1=female. (The data are available on the Wiley ftp site.)

  a)   Get summary statistics for physical functioning by gender.

  b)   Determine the least squares estimates.

  c)   Interpret a and b.

11.3   Yearly rainfall and yield of cotton were as follows:

Rainfall X (in.)	Yield Y (lb / acre)
7.12	1037
63.54	380
47.38	416
45.92	427
8.68	619
50.86	388
44.46	321

a) How do you think that the data were obtained? Do you think the sampling was done from the joint distribution of rainfall and yield, or from yields for fixed rainfall?

b) What model or models can be used for the data?

c) Write out the least squares regression line to predict the yield of cotton from yearly rainfall.

d) Draw a scatter diagram, and draw the sample regression line.

e) Obtain an ANOVA table.

f) Give a 95% confidence interval for (1) the regression coefficient β, (2) the mean yield of cotton for a yearly rainfall of 50 in.

g) Test whether ρ is zero using a t statistic.

h) Give a 95% confidence interval for ρ.

11.4 To predict the yield of rye Y from yearly rainfall X_1 and temperature X_2, data were collected as follows:

Yield of Rye (bushels/acre)	Rainfall (in.)	Temp (degF)	Yield of Rye (bushels/acre)	Rainfall (in.)	Temp (degF)
21.0	45	54.1	27.0	35	46.7
20.0	47	61.6	17.5	43	60.8
21.0	33	50.8	26.0	39	56.9
24.0	39	52.1	11.0	31	60.3
20.0	30	50.2	24.0	42	54.6
12.5	28	57.1	26.0	43	53.5
19.0	41	55.7	18.5	47	64.0
23.0	44	57.6	15.5	25	45.7
23.0	31	50.1	16.5	50	61.5
19.0	29	38.0	18.0	45	59.7
21.0	34	56.2	20.5	34	53.2
12.0	27	51.5	22.0	29	45.1
21.0	42	54.1			

a) Plot yield versus rainfall, yield versus temperature, and rainfall versus temperature.

b) Estimate the correlations between yield and rainfall, between yield and temperature, and between rainfall and temperature. Relate these correlations to the scatter plots constructed in part a.

c) Regress yield on rainfall. Construct a normal quantile plot of the residuals and plot residuals versus rainfall. Which assumptions, if any, of the random X model appear to be violated?

d) Regress yield on temperature. Construct a normal quantile plot of the residuals and plot residuals versus temperature. Which assumptions, if any, of the random X model appear to be violated?

11.5   In a study of the relation of age (in years) and physical strength for adults, strength of right-hand grip (in pounds) was measured for a sample of adult men. The data were as follows:

Age X	30	23	43	56	29	52	59	52	23	27
Grip strength Y	86	88	80	83	93	87	71	91	76	82

Age, X	59	24	24	37	62
Grip strength, Y	88	100	92	97	98

a)   Fit a straight line $\hat{Y} = a + bX$ predicting physical strength from age.

b)   What is an appropriate model for this problem.

c)   Give an estimate of σ^2.

d)   Test $H_0 : \beta = 0$.

e)   Give and interpret a 95% confidence interval for β.

11.6   The average yearly temperature Y (in °F) and the latitude X (in degrees) were determined for 15 selected cities in the United States. Data were as follows:

Latitude X	34	32	39	39	41	45	41	33
Temperature Y	56.4	51.0	36.7	37.8	36.7	18.2	30.1	55.7

Latitude, X	34	47	44	39	41	32	40
Temperature, Y	46.6	13.3	34.0	36.3	34.0	49.1	34. 5

a)   Plot the data.

b)   Find the least squares line.

c)   State a possible model, and discuss whether the model seems to be appropriate.

d)   Test $H_0 : \rho = 0$ under the assumption that the correlation model is appropriate.

e)   Find and interpret a 95% confidence interval for ρ.

11.7   For the cardiac rehabilitation study, regress physical functioning at the completion of 3 months of cardiac rehabilitation (mospost) on physical functioning at baseline (mospre) for women and men separately. (Data are available on the Wiley ftp site.)

a)   Determine the sample regression lines.

b)   Determine 95% confidence intervals for β. Do the confidence intervals include 0? Do the confidence intervals include 1? What do the intervals suggest about the relation between physical functioning before and after cardiac rehabilitation in men and women?

c)   Determine the sample (Pearson) correlation coefficients and Spearman correlation coefficients. Which of the two would you prefer to report? Why?

d)   Are the correlation coefficients equal for men and women?

11.8   (Note: This program works well as a group assignment.) Use the program bivariate.sas (from the Wiley ftp site) to generate samples of size 100 from bivariate normal distributions with differing values of μ_X, μ_Y, σ_X, σ_Y, and ρ as follows:

μ_X	μ_Y	σ_X	σ_Y	ρ
0.0	0.0	1.0	1.0	0.0
0.0	0.0	1.0	1.0	0.3
0.0	0.0	1.0	1.0	0.6
0.0	0.0	1.0	1.0	0.9
0.0	0.0	1.0	1.0	-0.3
0.0	0.0	10.0	10.0	0.0
0.0	0.0	10.0	10.0	0.3
0.0	0.0	10.0	10.0	0.6
0.0	0.0	10.0	10.0	0.9
10.0	10.0	1.0	1.0	0.3
10.0	10.0	1.0	1.0	0.6
10.0	10.0	1.0	1.0	0.9
10.0	10.0	10.0	10.0	0.3
10.0	10.0	10.0	10.0	0.6
10.0	10.0	10.0	10.0	0.9

Construct scatter diagrams. What do you conclude about the effect of the means, standard deviations, and correlation on the shape and location of the bivariate normal distribution?

11.9   (Note: This works well as a group assignment.) The program sim-corr.sas (from the Wiley ftp site) can be used to perform a simulation study to investigate properties of the sample correlation. For this program, vary sample size ($n = 10$ and $n = 100$) and $\rho = 0, 0.3, 0.6, 0.9$. Repeat each simulation 10,000 times. Write up a summary of the effects of sample size n and correlation ρ on:

a)   The bias of r. Is the average of the 1000 r's close to the specified value of ρ?

b)   The skewness of r. How symmetric is the distribution of r?

c)   The average length of the confidence interval for ρ.

d)   The percentage of times a 95% confidence interval for ρ covers ρ, i.e. is it close to the 95% that you would expect?

11.10   Verify the variance of $Y_i - \hat{Y}$. (This is a good problem for determining the variance of a linear combination when the two variables are not independent.) Note that the covariance between Y_i and $\hat{Y}_i$ is $\sigma^2[1/n + (X_i - \bar{X})^2 / \sum_{i=1}^{n} (X_i - \bar{X}]^2$.

REFERENCES

1. Ades, P.A., Maloney, A., Savage, P. and Carhart, R.L. [1999]. Determinants of Physical Functioning in Coronary Patients. *Archives of Internal Medicine*, 159, 2357–2360.

2. Altman, N.S. [1992]. An Introduction to Kernel and Nearest-Neighbor Nonparametric Regression. *The American Statistician*, 46, 175–185.

3. Belsey, D.A., Kuh, E., and Welsch, R.E. [1980]. *Regression Diagnostics: Identifying Influential Data and Sources of Collinearity*, New York: John Wiley & Sons, 11–21.

4. Birkes, D. and Dodge, Y. [1993]. *Alternative Methods of Regression*, New York: John Wiley & Sons.

5. Chatterjee, S. and Hadi, A.S. [1988]. *Sensitivity Analysis in Linear Regression*, New York: John Wiley & Sons, 71–127.

6. Conover, W.J. [1999]. *Practical Nonparametric Statistics*, New York: John Wiley & Sons, 332–342.

7. Cook, R.D. [1977]. Detection of Influential Observation in Linear Regression. *Technometrics*, 19, 15–18.

8. Dunn, O. J. and Clark, V. A. [1969]. Correlation Coefficients Measured on the Same Individuals, *Journal of the American Statistical Association*, 64, 366–377.

9. Dunn, O. J. and Clark, V.A. [1971]. Tests of Equality of Dependent Correlation Coefficients, *Journal of the American Statistical Association*, 66, 904–908.

10. Everitt, B.S. [1998]. *The Cambridge Dictionary of Statistics*, Cambridge, UK: Cambridge University Press.

11. Fox, J. [1991]. *Regression Diagnostics: An Introduction*, Sage University Paper Series on Quantitative Applications in the Social Sciences, 07-079, Newbury Park, CA: Sage, 21–39.

12. Hoaglin, D.C. and Welsch, R.E. [1978]. The Hat Matrix in Regression and ANOVA, *The American Statistician*, 17–22.

13. Neill, J.J. and Dunn, O.J. [1975]. Equality of Dependent Correlation Coefficients, *Biometrics*, 31, 531–543.

14. Stewart, A.L., Greenfield, S., Hays, R.D., Wells, K., Rogers, W.H., Berry, S.D. McGlynn, E.A., and Ware, J.E., Jr. [1989]. Functional Status and Well-being of Patients with Chronic Conditions: Results from the Medical Outcomes Study. *JAMA*, 262, 907–913.

15. Ware, J.E., Jr. and Sherbourne, C.D. [1992]. The MOS 36-Item Short-Form Health Survey (SF-36) 1. Conceptual Framework and Item Selection, *Medical Care*, 30, 473–483.

12

Multiple Regression

In Chapters 10 and 11, we studied two variables X and Y simultaneously; two general models were introduced — the fixed X and random X regression models. For both models, we distinguished between the two variables — Y as the dependent, response, outcome, or predicted, variable and X as the independent or predictor variable. We used simple linear regression either to investigate whether X and Y were related or to predict Y on the basis of an observed value of X. In this chapter, we consider multiple variables, $X_1, \ldots, X_k$, and we wish to investigate how these variables *in combination* are related to Y, or to predict Y on the basis of observed values of $X_1, \ldots, X_k$. Furthermore, we shall see a third application of multiple regression — the control or adjustment of variables.

The topic of regression was introduced in the context of the fixed X regression model. However, that model is seldom applied when there is more than a single X variable; instead, investigators routinely opt to perform ANOVA. Therefore, no chapter in this book is devoted exclusively to the fixed X model in multiple regression. This chapter addresses multiple regression and assumes that the random X or joint distribution model is applicable. (We note that much about regression is relevant to both models.)

In Section 12.1 we introduce a multiple regression example. In Section 12.2 we discuss how to fit a plane through a set of points using the method of least squares — a clear generalization of the least squares line — and address interpretation of the regression coefficients. In Section 12.3 we state the regression model formally. Section 12.4 addresses estimates of partial regression coefficients, their estimated standard errors, and confidence intervals. Hypothesis testing is covered in Section 12.5. Section 12.6 concerns how to determine whether the multiple linear regression model fits the data and Section 12.7 discusses what to do if they don't. The chapter is summarized in Section 12.8.

12.1 EXAMPLE

Suppose measurements were made for three variables from $n = 48$ adult subjects; the sampling unit was the individual subject. The Y variable is lung vital capacity, the volume of air which can be exhaled from the lungs after maximal inhalation, in liters. While vital capacity is a measure of lung function (the larger the volume, the better the lung function), we would also expect it to reflect the size of the individual (larger lungs, higher vital capacity) and their age (greater age, lower vital capacity). As an indicator of size, determinations were made on the height (in inches) of the individual, and age was assessed in years. The observed data are given in Table 12.1.

Table 12.1 Vital Capacity, Height, and Age for 48 Subjects

Vital Capacity	Age	Height	Vital Capacity	Age	Height
4.74	36	65	2.00	43	61
3.00	40	63	3.38	67	67
3.64	32	64	5.33	32	72
3.80	46	64	3.64	51	72
2.15	65	63	3.84	34	66
2.47	60	64	2.99	58	65
3.44	38	65	3.35	60	63
3.38	33	64	4.81	39	72
1.56	71	62	4.36	72	71
2.90	38	61	5.33	67	69
3.38	32	64	4.62	38	72
2.86	40	60	4.62	51	69
3.18	33	58	3.38	76	65
3.10	41	63	5.66	30	70
2.66	46	63	4.88	34	67
2.99	36	62	4.70	32	72
2.54	45	60	4.03	30	65
4.42	32	64	4.03	48	67
3.12	52	62	2.60	60	66
4.94	36	66	2.80	46	64
3.18	38	59	3.25	61	68
4.00	34	63	3.20	71	65
3.18	38	62	4.74	40	68
2.90	33	63	2.47	60	64

Let's first go back to the material presented in Chapters 10 and 11 and consider the regression of vital capacity on height and age separately. A

EXAMPLE   303

scatter diagram of vital capacity versus height suggests some linear relation between the two variables and that larger vital capacities tend to be found among taller individuals (Figure 12.1). Similarly, a plot of vital capacity versus age also suggests there is a linear relation and that lower vital capacities are found in older individuals (Figure 12.2). Sample regression lines are also drawn in these figures. Note that the slope of the line is indeed positive for height ($b = 0.18$) and negative for age ($b = -0.024$).

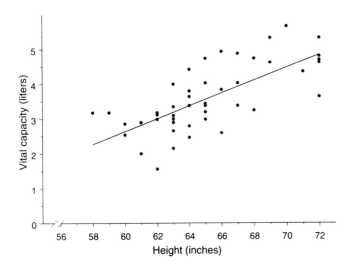

Fig. 12.1   Vital capacity versus height.

The linear relation between vital capacity and height appears stronger than the linear relation between vital capacity and age. This can be seen by comparing the spread of points in Figures 12.1 and 12.2. A more formal comparison can be made in terms of material obtained from Tables 12.2 and 12.3; the F value is higher and p value is lower for the test that the regression coefficient associated with height is 0. The square of the correlation coefficient between vital capacity and height ($r^2 = 0.49$) is higher than that between vital capacity and age ($r^2 = 0.12$); the residual sum of squares for the regression of vital capacity on height ($SS_r = 21.4$) is less than that on age ($SS_r = 37.0$); and the p value for the test of $H_0 : \beta = 0$ is smaller for height ($p < 0.0001$) than for age ($p = 0.015$).

We have considered the linear relations of vital capacity with height and with age separately, but have not considered the linear relation between height and age. The correlation between height and age is quite small ($r = 0.07$). The correlations among the three variables can be summarized in a 3 by 3

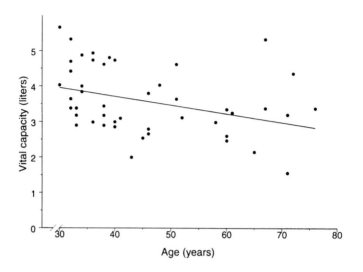

Fig. 12.2 Vital capacity versus age.

Table 12.2 ANOVA Table for the Regression of Vital Capacity on Height

Source of Variation	Sum of Squares	df	Mean Square	F Value	p Value
Regression	20.7	1	20.7	44.6	0.0001
Residual	21.4	46	0.46		
Total	42.1	47			

correlation matrix, with rows and columns ordered as vital capacity, height, age:

$$\begin{pmatrix} 1.00 & 0.70 & -0.35 \\ 0.70 & 1.00 & 0.07 \\ -0.35 & 0.07 & 1.00 \end{pmatrix}.$$

So far, we have only looked at the variables two at a time. This is simple and straightforward, but it doesn't allow us to investigate some of the questions we might have. For example, if we adjust for age, do we observe a significant linear relation between vital capacity and height? Similarly, if we adjust for height, do we observe a significant linear relation between vital capacity and

Table 12.3   ANOVA Table for the Regression of Vital Capacity on Age

Source of Variation	Sum of Squares	df	Mean Square	F Value	p Value
Regression	5.1	1	5.1	6.3	0.015
Residual	37.0	46	0.8		
Total	42.1	47			

age? Or, if our interests are in predicting vital capacity, are our predictions better if we combine the information in both age and height rather than trying to predict vital capacity on the basis of only one of the variables? Multiple regression allows us to investigate these and other questions.

12.2   THE SAMPLE REGRESSION PLANE

Let $X_1, \ldots, X_k$ and Y denote $k + 1$ variables, for which measurements are obtained on each of n units or individuals. For simplicity, let's consider the case of three variables, X_1, X_2, and Y and let's denote by X_{1l}, X_{2l}, Y the measurements obtained from the lth unit. Just as the data points could be plotted as a scatter diagram in two dimensions (the X, Y plane) when we considered a single X variable, so they can be plotted in three dimensions when there are three variables.

As a least squares line was fitted through the n points $(X_1, Y_1), \ldots, (X_n, Y_n)$ in the case of simple linear regression, so a least squares plane can be fitted through the n points $(X_{11}, X_{21}, Y_1), \ldots, (X_{1n}, X_{2n}, Y_n)$. We wish to determine, from the sample data, a least squares plane of the form

$$\hat{Y} = a + b_1 X_1 + b_2 X_2. \tag{12.1}$$

The least squares plane has the property that the sum of squared differences

$$Q = \sum_{l=1}^{n} (Y_l - \hat{Y}_l)^2 \tag{12.2}$$

is a minimum among all possible planes of the form given in Equation 12.1.

All points $(\hat{Y}_1, X_{11}, X_{21}), \ldots, (\hat{Y}_n, X_{1n}, X_{2n})$ fall on the least squares plane. The a is the Y-intercept, or value of $\hat{Y}$ when $X_1 = X_2 = 0$. The b_1 and b_2 are referred to as *partial regression coefficients* or as *slopes*.

While the interpretations are similar, the mechanics of obtaining the expression for the least squares plane are more involved than those applied for a single X variable, and formulas for a, b_1, and b_2 cannot be easily expressed in terms of the individual observations. The computations are extensive, and statistical packages are routinely used.

There are different ways to consider what the partial regression coefficients are indicating; each involves adjusting or controlling for the other predictor variables in the equation. Fortunately, the different ways of looking at the slope will provide equal estimates, so the interpretations are equivalent.

Perhaps the most straightforward way of thinking about the slope comes directly from the sample regression plane. The slope b_1 can be interpreted as follows: when X_1 changes by one unit and X_2 is held fixed, the height of the regression plane changes by b_1 units. When X_2 is constant, we are back to an expression for a straight line, $\hat{Y} = (a + b_2 X_2) + b_1 X_1$, with a Y-intercept which depends on the value of X_2 and a slope of b_1. The slope b_2 is defined similarly. In this context, we say that the slope b_1 tells us something about the linear relation between Y and X_1 when the effects of X_2 are adjusted by *holding X_2 constant.*

Alternatively, the slope b_1 can tell us something about the linear relation between Y and X_1 when the effects of X_2 are adjusted by *removing its linear effects on Y and X_1.* We have seen previously that we can remove effects of one variable on another by determining residuals. (For example, compare the scatter diagrams in Figure 10.4 that were used to illustrate what scatter diagrams should look like when all assumptions were satisfied. When Y was plotted against X, there was a linear relationship between the variables, and the slope of the line was positive. When the residuals were plotted against X, the slope of the line was zero.) In the present context, we can determine two sets of residuals — one from the regression of Y on X_2 and the other from the regression of X_1 on X_2; the linear effects of X_2 are removed from both variables. When the residuals for Y are regressed on the residuals for X_1, the slope of the regression line is equal to the partial regression coefficient b_1 obtained when Y is regressed on both independent variables.

Thus, whether we say we control or adjust for a variable by holding it fixed, or remove (the linear) effects of a variable, we are in fact doing the same thing. The two expressions can be used interchangeably.

Example. A plot of the sample regression plane is shown in Figure 12.3. The grid represents a plane in the three-dimensional space of age, height, and vital capacity. The way that the axes are drawn, age increases as our eyes move from left to right, height decreases as we look from left to right and vital capacity increases as we look up the page. Vital capacity tends to increase with height when age is constant and to decrease with increasing age when height is constant. Thus, on the basis of the figure, we would expect the partial regression coefficient associated with height to be positive and the partial regression coefficient associated with age to be negative.

The interpretation of the least squares plane is the same whether we examine the figure or the equation. The equation for the least squares plane that is fitted to the 48 points is

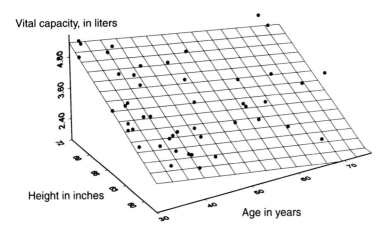

Fig. 12.3 Vital capacity versus height and age.

$$\widehat{\text{Vital capacity}} = -7.6 + 0.19 \times \text{ height} - 0.028 \times \text{ Age}$$

The partial regression coefficient for height is 0.19. This means that when age is fixed (at 30, 50, or 70 years or some other value), vital capacity is increased by 0.19 liters for every one inch increase in height. Similarly, the partial regression coefficient of -0.028 associated with age indicates that when height is fixed, vital capacity is decreased by 0.028 liters for every one year increase in age. In this example, the value of a of -7.6 is not of particular interest, as values of 0 for age and height are not possible. As the plot and plane were confined to values of height and age which were observed, we would be wary of extrapolating the plane beyond these values.

Interpretation of the partial regression coefficient associated with height as the change in vital capacity for a one inch change in height when the linear effects of age are removed can be illustrated as follows. When vital capacity (Y) is regressed only on age (X_2), the residual for the lth observation is calculated as $Y_l - 4.7 - (-0.024)X_{2l}$, and when height (X_1) is regressed on age, the residual for the lth individual is computed as $X_{1l} - 6.4 - 0.020X_{2l}$. When the 48 pairs of residuals are plotted against each other, as in Figure 12.4, the slope of the least squares line is 0.19. Note that this value is equivalent to the partial regression coefficient associated with height when the least squares plane was computed with both height and age.

How do these results compare with what we found when we considered the relationship between vital capacity and height only or age only? In this particular example, the slope associated with height was similar whether age was ignored ($b = 0.18$) or controlled ($b_1 = 0.19$). Likewise, it didn't make much of a difference to the slope associated with age whether height was ignored ($b = -0.024$) or controlled ($b_2 = -0.028$). In this example, there was little linear relation between height and age ($r = 0.07$), so it is reasonable that one would not have much effect on the change in vital capacity for a one unit change in the other. This is not true in general.

While the slopes were not greatly different, this doesn't mean that there were no gains achieved by considering both height and age in combination. The residual sum of squares $SS_r = \sum_{i=1}^{n}(Y_i - \hat{Y}_i)^2$ was equal to 14.6, a much smaller sum than that obtained when a least squares line was fitted which involved only height ($SS_r = 21.4$) or only age ($SS_r = 37.0$). This suggests that age and height in combination were better predictors of vital capacity than either variable by itself.

In this section, we have focused on two X variables, largely because this is the simplest case of multiple regression and we can visualize three-dimensional plots. What has been said, however, can be generalized to k variables. The only restriction to being able to fit a least squares plane through a set of points is that the number of X variables, k, must be less than or equal to $n - 1$.

It is not a good idea to have many variables and a small sample size. The resulting least squares equation may provide a very good fit to the data set being analyzed, but largely because random variation (peculiar to the data set) is being fitted. The resulting equation may provide an unsatisfactory representation of the relationships among the variables for a different sample. The model is said to be *overfitted*. To avoid this problem, a rule of thumb is to have a sample size n five times greater than the number of X variables, k.

As with the least squares line, the plane is the easiest surface to fit to a set of data; this doesn't necessarily mean that the plane is the best surface that could be used to summarize the relationship between the Y variable and the set of X variables.

12.3   THE MULTIPLE REGRESSION MODEL

One of the main objectives of fitting a plane to a set of data is to make inferences about underlying populations. The populations we are talking about are conditional distributions of Y given specific values of $X_1, \ldots, X_k$, that is the distributions of $Y|X_1, \ldots, X_k$. Assumptions are made in the context

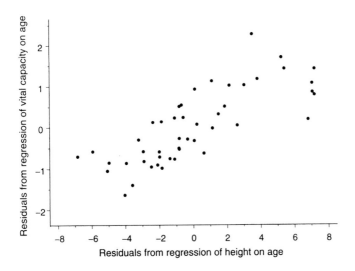

Fig. 12.4 Residuals for vital capacity (adjusted for age) versus residuals for height (adjusted for age).

of a multiple regression model, and inferences about its parameters will be considered.

In the context of the vital capacity example, we are making assumptions about the conditional distributions of vital capacity for specified levels of height and age, $Y|X_1, X_2$:

(1) The vital capacity measurements for persons of a specified height and specified age are normally distributed.

(2) Their means all lie on a plane, the population regression plane, in three dimensions. In symbols, this assumption is $E(Y|X_1, X_2) = \mu_{Y|X_1, X_2} = \alpha + \beta_1 X_1 + \beta_2 X_2$.

(3) Their variances are all equal: $\mathrm{Var}(Y|X_1, X_2) = \sigma^2$.

(4) All 48 vital capacity measurements are independent.

For a set of k variables, the model can be summarized as

$$Y|X_1, \ldots, X_k \sim \mathrm{IND}(\alpha + \beta_1 X_1 + \cdots + \beta_k X_k, \sigma^2), \qquad (12.3)$$

where IND indicates that the Y's for given $X_1, \ldots, X_k$ are independent and normally distributed. Alternatively, the model can be expressed as

$$Y_i = \alpha + \beta_1 X_1 + \cdots + \beta_k X_k + \varepsilon_i, \qquad i = 1, \ldots, n, \qquad (12.4)$$

where $\varepsilon_i \sim \text{IND}(0, \sigma^2)$, where IND means that the residuals are independent and normally distributed.

The model, as stated, is applicable whether the values of the X variables are selected by the researchers or are determined at random. That is, this regression model is applicable for both the fixed X and random X models. As a special case, it is appropriate if all variables are jointly normally distributed, as described in Chapter 13.

The X variables are typically referred to by a variety of terms, such as explanatory variables, covariates, predictor variables (particularly when regression is used for prediction), and independent variables. This use of the term "independent" should not be interpreted in terms of statistical independence or lack of correlation. The statement that X_1 and X_2 are independent variables provides no indication of a linear relation between them.

12.4   PARAMETERS, STANDARD ERRORS, AND CONFIDENCE INTERVALS

The parameters which are used in the specification of the regression model are α, $\beta_1, \ldots, \beta_k$, and σ^2. Depending on the application, investigators may want to make inferences about these parameters, or, if their interests are in prediction, they may focus more on inferences about the population regression plane itself, $E(Y|X_1, \ldots, X_k)$. To construct confidence intervals for these parameters, we need to obtain point estimates and estimates of their standard errors.

We first focus on the individual parameters of the regression model. The estimates of α and the β_i, the parameters of the population regression plane, are equivalent to the least squares estimates identified in Section 12.2. The variance σ^2 is estimated as $s^2 = \sum_{l=1}^{n}(Y_l - \hat{Y}_l)^2/(n - k - 1)$, or the residual mean square. This is the least squares sum of squared deviations divided by the number of degrees of freedom, ν, corresponding to the sample size n minus the number of parameters that are estimated for the least squares plane, $k+1$. These are all unbiased estimators of their respective parameters.

While we are neither deriving nor stating the expressions for the sample regression estimates in this chapter, one important characteristic that the estimates possess is that they are linear combinations of the Y_i. Thus, their variances and covariances can be written down in terms of σ^2, and their sample variances and sample covariances can be expressed in terms of s^2. The estimated standard errors of the sample regression coefficients, the square root of the variance estimates, are denoted here as $\text{se}(b_i)$. These estimates can be obtained directly from software programs.

In order to construct confidence intervals for each of the β_i, we make use of results that are consequences of the multiple regression model:

$$t = \frac{b_i - \beta_i}{\text{se}(b_i)} \sim t_{n-k-1}. \qquad (12.5)$$

That is, the t statistic is distributed as a t distribution with $n - k - 1$ degrees of freedom. Therefore, a $100(1 - \alpha)\%$ confidence interval for β_i has the form

$$b_i - t_{[1-\alpha/2;n-k-1]} \, \text{se}(b_i) \leq \beta_i \leq b_i + t_{[1-\alpha/2;n-k-1]} \, \text{se}(b_i) \qquad (12.6)$$

Example. Table 12.4 provides estimates of the partial regression coefficients for height and age, their estimated standard errors, and their corresponding 95% confidence intervals. The 97.5 percentile of a t distribution with 45 degrees of freedom, or $t = 2.014$, was used in the determination of the confidence interval.

12.4.1   Prediction of $E(Y|X_1, \ldots, X_k)$

To predict the point on the regression plane, $E(Y|X_1, \ldots, X_k)$, we use the point estimate

$$\hat{Y} = a + b_1 X_1 + \cdots + b_k X_k. \qquad (12.7)$$

As in simple linear regression, the variability of $\hat{Y}$ is smaller closer to the sample means for the X variables. We will denote the estimated standard error of $\hat{Y}$ by $\text{se}(\hat{Y})$. Most statistical software packages will provide estimates of standard errors of the $\hat{Y}$ as well as confidence intervals of $E(Y|X_1, \ldots, X_k)$.

12.4.2   Standardized Regression Coefficients

In trying to interpret a regression equation, research workers should not draw conclusions directly from the relative size of the regression coefficients. Besides depending on the set of variables included in the regression, the size of the coefficients depends on the units in which the variables are measured. This seems clear; in the vital capacity example, if heights were measured in feet instead of in inches, we would expect the sample regression coefficient associated with height to be larger, as the coefficient would reflect change in vital capacity for a one foot change in height instead of one inch. Similarly, if age were measured in months instead of in years, the sample regression coefficient associated with age would be smaller, as the coefficient would reflect a one month change in age instead of one year.

To obtain coefficients that are directly comparable, *standardized regression coefficients* are sometimes used. These can be obtained by first standardizing the data in order to make all means equal to zero and all standard deviations equal to one. This is accomplished by subtracting the mean from

Table 12.4 Point Estimates, Estimated Standard Errors, and 95% Confidence Intervals

Variable	Estimated Partial Regression Coefficient	Estimated Standard Error	95% Confidence Interval
Height	0.19	0.023	$0.15 \leq \beta_1 \leq 0.24$
Age	−0.028	0.0062	$-0.041 \leq \beta_2 \leq -0.016$

each observation and dividing by the standard deviation. So, for example, the observations on Y can be transformed by computing $(Y - \bar{Y})/s_y$. When the standardized Y variable is regressed on the standardized X variables, the intercept is zero, and the regression coefficients, because they have no units associated with them, can be directly compared.

By comparing the magnitude of the standardized regression coefficients, researchers can determine which explanatory variables have the strongest linear relations with the response variable when adjustment is made for the others. However, they have the disadvantage that they are more difficult to interpret than the usual partial regression coefficients; all statements about them must relate to the standardized variables rather than the original variables. For example, it is easier for most of us to think in terms of heights in inches and ages in years than in terms of standardized heights and standardized ages. Most statistical packages will either routinely report the standardized coefficients or provide them if requested; thus, it is not necessary for analysts to perform the transformations on their data.

Example. To illustrate how standardized data for vital capacity, height, and age could be computed, we need the sample mean and standard deviation for each variable. For example, the mean and standard deviation for vital capacity are 3.57 and 0.95 liters, respectively. If 3.57 were subtracted from each vital capacity measurement, and the difference divided by 0.95, the transformed observations would have a mean of zero and standard deviation of one. Similar transformations could be made on height and age. If (standardized) vital capacity were regressed on (standardized) height and age, the standardized regression coefficients would be 0.73 for height and −0.40 for age.

Since the standardized coefficient associated with height is larger in magnitude than that associated with age, the interpretation would be that, in this population, there is a stronger linear relation between vital capacity and height, when adjustment is made for age, than between vital capacity and age, when adjustment is made for height. (If we had a sample where the ages were more spread out, we would probably find a stronger association with age. In older populations, results generally are the reverse of what was found here, i.e., age tends to be a stronger predictor of vital capacity, when adjustment is made for height.)

12.5   HYPOTHESIS TESTING

When there are multiple X variables, there are a variety of questions that we may wish to investigate in the context of hypothesis testing.

12.5.1   Test That All Partial Regression Coefficients Are 0

One question of interest is whether all partial regression coefficients are equal to 0. This means that knowledge of neither X_1 nor X_2 nor $\cdots$ nor X_k provides statistically significant information about Y.

We can express the null and alternative hypothesis as follows:

$$
\begin{aligned}
H_0 &: E(Y|X_1, \ldots, X_k) = \alpha, \\
H_1 &: E(Y|X_1, \ldots, X_k) = \alpha + \beta_1 X_1 + \cdots + \beta_k X_k.
\end{aligned}
\tag{12.8}
$$

We will consider this hypothesis test in terms that we are well familiar with. The total sum of squares (SS_t) is separated into two parts, the sum of squares for the regression of Y on $X_1, \ldots, X_k$ (SS_{reg}) and a residual variation (SS_r), that is,

$$
\sum_{i=1}^{n}(Y_i - \bar{Y})^2 = \sum_{i=1}^{n}(\hat{Y}_i - \bar{Y})^2 + \sum_{i=1}^{n}(Y_i - \hat{Y}_i)^2.
\tag{12.9}
$$

As before, the $SS_t = \sum_{i=1}^{n}(Y_i - \bar{Y})^2$, $SS_{reg} = \sum_{i=1}^{n}(\hat{Y}_i - \bar{Y})^2$, and $SS_r = \sum_{i=1}^{n}(Y_i - \hat{Y}_i)^2$.

After identifying the sources of variation in the Y, and quantifying them in terms of the sums of squares, we can summarize everything that is needed to perform the hypothesis test in terms of an ANOVA table. See Table 12.5. There are $n - 1$ degrees of freedom associated with SS_t, k degrees of freedom associated with SS_{reg} and $n - k - 1$ degrees of freedom associated with SS_r.

The test statistic, $F = MS_{reg}/MS_r$ follows an F distribution with k and $n - k - 1$ degrees of freedom when H_0 is true, that is, $E(Y|X_1, \ldots X_k) = \alpha$.

Example. The ANOVA table for testing the null hypothesis that the partial regression coefficients for height and age are both 0 is given in Table 12.6.

The sums of squares were computed as in Table 12.5. Since there are two X variables, the degrees of freedom for regression are $k = 2$. The degrees of freedom associated with the total sum of squares are $n - 1 = 48 - 1 = 47$. By subtraction, the degrees of freedom associated with the residual sum of squares are $47 - 2 = 45$. The ratio of the two mean squares is $F = 42.3$. Since the chance of getting a value of F greater than 42.3 when both partial regression coefficients are equal to 0 is so small ($p < 0.0001$), the hypothesis that the partial regression coefficients relating vital capacity with height and age are both 0 is rejected.

Table 12.5   ANOVA Table for Testing That All Partial Regression Coefficients Are 0

Source of Variation	Sum of Squares	df	Mean Square	F
Regression of Y on $X_1, \ldots, X_k$	SS_{reg}	k	MS_{reg}	MS_{reg}/MS_r
Residual	SS_r	$n - k - 1$	MS_r	
Total	SS_t	$n - 1$		

12.5.2   Tests that One Partial Regression Coefficient is 0

Like tests that all partial regression coefficients are 0, tests that one partial regression coefficient is 0 are standard output from regression programs. For each of the k variables included in a regression model, we can investigate whether the partial regression coefficient associated with each X variable is 0 when the other $k - 1$ variables are included in the model. That is, if the $k - 1$ other variables have been adjusted or controlled for, does knowing the value of X_k provide any information about the (mean) value of Y? The null and alternative hypotheses that, say, $\beta_k = 0$ may be expressed as

$$\begin{aligned} H_0 : E(Y|X_1, \ldots, X_k) &= \alpha + \beta_1 X_1 + \cdots + \beta_{k-1} X_{k-1}, \\ H_1 : E(Y|X_1, \ldots, X_k) &= \alpha + \beta_1 X_1 + \cdots\cdots + \beta_k X_k. \end{aligned}$$

The test statistic may be expressed as a t statistic or as an F statistic. We first consider the test as a t test. In this case, the test statistic is expressed as

$$t = \frac{b_k}{se(b_k)}. \tag{12.10}$$

Table 12.6   Test that Partial Regression Coefficients for Height and Age Are 0

Source of Variation	SS	df	MS	Calculated F	p Value
Regression of vital capacity on height and age	27.5	2	13.7	42.3	< 0.0001
Residual	14.6	45	0.324		
Total	42.1	47			

When H_0 is true, the test statistic follows a t distribution with number of degrees of freedom equal to $n - k - 1$, the number used in the calculation of MS_r.

As usual, a confidence interval for β_i can serve to test the null hypothesis $H_0 : \beta_i = \beta_{i0}$. The corresponding test statistic is

$$t = \frac{b_i - \beta_{i0}}{\text{se}(b_i)}. \tag{12.11}$$

When H_0 is true, it is assumed that the test statistic follows a t distribution with $n - k - 1$ degrees of freedom. Most statistical software packages routinely provide tests that individual partial regression coefficients are 0 as t tests and give the estimated standard error of the coefficients.

If there are k X variables in the regression equation, it is likely that interest is in making the k inferences. Since the t ratios have no units associated with them, their magnitudes can be compared when assessing the relative strength of the linear relationship between the Y and each X variable, when the effects of the other X variables are controlled. Their relative magnitudes always coincide with those of the standardized partial regression coefficients.

One question that may arise when multiple inferences such as these are made is whether or not adjustments for multiple comparisons should be made. Generally, such adjustments are not made. However, it is straightforward to make a Bonferroni adjustment to the level of significance, by redefining it as α/k.

Example. In Table 12.4, estimates of the partial regression coefficients associated with height and weight, their estimated standard errors, and 95% confidence intervals for the partial regression coefficients were provided. Here, in Table 12.7, we repeat the point estimates and their estimated standard errors, and report the calculated t values and corresponding p values appropriate for making two-sided tests without adjustment for multiple comparisons.

In this example, we conclude that when adjustment is made for (the linear effects of) age, the partial regression coefficient for height is not 0. Similarly, when adjustment is made for (the linear effects of) height, the partial regression coefficient for age is not 0. The t statistic for height is larger in

Table 12.7   Tests That One Partial Regression Coefficient Is 0

Variable	Est. Partial Reg. Coef.	Est. se	t	p
Intercept	−7.64	1.51	−5.05	< 0.0001
Height	0.19	0.023	8.30	< 0.0001
Age	−0.028	0.0062	−4.56	< 0.0001

magnitude than that for age. This indicates that after controlling for age, we see a stronger linear relation between vital capacity and height than that between vital capacity and age after controlling for height. For completeness, we have included the test that the intercept α is 0. This is not of interest in this example. The null hypothesis is $H_0 : E(Y|X_1,\ldots,X_k) = \beta_1 X_1 + \beta_2 X_2$. The interpretation of this is is $H_0 : E(Y|X_1,\ldots,X_k) = 0$ when $X_1 = X_2 = 0$. Heights and ages of 0 are not meaningful.

The test that one partial regression coefficient is equal to 0 can be made equivalently as an F test and involves breaking the total sum of squares into three parts in an ANOVA table.

But first, let's clarify some notation. $\hat{\hat{Y}}$ is the fitted value for Y when Y is regressed on $X_1,\ldots,X_{k-1}$, that is,

$$\hat{\hat{Y}} = a^* + b_1^* X_1 + \cdots + b_{k-1}^* X_{k-1}, \tag{12.12}$$

and, as before, $\hat{Y}$ is the fitted value for Y when Y is regressed on $X_1,\ldots,X_k$, that is.

$$\hat{Y} = a + b_1 X_1 + \cdots + b_k X_k. \tag{12.13}$$

For observation l, we make use of the identity

$$Y_l - \bar{Y} = (\hat{\hat{Y}}_l - \bar{Y}) + (\hat{Y}_l - \hat{\hat{Y}}_l) + (Y_l - \hat{Y}_l). \tag{12.14}$$

Squaring both sides of Equation 12.14 and summing over the observations, we have

$$\sum_{i=1}^{n}(Y_i - \bar{Y})^2 = \sum_{i=1}^{n}(\hat{\hat{Y}}_i - \bar{Y})^2 + \sum_{i=1}^{n}(\hat{Y}_i - \hat{\hat{Y}}_i)^2 + \sum_{i=1}^{n}(Y_i - \hat{Y}_i)^2, \tag{12.15}$$

where the cross-product terms have summed to zero, as usual.

The total sum of squares has been broken into three parts. The first part describes the regression of Y on $X_1,\ldots,X_{k-1}$, the X variables included in the null model; it is frequently referred to as the sum of squares for the regression of Y on $X_1,\ldots,X_{k-1}$; here it is denoted $SS_{reg}(X_1,\ldots,X_{k-1})$. The second part is computed as the sum of squared differences between the fitted values for the alternative and null models; it is frequently referred to as the sum of squares for the regression of Y on X_k after $X_1,\ldots,X_{k-1}$, or simply as $SS(X_k|X_1,\ldots,X_{k-1})$. It can also be regarded as a *difference in the residual sums of squares* between the null and alternative models. The third part is the usual residual sum of squares for the alternative model, SS_r. These sums of squares form a piece of an ANOVA table, as in Table 12.8. The F statistic follows an F distribution with 1 and $n-k-2$ degrees of freedom when $\beta_k = 0$.

Table 12.8   ANOVA table for testing $\beta_k = 0$

Source of Variation	Sum of Squares	df	Mean Square	F Value
Regression on $X_1, \ldots, X_{k-1}$	$\mathrm{SS}_{reg}(X_1, \ldots, X_{k-1})$	$k - 1$	MS_{reg}	
Regression on $X_k \vert X_1, \ldots X_{k-1}$	$\mathrm{SS}(X_k \vert X_1, \ldots X_{k-1})$	1	MS	$\dfrac{\mathrm{MS}(X_k \vert X_1, \ldots X_{k-1})}{\mathrm{MS}_r}$
Residual	SS_r	$n - k - 1$	MS_r	
Total	SS_t	$n - 1$		

The first two sums of squares are referred to as sequential or Type I sums of squares in many statistical packages. They have the characteristic that they sum to SS_{reg} as in Table 12.5. Note that this ANOVA table can only be used to test that one of the partial regression coefficients is equal to 0.

We would likely be interested in testing that each of the partial regression coefficients is zero, when adjustment has been made for all of the other X variables in the alternative model. To perform each of these tests, we need to know the sum of squares for each X after adjustment has been made for the other $k - 1$ variables (or the difference in residual sums of squares between each appropriate null model and the alternative model). These k sums of squares are referred to as *Type III* or *adjusted sums of squares* by many of the statistical packages. The k adjusted sums of squares do not add up to SS_{reg} for the k-variable regression model.

Example. The total sum of squares for the lung function example can be broken into three parts. Suppose that the three parts of interest are (1) regression of vital capacity on height, (2) regression of vital capacity on age after fitting height, and (3) residual after fitting both height and age. The corresponding ANOVA table is shown in Table 12.9. As the table is presented, it is used to test that the partial regression coefficient for age is 0 (when adjustment is made for height).

Table 12.10 presents the Type III or adjusted sums of squares as well as the calculated F and t statistics. Note that the sum of squares for the regression of age after height, given in Table 12.9, is a difference of residual sums of squares, and is equivalent to the sum of squares given in Table 12.10, 6.8. Recall from Table 12.2, that $\mathrm{SS}_r = 21.4$ when vital capacity was regressed on height. In Table 12.6, $\mathrm{SS}_r = 14.6$ when vital capacity was regressed on height and age. The difference in residual sums of squares is $21.4 - 14.6 = 6.8$. Similarly, the F and p values are equal. For each variable, the calculated F statistic is equal to the square of the t statistic, and the p values are equal.

Table 12.9   ANOVA Table for Testing that the Partial Regression Coefficient Associated with Age Is Zero

Source of Variation	SS	df	MS	F	p
Regression on height	20.7	1	20.7		
Regression on age after height	6.8	1	6.8	20.8	< 0.0001
Residual	14.6	45	0.325		
Total	42.1	47			

Table 12.10   Adjusted or Type III Sums of Squares, F Tests and t Tests for Testing That Each Partial Regression Coefficient Is Zero

Variable	Type III Sum of Squares	F	t	p
Height	22.4	69.0	8.30	< 0.0001
Age	6.8	20.8	−4.56	< 0.0001

Further comparisons of Table 12.9 with other tables in this chapter demonstrate that different ways of breaking apart a total sum of squares can be used to achieve different ends. For example, suppose the sums of squares in the first two rows of the table are summed. The total sum of squares is then broken into two parts, and an ANOVA table equivalent to that given in Table 12.6 is formed, which can be used to test the hypothesis that the partial regression coefficients for height and age are both zero. Suppose the sums of squares in the second and third rows are summed. The total sums of squares is then broken into two parts, and an ANOVA table equivalent to that given in Table 12.2, is formed which can be used to test whether the regression coefficient for height is zero, while ignoring age.

Since the total sums of squares can be broken apart in many different ways to perform different F tests, it can be seen that only two special cases have been considered here: tests that all partial regression coefficients are zero and that only one is zero. While these are the most common tests that are made, by breaking apart the sums of squares differently, tests that general subsets of the partial regression coefficients can also be made. More generally, we wish to compare two models, a null model H_0 (with some of the partial regression coefficients constrained to be zero) and an alternative model H_1 (without the constraints on the partial regression coefficients).

Suppose altogether there are k X variables and we wish to test that the partial regression coefficients associated with $k', \ldots, k$ are equal to 0, where $0 \leq k' \leq k - 1$. The null and alternative models are specified as:

$$H_0 : E(Y|X_1, \ldots, X_k) = \alpha + \beta_1 X_1 + \cdots + \beta_{k'} X_{k'}$$
$$H_1 : E(Y|X_1, \ldots, X_k) = \alpha + \beta_1 X_1 + \cdots + \beta_k X_k$$

Assuming H_0, a sample regression plane is fit and the residual sums of squares and corresponding degrees of freedom are defined. The equation for this plane is:

$$\hat{Y} = a^* + b_1^* X_1 + \cdots + b_{k'}^* X_{k'}. \tag{12.16}$$

The residual sum of squares, computed as $\sum_{l=1}^{n}(Y_l - \hat{Y}_l)^2$, is SS_r under H_0 and the corresponding degrees of freedom, $n - k' - 1$, is df under H_0.

Similarly, assuming H_1, a sample regression plane is fit and the residual sums of squares and corresponding degrees of freedom $(n - k - 1)$ are defined. The equation for this plane is:

$$\hat{Y} = a + b_1 X_1 + \cdots + b_k X_k. \tag{12.17}$$

The corresponding residual sum of squares, computed as $\sum_{l=1}^{n}(Y_l - \hat{Y}_l)^2$, is SS_r under H_1 and the corresponding degrees of freedom, $n - k - 1$ is df under H_1.

The F test can then be expressed as:

$$F = \frac{(SS_r \text{ under } H_0 - SS_r \text{ under } H_1)/(df_r \text{ under } H_0 - df_r \text{ under } H_1)}{SS_r \text{ under } H_1/df_r \text{ under } H_1}. \tag{12.18}$$

When H_0 is true (i.e. the subset of partial regression coefficients restrained to be 0 are indeed all equal to 0), the F statistic follows an F distribution with $\nu_1 = (df_r \text{ under } H_0 - df_r \text{ under } H_1) = k - k'$ and $\nu_2 = n - k - 1$. Alternative ways of expressing this F statistic which may or may not be appropriate in various situations are described in [13].

The two extremes are the testing situations we considered previously - that all k partial regression coefficients are zero (i.e. $k' = 0$) as discussed in Section 12.5.1 and that one partial regression coefficient is zero (i.e. $k' = k$) as described in Section 12.5.2.

12.6 CHECKING IF THE DATA FIT THE MULTIPLE REGRESSION MODEL

One measure of fit of the multiple regression model is the coefficient of determination, R^2, which was defined in Chapter 10 as the ratio of the regression sum of squares to the total sum of squares. This is interpreted as the proportion of variation in the dependent variable Y that is explained by the linear relation between Y and the linear combination of $X_1, \ldots, X_k$. There are a variety of ways of expressing R^2 in addition to the one used here. One alternative is $R^2 = 1 - SS_r/SS_t$. Anderson-Sprecher recommends this formulation [2], as the R^2 can be seen as 1 minus the ratio of two residual sums of squares: the SS_e is the residual sum of squares when the model $Y_i = \alpha + \beta_1 X_1 + \beta_2 X_2 + \cdots + \beta_k X_k + \varepsilon_i$ is fit and the SS_t is the residual sum of squares when the model $Y_i = \alpha + \varepsilon_i$ is fit. From this perspective, the R^2 involves the comparison of two models. A high R^2 indicates that the model with the k X variables provides a better fit than the model with only the intercept term, α. See [2, 11] for alternative ways of writing and interpreting the coefficient of determination.

To further evaluate the fit of the multiple regression model, we are concerned with the same assumptions that we were concerned with in Chapters 10 and 11 — looking for outliers, high leverage points, and influential points and checking for linearity, equal variances, and normality of errors. The procedures are mostly extensions or generalizations of what we've already described in Chapters 10 and 11. More complete coverage of these topics can be found elsewhere (for example, [3, 4, 5, 6, 8, 9]).

In this section, we focus on what is different when there are k X variables instead of just one. While it is always useful to use graphical or numerical summaries of data for one or two variables at a time, scatter diagrams of Y versus each of the k X's are less informative for checking the appropriateness of a multiple regression model. This is because we are interested in evaluating the relationship between Y and each X when we control for the linear effects of the other X variables, rather than the relationship between Y and each X when the other X variables are ignored. (Nevertheless, simple pairwise scatter plots of each X variable with each other X variable as well as of each X variable with the Y are useful an an initial screening tool. They are readily available in many software packages and can be examined for obvious outliers, linearity, and high correlations between two X variables.) However, we can still make extensive use of the residuals obtained from fitting a model.

12.6.1   Checking for Outlying, High Leverage and Influential Points

We search for outliers in the same way we did previously (Chapters 10 and 11), by examining unusual values of residuals, standardized residuals, or Studentized residuals (Section 11.5.1).

A commonly used measure of leverage in multiple regression is the hat-value (Section 11.5.1). There is still one hat value associated with each of the n observations; now, a large value indicates that at least one of the k X values is an outlier.

The identification of influential points can still be made using measures such as Cook's distance (Section 11.5.1). Plots of residuals, as in Figure 12.4, were used in Section 12.2 to interpret a partial regression coefficient, but they can also be used to identify influential points. For example, suppose we were to plot the residuals of Y (obtained by removing the linear effects of $X_2, \ldots, X_k$ on Y) versus the residuals of X_1 (obtained by removing the linear effects of $X_2, \ldots, X_k$ on X_1). Points that stand out, with large residuals for Y and large residuals for X_1, have more influence on the slope of the sample regression line than points that are very close to the line. Separate plots would need to be generated to evaluate influential points for each of the X variables. The plots are sometimes referred to as *partial regression plots* or as *added variable plots*.

Example. Going back to Figure 12.4, we see that there are no points that stand out as particularly unusual on this plot. For completeness, the plot of the residuals for vital capacity (adjusted for height) versus age (adjusted for height) should also be examined. However, no points were identified as standing out, and so the graph is not presented here.

12.6.2 Checking for Linearity

If the multiple regression model fits, the k plots of residuals ($e_i = Y - \hat{Y}$) versus each X should show no apparent patterns in the points. This is what we used in previous chapters, only now there are k plots to examine instead of one, since there are k independent variables. Standardized or Studentized residuals can also be used.

Example. To check that the assumption of linearity is satisfied in the vital capacity example, the residuals are plotted against height and against age, as in Figures 12.5 and 12.6. Since there are no apparent patterns in the data points, we can conclude that the assumption of linearity is satisfied.

12.6.3 Checking for Equality of Variances

As before, the plots that were used to check for linearity can also be used to check for equality of variances. There should be no trend of increasing or decreasing spread as values of each X are increased or decreased. Similarly, the plot of residuals e_i versus the fitted values $\hat{Y}$ should also show no trend. Standardized or Studentized residuals can also be used.

Example. The two plots that were used to check for linearity can also be used to check for equality of variances (see Figures 12.5 and 12.6). Since there is no apparent trend in the spread of the points, these plots suggest

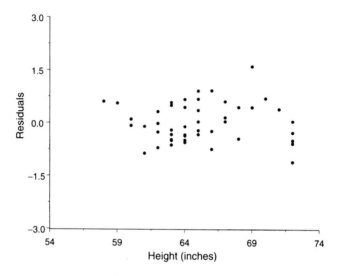

Fig. 12.5   Residuals versus height.

that the variance of vital capacity measurements does not change with values of either height or age. Similarly, there is also no trend in the spread of points when residuals are plotted against fitted values in Figure 12.7. This suggests that the variance of vital capacity measurements (for given height and age) does not change with values of vital capacity. There is no indication that the assumption of equality of variances is not satisfied.

12.6.4   Checking for Normality of Errors

We investigate whether the errors are normally distributed in exactly the same way that we did in Chapters 10 and 11. We can look for a straight line on a normal quantile plot or on a normal, bell-shaped stem and leaf diagram or histogram.

12.6.5   Other Potential Problems

In the example we have discussed in this chapter, there were no missing data. However, missing data can become a problem when there are many X variables included in the analysis. Each variable by itself might not have a lot of missing values, but the observations that are missing for one variable might not be the same as those missing for another variable. Because regression analyses are restricted to complete cases, any case with at least one missing value is eliminated. Thus, it is possible that a large proportion of the cases are not included in the analysis and this can make the analysis suspect.

It is always important to check the number of cases that are actually included in the regression analysis and to report that number. If one X has numerous missing values and is not essential to the regression analysis, it may be sensible simply not to include that variable in the set that is used for the analysis. Note that most statistical packages will allow the user to control what variables can be entered into the regression analysis. For further discussion of performing regression analyses with missing values, see Little [12]. A highly readable introduction to missing values is given by Allison [1]. Horton and Lipsitz provide a review of the various statistical packages that are used to replace missing values in regression analyses [10]. The replacement of missing values with data derived from other data in the sample (imputation) is one of the most commonly used methods.

Sometimes, when many X variables are included in a model or when the X variables are highly correlated with each other, the estimated standard errors of the sample partial regression coefficients can become large. Consequently, confidence intervals for the partial regression coefficients can become so wide that they aren't meaningful and test statistics for the individual partial regression coefficients are small. It is difficult to estimate the standard errors when the X variables are highly correlated. There isn't a problem with the overall test that all partial regression coefficients are zero; this test does not

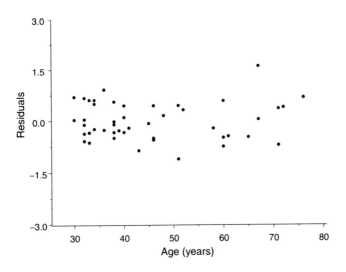

Fig. 12.6 Residuals versus age.

depend on the ability to estimate the standard errors. It is not unusual to obtain a significant overall test but find that none of the individual partial regression coefficients are significantly different from 0. When this occurs, there are likely too many variables included in the regression model.

Statistical packages usually print out the correlation of each X variable with every other X variable. Either these correlations or the pairwise scatter plots should be checked to see if two or more X's are highly correlated. If two X's are highly correlated, the simplest solution is to omit one of them. Many statistical packages also print out a factor called *tolerance*, a measure of how highly correlated an X variable is with the other X variables in the regression equation. If the tolerance is less than 0.01, a problem with collinearity (sometimes called multicollinearity) may exist. This may lead to inaccurate regression coefficients and large estimated standard errors. One simple method for improving the accuracy of regression coefficients is to compute the standardized coefficients [7]. This tends to reduce the effect of roundoff error.

12.7   WHAT TO DO IF THE DATA DON'T FIT THE MODEL

If large violations of the assumptions of the multiple regression model are detected, transforming the data is a commonly used solution. Common transformations include the log and square root transformation. We refer the reader

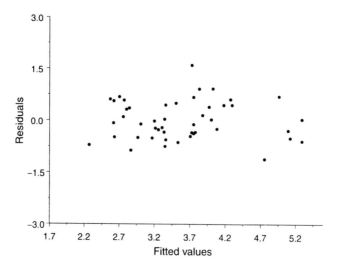

Fig. 12.7 Residuals versus fitted values.

to discussions of transformations in earlier chapters, such as Chapters 1 and 10. Generally, it is preferable to transform an X variable rather than the Y; a transformation in Y can affect its relationship with each of the X variables and influence the distribution of the errors [8]. It is always a good idea to recheck whether the assumptions of the multiple regression model are satisfied after making transformations.

12.8 SUMMARY

In this chapter, we extended simple linear regression (regression with only one X variable, as described in Chapters 10 and 11) to multiple regression (regression with more than one X variable). We introduced the subject in terms of an example with two X variables. In this context, we considered how to estimate a sample regression plane, and we described alternative ways of interpreting the *partial* regression coefficients.

We introduced the multiple regression model and its accompanying assumptions. Once this model was specified, we discussed how to make inferences about the partial regression coefficients and the population regression plane. We described how to construct and interpret confidence intervals and how to make hypothesis tests. With multiple X variables, there is a greater number of hypothesis tests which may be of interest. We described an overall F test for testing that all of the partial regression coefficients are 0, and both t and F tests for testing that a single partial regression coefficient is 0.

We described and illustrated ways to check the appropriateness of the multiple regression model through identifying outliers and high leverage and influential points and through checking the assumptions of linearity, equality of variances, and normality of the distribution of errors. Most of these procedures depended on the residuals obtained from fitting the models. We focused on transforming variables as a means of respecifying the multiple regression model so that its assumptions are more nearly satisfied.

Though we included many expressions and formulas in Chapters 10 and 11, there was very little use of these in this chapter. This is because the concepts were easier to understand in the context of simple linear regression and the appropriate expressions are generalizations of what was specified in the earlier chapters. Our objective was to gain understanding of the concepts in the simpler case, and to rely on the computer to produce appropriate analyses in the more complex cases.

In the next chapter, we extend the concept of correlation from two variables to multiple variables.

Problems

12.1 On the basis of eight patients who underwent a thyroid operation, an attempt was made to determine factors related to blood loss. Measurements of weight, duration of operation, and blood loss for the eight cases were as follows:

X_1 Weight (kg)	X_2 Duration (min)	Y Blood Loss (ml)
44.3	105	503
40.6	80	490
69.0	86	471
43.7	112	505
50.3	109	482
50.2	100	490
35.4	96	513
52.2	120	464

a)   Plot blood loss versus weight and blood loss versus duration.

b)   What do the two scatter diagrams suggest about the relation between blood loss and 1) weight and 2) duration?

c)   Find the sample regression plane, fitting blood loss to weight (kg) and duration (min). Interpret the partial regression coefficients for weight and duration. Determine the standardized sample regression coefficients.

d)   Regress blood loss on duration of operation, and compute residuals for blood loss (with linear effects of duration of operation removed). Regress weight on duration of operation, and compute residuals for weight (with linear effects of duration of operation removed). Construct a scatter diagram of the residuals for blood loss versus the residuals for weight. Determine the same regression line, and verify that the slope of this line is equal to the partial regression coefficient for weight, determined in the previous subproblem.

e)   Transform weight in kilograms to weight in pounds (1 kg = 2.2046 lb). Find the sample regression plane, fitting blood loss to weight (lb) and duration of operation (min). Interpret the partial regression coefficients for weight and duration. Determine the standardized sample regression coefficients.

f)   Compare and contrast regression output (such as sample regression coefficients, F and t statistics, percentage of variation explained by the linear regression of Y on X_1 and X_2, standardized sample regression coefficients) when analyses were performed with weight measured in (a) kilograms and (b) pounds.

12.2   It was of interest to predict the change of hemoglobin resulting from thyroid operations. Blood loss (in milliliters), duration of operation (in minutes), and hemoglobin percentage change recorded on eight patients were as follows:

X_1 Blood Loss (ml)	X_2 Duration (min)	Y Hemoglobin Change (%)
405	140	-7.0
401	90	-6.2
710	99	-0.5
280	112	-1.1
502	97	-4.3
691	108	-1.0
370	120	-5.9
486	65	-10.2

a) Regress hemoglobin change on blood loss and duration of operation. Obtain an ANOVA table, and test $H_0 : E(Y|X_1, X_2) = \alpha$. Test $H_0 : E(Y|X_1, X_2) = \alpha + \beta_1 X_1$ with a t test (use level of significance, $\alpha = 0.05$).

b) Regress hemoglobin change on blood loss. Using the residual sums of squares obtained from this part and part (a), test $H_0 : E(Y|X_1, X_2) = \alpha + \beta_1 X_1$ with an F test. Verify that the square of the t statistic obtained in the previous subproblem is equal to the F statistic calculated here, namely, $t^2 = F$.

12.3 This problem makes use of the rye yield, yearly rainfall, and temperature data given in Problem 11.4. To predict the yield of rye Y from yearly rainfall X_1 and temperature X_2, data were collected as follows:

a) State the multiple regression model, including all assumptions, in terms of this problem.

b) Compute the sample regression plane fitting rye yields to rainfall and temperature.

c) Predict the rye yield at $X_1 = \bar{X}_1 = 37.32$ and $X_2 = \bar{X}_2 = 54.01$. Compute a 95% confidence interval for average rye yield, and calculate the length of the interval.

d) Predict the rye yield at $X_1 = 25$ and $X_2 = 38$. Compute a 95% confidence interval for average rye yield at these values of rainfall and temperature and calculate the length of the interval. Why is this confidence interval wider than the one computed in part(c)?

e) Evaluate the appropriateness of the assumptions of the multiple regression model. Construct a normal quantile plot of the residuals. Plot residuals versus rainfall and residuals versus temperature. Are there any outliers? What assumptions, if any, of the multiple regression model may be violated?

12.4 Data on altitude, longitude, latitude, and mean temperature were recorded for 16 cities:

X_1 Altitude (ft)	X_2 Longitude (deg)	X_3 Latitude (deg)	Y Temperature (°F)
1083	112	33	55.7
457	86	38	37.8
312	118	34	56.4
305	90	32	51.0
5221	105	40	34.5
2842	116	44	34.0
807	94	41	36.7
4260	112	41	33.4
815	83	40	32.6
3920	106	32	49.1
1054	84	34	46.6
4397	120	39	36.3
830	93	45	18.2
465	90	39	36.7
1162	92	47	13.3
787	82	41	30.1

a)   Find the least squares plane fitting temperature to altitude, longitude, and latitude. Predict the temperature for a city whose latitude is 1700 ft, whose longitude is 100 degree and whose latitude is 40 degree. Determine a 95% confidence interval for the mean temperature for such a city.

b)   Break the total variation in temperature into four parts: (1) variation due to regression of temperature on latitude, (2) variation due to longitude after latitude, (3) variation due to altitude after longitude and latitude, and (4) residual. Complete the ANOVA table.

c)   Make the several F tests which your completed ANOVA table enables you to make. For each test, state the assumptions and the null and alternative hypotheses in terms of $E(Y|X_1, X_2, X_3)$.

12.5   Use the cardiac rehabilitation data given on the Wiley ftp site to investigate the relationship between self-reported physical functioning after completion of the cardiac rehabilitation program (mospost) and age, sex, and self-reported physical functioning before rehabilitation (mospre).

a)   Describe the distributions of mospre, mospost, and age. Do they appear to be normal?

b)   Regress self-reported physical functioning after cardiac rehabilitation (mospost) on (1) age alone, (2) sex alone, (3) mospre alone. What percentage of the variation in mospost is explained by the linear relation between mospost and (1) age, (2) sex, and (3) mospre?

c)   Regress self-reported physical functioning after cardiac rehabilitation (mospost) on age, sex, and mospre. What percentage of the variation in mospost is explained by the linear relation between mospost and age, sex, and mospre?

d)   Check the sample size that was used in the regression analyses performed in the two previous subproblems. What does this suggest about a problem that can occur when many X variables are included in a multiple regression model?

REFERENCES

1. Allison, P.D. [2002]. *Missing Data*, Sage University Paper 136, Thousand Oaks, CA: Sage Publications Inc., 1–55.

2. Anderson-Sprecher, R. [1994]. Model Comparisons and R^2, *The American Statistician*, 48, 113–116.

3. Belsey, D.A., Kuh, E., and Welsch, R.E. [1980]. *Regression Diagnostics: Identifying Influential Data and Sources of Collinearity*, New York: John Wiley & Sons, 6–84.

4. Birkes, D. and Dodge, Y. [1993]. *Alternative Methods of Regression*, New York: John Wiley & Sons.

5. Chatterjee, S. and Hadi, A.S. [1988]. *Sensitivity Analysis in Linear Regression*, New York: John Wiley & Sons, 71–127.

6. Cook, R.D. [1977]. Detection of Influential Observation in Linear Regression, *Technometrics*, 19, 15–18.

7. Dillon, W.R. and Goldstein, M. [1984]. *Multivariate Analysis: Methods and Applications*, New York: John Wiley & Sons, 281–282.

8. Fox, J. [1991]. *Regression Diagnostics: An Introduction*, Sage University Paper Series on Quantitative Applications in the Social Sciences, 07-079. Newbury Park, CA: Sage, 58–59.

9. Hoaglin, D.C. and Welsch, R.E. [1978]. The Hat Matrix in Regression and ANOVA, *The American Statistician*, 32, 17–22.

10. Horton, N.J. and Lipsitz, S.R. [2001]. Multiple Imputation in Practice: Comparison of Software Packages for Regression Models with Missing Variables, *The American Statistician*, 55, 244–254.

11. Kvalseth, T.O. [1985]. Cautionary Note About R^2, *The American Statistician*, 39, 279–285.

12. Little, R.J.A. [1992]. Regression with Missing X's: A Review, *Journal of the American Statistical Association*, 87, 1727–1737.

13. Peixoto, J.L. [1993]. Incorrect F Formulas in Regression Analysis, *The American Statistician*, 47, 194–197.

13

Multiple and Partial Correlation

In this chapter, the methods of Chapter 11 are extended from two to more than two variables. Recall that the simple correlation between two variables is a measure of the strength of linear relation between them. There are a variety of ways to extend the simple correlation, and we consider two here. One involves the correlation between a single variable and a linear combination of the others; this is referred to as *multiple correlation*. The second concerns the correlation between two variables when adjustment is made for the linear effects of other variables; this is called *partial correlation*.

There is much in common between the contents of this chapter and Chapter 12 on multiple regression, but there are also important conceptual differences. In regression, a greater distinction is made between a Y variable and a set of X variables. Correlation analyses are also relevant for sets of variables which are regarded equally, without distinction as to being dependent or independent. For example, if investigators have made determinations of multiple blood chemistry measures or of multiple measures of water quality, they may want to study how these variables are interrelated, not only how one variable in particular is related to the others. The focus of correlation analyses is more on determining the strengths of the linear associations among all the variables. Often, investigators are interested in performing both regression and correlation analyses.

Because of the large overlap between regression and correlation, the majority of statistical software packages do not have separate procedures for the.. Regression procedures typically offer options for performing correlation analyses.

In Section 13.1 a data example in which both multiple and partial correlation are relevant is introduced. The concept of multiple correlation is considered in Section 13.2 and, the concept of partial correlation in Section 13.3. In Section 13.4 the joint distribution model is presented; the parameters that define this distribution are expressed in terms of both multiple and partial correlations. In Section 13.5 inferences about the multiple correlation are described, and in Section 13.6 inferences about partial correlation coefficients are considered. These are followed by brief sections on checking whether the joint distribution model is appropriate (Section 13.7) and what to consider if the model is not appropriate (Section 13.8). The chapter is summarized in Section 13.9.

13.1 EXAMPLE

The example that was used in Chapter 12 is also an appropriate illustration for this chapter on correlation. Recall that observations were made on lung function, age, and height for $n = 48$ individuals. The simple correlations among the three variables can be summarized in a 3 by 3 correlation matrix, with rows and columns ordered as vital capacity, height, age:

$$\begin{pmatrix} 1.00 & 0.70 & -0.35 \\ 0.70 & 1.00 & 0.07 \\ -0.35 & 0.07 & 1.00 \end{pmatrix}.$$

Now, we want to make use of all the variables simultaneously, rather than just two at a time. We consider two ways to do this. First, what is the correlation between vital capacity and a linear combination of height and age? This is referred to as the multiple correlation of vital capacity with height and age. We anticipate that the correlation of vital capacity with both height and age should be at least as strong as its correlation with height or with age alone. Second, what is the correlation between vital capacity and height if we remove the effects of or control for age? This is referred to as the partial correlation between vital capacity and height when adjustment is made for age. The matrix of the simple correlations indicates that vital capacity is fairly highly correlated with height and moderately correlated with age, whereas height and age are essentially uncorrelated. We anticipate that removing effects of age on height would likely have little effect, because of the small correlation between height and age; we may anticipate greater effect of removing effects of age on vital capacity, as these are more highly correlated.

In this example, there is particular interest in vital capacity as the outcome and in its relation to height and age. As in the previous chapter, we refer to vital capacity as the Y variable and to height and age as the X variables. (Note that if we weren't making any distinction between dependent and independent variables as we are in this example, alternative notation, such as X_1, X_2, X_3, could have just as easily been used.)

13.2   THE SAMPLE MULTIPLE CORRELATION COEFFICIENT

We now wish to generalize the concept of the correlation coefficient to the situation with measures on $X_1, \ldots, X_k$ and Y. To obtain an idea of the strength of the linear relationship between Y and $X_1, \ldots, X_k$, we might calculate the simple correlation coefficients $r_{X_1 Y}, \ldots, r_{X_k Y}$; as a set, however, these seem to be difficult to interpret, and we look instead for a single statistic.

We will use the properties of the simple correlation between one X and Y to explain the sample multiple correlation coefficient. The simple correlationbetween X and Y is estimated as

$$ r = \frac{\sum_{i=1}^{n} (Y_i - \bar{Y})(X_i - \bar{X})}{\sqrt{\sum_{i=1}^{n}(Y_i - \bar{Y})^2 \sum_{i=1}^{n}(X_i - \bar{X})^2}}. $$

Now, consider the correlation calculated between Y (the observed values of Y) and $\hat{Y} = a + bX$, $r_{Y,\hat{Y}}$. [Note that $\bar{\hat{Y}} = \bar{Y}$ and $\hat{Y}_i - \bar{Y} = b(X_i - \bar{X})$]:

$$ r_{Y,\hat{Y}} = \frac{\sum_{i=1}^{n}(Y_i - \bar{Y})[b(X_i - \bar{X})]}{\sqrt{\sum_{i=1}^{n}(Y_i - \bar{Y})^2 \sum_{i=1}^{n}[b(X_i - \bar{X})]^2}} $$

$$ = \frac{br}{|b|} $$

$$ = |r|. $$

Thus, the magnitude of the correlation between Y and X is the same as the correlation between Y and $a + bX$. However, the signs may or may not be equal. The correlation between the observed and predicted values of Y can range from 0 to 1; thus $r_{Y,\hat{Y}} = |r_{X,Y}|$. (Recall that the slope b has the same sign as the correlation r. If the correlation between Y and X is positive, the correlation between Y and $a + bX$ is also positive. If the correlation between Y and X is negative, the correlation between the observed and predicted values of Y is positive.)

Extending this idea further, the *sample multiple correlation* of Y with $X_1, \ldots, X_k$ is defined as the simple correlation coefficient between Y and its fitted value $\hat{Y}$, determined from the least squares regression plane. It is denoted here by $R_{Y|X_1 \ldots X_k}$ or simply by R. Thus we have

$$ R_{Y|X_1 \ldots X_k} = r_{Y,\hat{Y}} \qquad \text{where} \quad \hat{Y} = a + b_1 X_1 + \cdots + b_k X_k. $$

That is, after fitting a least squares plane using a sample of size n, the multiple correlation can be calculated as the simple correlation between the observed and fitted values. The multiple correlation coefficient, as we have estimated it, is the *maximum* correlation between Y and any linear combination of the X.

Because $R_{Y|X_1 \ldots X_k} = r_{Y,\hat{Y}}$, the multiple correlation coefficient reduces to the simple correlation coefficient between X_1 and Y (except for a possible sign difference), when k is 1.

Example. The sample regression plane obtained when vital capacity was regressed on both height and weight was $\hat{Y} = -7.6 + 0.19 \times \text{height} - 0.028 \times \text{age}$. A plot of the observed versus predicted value of vital capacity is given in Figure 13.1. The simple correlation between vital capacity Y and its predicted value $\hat{Y}$ is 0.81. Thus, the multiple correlation between vital capacity and the linear combination of height and weight is $R = 0.81$. This multiple correlation is greater in magnitude than the simple correlation of vital capacity with height (0.70) or with age (−0.35).

The square of the sample multiple correlation, R^2, also has an interpretation. This statistic can be expressed as the ratio of SS_{reg} to SS_t, obtained from the regression of Y on $X_1, \ldots, X_k$:

$$R^2 = \frac{\text{SS}_{reg}}{\text{SS}_t} = 1 - \frac{\text{SS}_r}{\text{SS}_t}.$$

This is the same expression as for the square of the coefficient of determination defined in Section 10.7. Thus, R^2 is also the proportion of the variation in Y

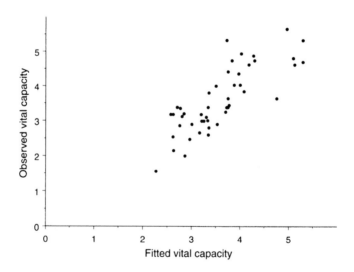

Fig. 13.1 Scatter diagram of observed vital capacity versus vital capacity predicted from height and age.

(SS_t) explained by the linear relation between Y and the linear combination of the X variables (SS_{reg}).

Example. The square of the sample correlation coefficient is $(0.81)^2 = 0.65$. From the ANOVA table given in Table 12.6, the ratio of the SS_{reg} to SS_t is $27.5/42.1 = 0.65$. That is, 65% of the variation in vital capacity is explained by the linear regression of vital capacity on height and age.

13.3   THE SAMPLE PARTIAL CORRELATION COEFFICIENT

There are many ways that investigators have chosen to explain the linear relationship between two variables. One approach is to ignore any other variables and focus only on the two. This approach has the advantage of simplicity but seems unsatisfactory and can in fact be misleading. When considering a correlation coefficient that has been calculated between two variables, say Y and X_1, we often wonder whether r_{X_1Y} can be explained in terms of another variable X_2. This is a natural question if we are trying to explain an apparent relationship. For example, if we obtained a correlation of 0.8 between mental age and height among children, an early thought in interpreting this correlation (rather than plunging into discussions of whether height affects intelligence or intelligence affects height) would be that both variables might be correlated with chronological age. Would there be any correlation between mental age and height if we took children of the same chronological age?

To examine the correlation between mental age and height while controlling for chronological age, we remove the *linear effects* of chronological age from our data on mental age and on height and correlate what is left over. To do this, we regress mental age on chronological age ($\hat{Y} = a + b_2X_2$) and we regress height on chronological age ($\hat{X}_1 = a^* + b_2^*X_2$). The linear effects of chronological age on mental age can be obtained by determining the residuals $Y - \hat{Y}$, and the linear effects of chronological age on height can be obtained by determining the residuals $X_1 - \hat{X}_1$. Having removed the linear effect of chronological age, we correlate the residuals. The correlation between the residuals is the *sample partial correlation*. In particular, it is the sample partial correlation between chronological age and height when the linear effects of mental age are removed. It is denoted here by $r_{YX_1|X_2}$.

Example. The partial correlation between vital capacity and height when the linear effects of age are removed is 0.78. To verify this, we can regress vital capacity on age and regress height on age, determine the residuals, and compute the simple correlation of the residuals. The sample regression line estimated when vital capacity Y is regressed on age (X_2) is

$$\hat{Y} = 4.7 - 0.024X_2,$$

and the residuals are computed as $Y - \hat{Y}$. Similarly, the sample regression line estimated when height (X_1) is regressed on age (X_2) is

$$\hat{X}_1 = 64.2 + 0.02X_2$$

and the residuals are computed as $X_1 - \hat{X}_1$. Figure 13.2 displays a scatter diagram of the residuals for vital capacity versus the residuals for height. The simple correlation of the 48 pairs of residuals (i.e., the sample partial correlation between vital capacity and height when adjustment is made for age) is 0.78. (Recall that the simple correlation between vital capacity and height, with no adjustment for age is slightly lower, 0.70.)

The sample partial correlation can be expressed in terms of the simple correlations among the variables. For example, the sample partial correlation $r_{X_1Y|X_2}$ can be expressed as

$$r_{X_1Y|X_2} = \frac{r_{X_1Y} - r_{X_2Y}r_{X_1X_2}}{\sqrt{(1 - r^2_{X_2Y})(1 - r^2_{X_1X_2})}}. \tag{13.1}$$

Examining this formula is instructive, as it can provide some insight into why a partial correlation may be greater than, less than, or equal to the simple correlation between two variables. For example, when r_{X_2Y} and $r_{X_1X_2}$ are

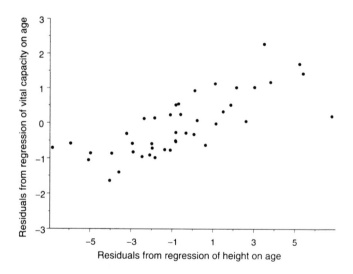

Fig. 13.2 Residuals from the regression of vital capacity on age versus residuals from the regression of height on age.

both equal to 0, $r_{X_1Y|X_2}$ is equal to r_{X_1Y}. This makes sense, as knowing the value of X_2 provides no information about Y or X_1.

We would also like to know under what conditions a partial correlation is larger (in magnitude) than a simple correlation. In this case, by not adjusting for a third variable, a researcher could be misled into thinking that the strength of the linear relationship between the two is lower than it is. Similarly, we would like to know under what conditions a partial correlation is smaller (in magnitude) than a simple correlation. Here, by not controlling for the third variable, a researcher could be misled into thinking that the strength of the linear relationship between the two is greater than it actually is. Unfortunately, there are no definite answers to these questions, but general statements can be made.

Suppose r_{X_1Y} is positive and $r_{X_1X_2} = 0$ (that is, the simple correlation between the two X variables is 0). Then the simple correlation between X_1 and Y is divided by $\sqrt{1 - r_{X_2Y}^2}$, a number between 0 and 1. Thus, adjustment for X_2 has the effect of increasing the strength of the correlation; the partial correlation between X_1 and Y is further from 0 than the simple correlation. Similarly, suppose r_{X_1Y} is negative and $r_{X_1X_2} = 0$. Then adjustment for X_2 has the effect of increasing the strength of the correlation; the partial correlation is more negative than the simple correlation.

It is usually the case that when all variables are positively correlated with each other, the partial correlation $r_{X_1Y|X_2}$ is less than the simple correlation r_{X_1Y}. This seems reasonable, as the effect of a common variable has been removed in a linear fashion. But if one of the correlations, say $r_{X_1X_2}$ is negative, then $r_{X_1Y|X_2}$ is greater than the simple correlation r_{X_1Y}. (These statements are general, and counterexamples can be found; they depend on the relative sizes of the numerator and denominator of Equation 13.1. Of course, it is more difficult to make statements such as these when adjustment is made for more than one variable.)

Example. This lung function example illustrates how a partial correlation can be greater in magnitude than a simple correlation. The simple correlation between vital capacity and height is 0.7, and the partial correlation between vital capacity and height (adjusted for age) is 0.78. We note that the correlation between vital capacity and age is negative (-0.35) while the correlation between height and age is positive (0.07). The simple correlation between vital capacity and age is -0.35, and the partial correlation between these two variables (adjusted for height) is -0.56. We note that the correlation between vital capacity and height is positive (0.70) as is the correlation between age and height (0.07).

It is not surprising that the partial correlations would be greater in magnitude than the simple correlations when we look at Equation 13.1. The numerators are little changed by the subtraction of the product of the simple correlations (the simple correlation between age and height was 0.07, essentially 0), but the denominators are less than 1 because of the correlations with vital capacity. The positive correlation between vital capacity and height is inflated when adjustment is made for age as is the negative correlation between vital capacity and age when adjustment is made for height.

The square of a sample partial correlation coefficient also has an interpretation. It can be expressed in terms of residual sums of squares obtained when an additional variable has and has not been included in a model. For example, suppose we are interested in the square of the partial correlation between X_1 and Y, when adjustment for $X_2, \ldots, X_k$ is made. Then we can verify that

$$r^2_{X_1 Y | X_2 \ldots X_k} = \frac{\mathrm{SS}_r(X_2, \ldots X_k) - \mathrm{SS}_r(X_1, \ldots, X_k)}{\mathrm{SS}_r(X_2, \ldots, X_k)}. \tag{13.2}$$

where $\mathrm{SS}_r(X_2, \ldots, X_k)$ denotes the residual sum of squares obtained when Y is regressed on $X_2, \ldots, X_k$, and $\mathrm{SS}_r(X_1, \ldots, X_k)$ denotes the residual sum of squares when Y is regressed on $X_1, X_2, \ldots, X_k$. Here $\mathrm{SS}_r(X_2, \ldots, X_k)$ is always at least $\mathrm{SS}_r(X_1, \ldots, X_k)$, so it is clear that the square of the sample partial correlation ranges between 0 and 1 and can be interpreted as a proportion. It is the proportion of the variation in Y that is explained by the regression of Y on $X_1, \ldots, X_k$, after adjustment has been made for the regression of Y on $X_2, \ldots, X_k$. Equivalently, it can be interpreted as the reduction in the residual sum of squares when X_1 has been added to a model that already included $X_2, \ldots, X_k$.

Note that we can also calculate the partial correlation between any two variables after removing the linear effects of two or more other variables. Here the residuals are calculated as deviations from the regression planes on the variables whose effects the investigator wishes to remove. The partial correlation is still a simple correlation between the residuals.

Example. The square of the sample partial correlation between vital capacity and height, when age is fixed, is $(0.78)^2$, or 0.61. In Chapter 12, the SS_r obtained from the regression of vital capacity on age was 37.0, and the SS_r obtained from the regression of vital capacity on height and age was 14.6. Thus, $r^2_{X_1 Y | X_2}$ is $(37.0 - 14.6)/37.0 = 0.61$. In addition to being the square of the sample partial correlation coefficient, we would say that after adjustment for age, 61% of the variation in vital capacity is explained by the linear relation between vital capacity and height.

13.4   THE JOINT DISTRIBUTION MODEL

In Chapter 11, the joint distribution model was introduced in the context of a single Y and single X variable. The two variables were assumed to be jointly normally distributed. From this assumption, the conditional distribution of $Y|X$ could be determined as a normal distribution with mean

$$E(Y|X) = \mu_{Y|X} = \mu_Y + \frac{\rho \sigma_Y}{\sigma_X}(X - \mu_X) \tag{13.3}$$

and variance

$$\text{Var}(Y|X) = \sigma_{Y|X}^2 = \sigma^2(1 - \rho^2). \tag{13.4}$$

Both the mean and variance could be expressed in terms of ρ.

In this chapter, there is a Y variable and a set of X variables, $X_1, \ldots, X_k$, which are jointly normally distributed. Each of these $k + 1$ variables is then normally distributed with some mean and variance. The joint distribution is defined in terms of the means of these $k + 1$ variables $(\mu_Y, \mu_{X_1}, \ldots, \mu_{X_k})$, the variances of these $k + 1$ variables $(\sigma_Y^2, \sigma_{X_1}^2, \ldots \sigma_{X_k}^2)$, and the $k(k + 1)/2$ covariances or correlations between the variables. As in the context of regression, we are interested in the conditional distribution $Y|X_1, \ldots, X_k$, which is normally distributed with a mean and a variance which can be expressed in terms of the population multiple and partial correlations.

For simplicity, consider the special case of $k = 2$. So there are three variables, X_1, X_2, Y. The $Y|X_1, X_2$ is normally distributed with mean

$$
\begin{aligned}
E(Y|X_1, X_2) &= \mu_{Y|X_1, X_2} \\
&= \mu_Y + \frac{\rho_{X_1 Y|X_2} \sigma_{Y|X_2}}{\sigma_{X_1|X_2}}(X_1 - \mu_{X_1}) \\
&\quad + \frac{\rho_{X_2 Y|X_1} \sigma_{Y|X_1}}{\sigma_{X_2|X_1}}(X_2 - \mu_{X_2})
\end{aligned}
\tag{13.5}
$$

and variance

$$\text{Var}(Y|X_1, X_2) = \sigma_{Y|X_1, X_2}^2 = \sigma_Y^2(1 - \rho_{Y|X_1 X_2}^2). \tag{13.6}$$

Here, the population multiple correlation coefficient is denoted $\rho_{Y|X_1 X_2}$ and the partial correlation coefficients are denoted $\rho_{X_1 Y|X_2}$ and $\rho_{X_2 Y|X_1}$. These parameters will be described in Sections 13.4.1 and 13.4.2.

The conditional variance can also be expressed in terms of the population partial correlation coefficients:

$$
\begin{aligned}
\text{Var}(Y|X_1, X_2) &= \sigma_{Y|X_1, X_2}^2 \\
&= \sigma_{Y|X_1}^2(1 - \rho_{X_2 Y|X_1}^2) \\
&= \sigma_{Y|X_2}^2(1 - \rho_{X_1 Y|X_2}^2).
\end{aligned}
\tag{13.7}
$$

More generally, for k X variables,

$$E(Y|X_1,\ldots,X_k) = \mu_{Y|X_1\ldots X_k}$$

$$= \mu_Y + \frac{\rho_{X_1Y|X_2\ldots,X_k}\sigma_{Y|X_2,\ldots,X_k}}{\sigma_{X_1|X_2,\ldots,X_k}}(X_1 - \mu_{X_1}) + \cdots$$

$$+ \frac{\rho_{X_kY|.X_1,\ldots,X_{k-1}}\sigma_{Y|X_1,\ldots,X_{k-1}}}{\sigma_{X_k|X_1,\ldots,X_{k-1}}}(X_k - \mu_{X_k}) \quad (13.8)$$

and

$$\mathrm{Var}(Y|X_1,\ldots,X_k) = \sigma^2_{Y|X_1,\ldots,X_k} = \sigma^2_Y(1 - \rho^2_{Y|X_1,\ldots,X_k}). \quad (13.9)$$

13.4.1   The Population Multiple Correlation Coefficient

The population multiple correlation coefficient corresponding to $R_{Y|X_1\ldots X_k}$ is denoted by $\rho_{Y|X_1\ldots X_k}$. It is defined by

$$\rho^2_{Y|X_1\ldots X_k} = 1 - \frac{\sigma^2_{Y|X_1,\ldots,X_k}}{\sigma^2_Y}, \quad (13.10)$$

where $\sigma^2_{Y|X_1,\ldots,X_k}$ is the variance of a population of Y's conditioned on $X_1,\ldots,X_k$, and σ^2_Y is the variance of the population of all possible Y's.

From examining Equation 13.10, we can determine some properties of $\rho^2_{Y|X_1,\ldots,X_k}$. First, it can vary between 0 and 1. Similarly, the σ^2, the variance of the Y distributions for given values of $X_1,\ldots X_k$ (or about the population regression plane) must always be less than or equal to the variance of all possible Y's. $\rho^2_{Y|X_1,\ldots,X_k}$ is equal to 1 when σ^2 is 0. That is, once $X_1,\ldots,X_k$ are specified, Y is known without error; all possible observations must fall on the population regression plane. At the other extreme, $\rho^2_{Y|X_1,\ldots,X_k}$ is equal to 0 when σ^2 is equal to σ^2_Y. This situation will arise when $X_1,\ldots,X_k$ provides no information about Y.

13.4.2   The Population Partial Correlation Coefficient

The partial regression coefficients for the population regression line are expressed as functions of the population partial correlation coefficients and conditional standard deviations. For example, for X_1,

$$\beta_1 = \frac{\rho_{X_1Y|X_2,\ldots,X_k}\sigma_{Y|X_2,\ldots,X_k}}{\sigma_{X_1|X_2,\ldots,X_k}}.$$

Similarly, the population partial correlation coefficients can be expressed in terms of the partial regression coefficients and conditional standard deviations. For example,

$$\rho_{X_1 Y | X_2, \ldots, X_k} = \frac{\beta_1 \sigma_{X_1 | X_2, \ldots, X_k}}{\sigma_{Y | X_2, \ldots, X_k}}.$$

From these equations, it is apparent that the partial correlation between X_1 and Y must have the same sign as the partial regression coefficient; the standard deviations must be nonnegative.

13.5   INFERENCES FOR THE MULTIPLE CORRELATION COEFFICIENT

Inferences for the multiple correlation coefficient are based on the assumptions of the joint distribution model, as given in Section 13.4. Most regression programs routinely report hypothesis tests, but confidence intervals for correlation coefficients are not generally available.

An inference that a multiple correlation coefficient is greater than 0 suggests that a linear combination of the X variables is linearly related to Y. Knowing the measured values of the X variables can provide some indication of the value of Y. This doesn't mean that the X variables are causally related to Y.

As indicated above by Equation 13.10, the population multiple correlation coefficient is equal to 0 when $\sigma^2_{Y | X_1, \ldots, X_k}$ is equal to σ^2_Y. That is, knowing $X_1, \ldots, X_k$ provides no indication about Y. So the null hypothesis

$$H_0 : \rho_{Y | X_1, \ldots, X_k} = 0$$

is equivalent to the null hypothesis that all partial regression coefficients $\beta_1, \ldots, \beta_k$ are equal to 0. The sums of squares and mean squares given in Table 12.5 in Chapter 12 can be reexpressed in terms of the sample multiple correlation, as in Table 13.1.

The null hypothesis that $\rho_{Y | X_1, \ldots, X_k} = 0$ is sometimes expressed as $\rho^2_{Y | X_1, \ldots, X_k} = 0$. If the hypothesis is rejected, the conclusion is that the multiple correlation coefficient (or its square) is greater than 0; unlike other correlations, $\rho_{Y | X_1 \ldots X_k}$ can assume values only between 0 and 1.

As throughout the book, the hypothesis is rejected for large values of F. From the expression for the F statistic — a function of R^2 — this makes sense. Higher values of R^2 would be associated with higher values of the statistic. When H_0 is true, the test statistic follows an F distribution with k and $n - k - 1$ degrees of freedom.

Examination of this ANOVA table also provides insight into the interpretation of R^2. From the sum of squares column, we can see that

$$R^2 = \frac{\text{SS}_{reg}}{\text{SS}_t} = 1 - \frac{\text{SS}_r}{\text{SS}_t}.$$

Here R^2, the square of the sample multiple correlation coefficient, is the proportion of the variation in Y (SS_t) explained by the linear relation between Y and the linear combination of the X variables (SS_{reg}).

Example. Since the test that the multiple correlation coefficient is 0 is equivalent to the test that all partial regression coefficients are 0, the same ANOVA table that was constructed to test that the partial regression coefficients for height and age were both 0 in Section 12.5.1, is repeated here as Table 13.2.

For this example, if the population multiple correlation were 0, the F statistic would follow an F distribution with $k = 2$ and $n - k - 1 = 45$ degrees of freedom. With the calculated F of 42.3, the hypothesis is rejected. The p value, the probability that a value of F of 42.3 or larger would be obtained if $\rho_{Y|X_1 X_2}$ were 0, is < 0.0001. This F value is quite unlikely to have occurred by chance, and we conclude that the population multiple correlation is > 0.

13.6   INFERENCES FOR PARTIAL CORRELATION COEFFICIENTS

Inferences for the population partial correlation coefficients are based on the assumptions of the joint distribution model, as given in Section 13.4. Statistical packages routinely provide tests that population partial correlation coefficients are equal to 0. Confidence intervals are less available. Inferences based on both confidence intervals and hypothesis are discussed in this chapter.

As with multiple correlation, caution should be used when making inferences about partial correlation coefficients. A partial correlation between two variables that is unequal to 0 simply means that when adjustment is made for other variables, there is a linear relationship between the two. Knowledge of the value of one of them can provide some information about the value of the other. We cannot conclude there is a causal relationship between them.

Table 13.1   ANOVA Table

Source of Variation	Sum of Squares	df	Mean Square	F
Regression of Y on $X_1,\dots,X_k$	$R^2 SS_t$	k	MS_{reg}	$\frac{R^2/k}{(1-R^2)/(n-k-1)}$
Residual	$(1-R^2)SS_t$	$n-k-1$	MS_r	
Total	SS_t	$n-1$		

Table 13.2 Test That Population Multiple Correlation Coefficient Is 0

Source of Variation	Sum of Squares	df	Mean Square	Calculated F	p Value
Regression of vital capacity on height and age	27.5	2	13.7	42.3	< 0.0001
Residual	14.6	45	0.32		
Total	42.1	47			

13.6.1 Confidence Intervals for Partial Correlation Coefficients

Confidence intervals for $\rho_{X_1Y|X_2,\ldots,X_k}$ are obtained using the same methods as those given in Chapter 11 for ρ. A confidence interval for

$$\mu_Z = \frac{1}{2} \log \frac{1 + \rho_{X_1Y|X_2,\ldots,X_k}}{1 - \rho_{X_1Y|X_2,\ldots,X_k}}$$

is made first. The distribution of the statistic

$$Z = \frac{1}{2} \log \frac{1 + r_{X_1Y|X_2,\ldots,X_k}}{1 - r_{X_1Y|X_2,\ldots,X_k}}$$

is approximately known:

$$Z \sim \mathrm{ND}\left(\mu_Z, \frac{1}{n - 3 - (k - 1)}\right),$$

where $k - 1$ is the number of variables whose linear effects are controlled, indicated here by $X_2, \ldots, X_k$. Recall that in Chapter 11, the variance of Z was $1/(n - 3)$; no variables were controlled for the simple correlation.

Once the interval for μ_Z is determined, it is transformed to an interval for $\rho_{X_1Y|X_2,\ldots,X_k}$. The resulting confidence interval can be used either as an interval estimate of the population parameter or for a hypothesis test.

Example. First, let's obtain 95% confidence intervals for $\rho_{X_1Y|X_2}$, the partial correlation between vital capacity and height, when adjustment is made for age. As we have seen before, the point estimate is $r_{X_1Y|X_2} = 0.78$. Transforming this partial correlation using Fisher's Z transformation gives the point estimate $\mu_Z = 0.5 \log_e[(1 + 0.78)/(1 - 0.78)] = 1.04$; its variance estimate is $1/(48 - 3 - 1) = 1/44 = 0.023$, and its estimated standard error is $1/\sqrt{44} = 0.15$. The 95% confidence interval for μ_Z is

$$1.04 - 1.96(0.15) \;<\mu_Z<\; 1.04 + 1.96(0.15),$$
$$0.71 \;<Z<\; 1.37.$$

Transforming this to an interval for $\rho_{XY|X_2}$, either using Table B.5 or by hand, we obtain

$$0.63 < \rho_{X_1Y|X_2} < 0.87.$$

We are 95% confident that this population partial correlation coefficient lies between 0.63 and 0.87. Since the interval does not include 0, we can also conclude that $\rho_{X_1Y|X_2}$ is not equal to 0. Note that this confidence interval, like ones obtained for correlations in Chapter 11, is not symmetric about its point estimate.

Let's calculate the 95% confidence interval for $\rho_{X_2Y|X_1}$, the population correlation between vital capacity and age when adjustment is made for height. The point estimate is $r_{X_2Y|X_1} = -0.56$ and the transformed value is $Z = -0.64$. Performing the required calculations gives

$$-0.93 \quad < \mu_Z < \quad -0.34$$
$$-0.73 \quad < \rho_{X_2Y|X_1} < \quad -0.33$$

We are 95% confident that $\rho_{X_2Y|X_1}$ is between -0.73 and -0.33. Since the entire interval lies below 0, we can conclude that $\rho_{X_2Y|X_1}$ is not 0, indicating that when adjustment is made for height, there still is correlation between vital capacity and age. Note also that the interval is wider than the interval calculated for $\rho_{X_1Y|X_2}$ (0.40 versus 0.24), even though the estimated standard error of the transformed statistic z is the same. The length of the interval depends on the value of the point estimate. The larger the estimate (in magnitude), the shorter the confidence interval.

13.6.2   Hypothesis Tests for Partial Correlation Coefficients

The relationship between the population partial regression and partial correlation coefficients, as described in Section 13.4.2, suggests that the test that a partial correlation coefficient is equal to 0 is equivalent to a test that a partial regression coefficient is 0. In Chapter 12, we saw there were two equivalent ways to test that a partial regression coefficient was 0 — a t test and an F test. So, to test the hypothesis

$$\rho_{X_1Y|X_2,\ldots,X_k} = 0.$$

the same t and F tests can be applied.

The expression for the t statistic can be written in terms of the partial regression coefficient, as in Equation 12.10, or in terms of the partial correlation coefficient. In the latter case, the expression in quite similar to the t statistic for testing $H_0 : \rho = 0$ is Chapter 11:

$$t = \frac{r_{X_1Y|X_2}\sqrt{n-k-1}}{\sqrt{1 - r_{X_1Y|X_2}^2}}. \tag{13.11}$$

When H_0 is true, the test statistic follows a t distribution with $n - k - 1$ degrees of freedom.

An F statistic can be calculated. Recall in Equation 13.2 that the square of the sample partial correlation could be expressed in terms of residual sums of squares:

$$r^2_{X_1 Y | X_2 \ldots X_k} = \frac{SS_r(X_2, \ldots X_k) - SS_r(X_1, \ldots, X_k)}{SS_r(X_2, \ldots, X_k)}.$$

This expression looks a lot like the F statistic used in Table 12.8 for testing $H_0 : \beta_1 = 0$. It can be converted to the F statistic by dividing the sums of squares by their appropriate numbers of degrees of freedom: 1 for the numerator and $n - k - 1$ for the denominator.

Example. Let's first calculate the t ratios for testing that $H_0 : \rho_{X_2 Y | X_1} = 0$ and that $H_0 : \rho_{X_1 Y | X_2} = 0$.

The partial correlation between between vital capacity and age, when adjustment is made for height, is $r_{Y X_2 | X_1} = -0.5622$. Substituting into Equation 13.11, we obtain

$$t = \frac{-0.56\sqrt{45}}{\sqrt{1 - (-0.56)^2}} = -4.56.$$

Similarly, the partial correlation between vital capacity and height, when adjustment is made for age, is $r_{X_1 Y | X_2} = 0.78$. The computed t is 8.30. Note that these computed t values are the same as those obtained from testing $H_0 : \beta_2 = 0$ and $H_0 : \beta_1 = 0$ in Chapter 12. See Table 12.7.

Since the F tests for the partial correlation coefficients are identical to the tests for the partial regression coefficients in Chapter 12, they are not repeated here for this example.

The test of the hypothesis that a partial correlation coefficient is equal to 0 can also be expressed in terms of the multiple correlation coefficient, that is,

$$H_0 : \rho_{X_1 Y | X_2} = 0$$

is equivalent to

$$H_0 : \rho_{Y | X_1 X_2} = \rho_{Y | X_2}.$$

That is, after adjustment is made for X_2, is anything gained by including X_1 in the correlation model? If there is, the partial correlation $\rho_{X_1 Y | X_2}$ is greater than 0, and the multiple correlation $\rho_{Y | X_1 X_2}$ should be greater than $\rho_{Y | X_2}$.

13.7   CHECKING IF THE DATA FIT THE JOINT NORMAL MODEL

An important consequence of the joint normal model concerns the conditional distributions; both of these were discussed in Section 13.4. That is, for the conditional model, the partial regression coefficients which contribute to the conditional mean are functions of the partial correlation coefficients, and the conditional variance can be expressed in terms of the partial or multiple correlations. Thus, if the joint normal model holds, we do not need to be concerned about the interpretation of the statistics in terms of correlations or the appropriateness of the inferences. If all of the variables measured are determined at random, then each one can be evaluated individually to assess whether it is normally distributed. As indicated in Chapter 11, normality of each of the variables does not guarantee that the variables are jointly normally distributed, but this is frequently the case. For application of testing for univariate normality to the testing of multivariate normality see [5]. Scatter diagrams for all pairs of variables are also useful. The plots should show that the data points fall roughly into an elliptical shape. For further discussion of graphical methods for three variables see [1, 2, 4]. For a general reference on regression analysis, see [3, 6, 7].

If joint normality holds, then the assumptions of the multiple regression model hold, but the reverse isn't necessarily true. Of course, checking the assumptions of the multiple regression model can be useful, as departures may suggest ways to transform variables so that joint normality is satisfied. Some of these procedures were discussed in Chapter 12 and are not repeated here.

If the X variables are fixed rather than random, then it isn't appropriate to discuss correlation. In previous chapters, we referred to R^2 in terms of the ratio of SS_{reg} to SS_t for the fixed X regression model or of the ratio of SS_{factor} to SS_t for ANOVA models, but we did not refer to these R^2's as correlations. Thus, the design of the study is an important determinant in whether to proceed with a correlation analysis.

Based on earlier work with our example in Chapter 12, we are not concerned about violation of the assumptions. We assume that the three variables have a trivariate normal distribution; pairwise scatter diagrams indicate that there are linear relationships between each pair of variables. An illustrative example of checking if the data fit the model is omitted from this section.

13.8   WHAT TO DO IF THE DATA DON'T FIT THE MODEL

If the joint normal model does not fit the data, we have several options. One approach is to transform variables so that the data fit. Attempting to transform the variables can be difficult, particularly when many variables are included in the analysis. Interpretations of the correlations can be difficult also because they must be made in terms of the transformed variables. Nevertheless, this is a reasonable option. For some variables, investigators become very accustomed to working with the transformed ones. This is particularly the case when the use of a transformation has become well established in the investigator's field.

Instead of making the model fit, an alternative approach is to accept that nonlinear relationships exist among the variables. If alternative models seem more appropriate, then investigators would likely not want to pursue correlation analyses, as correlations are measures of linear relationships.

13.9   SUMMARY

In this chapter, we extended the concept of correlation to the multivariate setting in two ways: multiple correlation and partial correlation. These correlations were described as measures of the strengths of linear associations among variables: multiple correlation as the strength of the linear relation between a Y variable and a linear combination of X variables, and partial correlation as the strength of the linear relation between two variables when adjustment has been made for linear effects of other variables. Characteristics and interpretations of the estimates and their squares were made. Inferences (both confidence intervals and hypothesis tests) for both types of correlations were discussed.

Problems

13.1   This problem uses the same small data set as that given in the first problem of Chapter 12 (involving weight, duration of operation, and blood loss).

   a)   Determine the simple correlations r_{X_1Y}, r_{X_2Y}, and $r_{X_1X_2}$. What do the values suggest about the bivariate relationships between the variables?

   b)   Regress blood loss on weight and duration of operation, and save the fitted values. Calculate R as the simple correlation between the observed and fitted values of blood loss. Calculate R^2.

   c)   Verify that R^2 is equal to SS_{reg}/SS_t. Interpret R^2.

   d)   For the regression model that was fitted in part (b), break the total sum of squares into three parts: SS(duration), SS(weight | duration), and SS_r. [Make use of either sequential (Type I) or adjusted (Type III) sums of squares.] Calculate $r^2_{X_1Y|X_2}$ as SS(weight | duration) / SS_r. Interpret this value.

   e)   If you were to calculate $r^2_{X_1Y|X_2}$ in terms of residual sums of squares, which two regression models would you fit? Fit the models and determine $r^2_{X_1Y|X_2}$.

f)   Regress blood loss on duration of operation, and save the residuals; regress weight on duration of operation, and save the residuals. Verify that $r_{X_1Y|X_2}$ is the simple correlation between the two sets of residuals.

g)   For the regression model that was fitted in part(b), break the total sum of squares into three parts: SS(weight), SS(duration | weight) and SS$_r$. [Make use of either sequential (Type I) or adjusted (Type III) sums of squares.] Calculate $r^2_{X_2Y|X_1}$ as SS(duration | weight) / SS$_r$. Interpret this value.

h)   If you were to calculate $r^2_{X_2Y|X_1}$ in terms of residual sums of squares, which two regression models would you fit? Fit the models and determine $r^2_{X_2Y|X_1}$.

i)   Regress blood loss on weight, and save the residuals; regress duration of operation on weight, and save residuals. Verify that $r_{X_2Y|X_1}$ is the simple correlation between the two sets of residuals.

13.2   This problem uses the same small data set as that given in the second problem in Chapter 12 (involving blood loss, duration of operation, and hemoglobin change).

a)   Determine the simple correlations r_{X_1Y}, r_{X_2Y}, and $r_{X_1X_2}$. What do the values suggest about the bivariate relationships between the variables?

b)   Estimate $\rho_{Y|X_1X_2}$.

c)   Test the hypothesis $H_0 : \rho_{Y|X_1X_2} = 0$ (using $\alpha = 0.05$). What do you conclude from this test?

d)   Estimate $\rho_{X_2Y|X_1}$. Determine a 95% confidence interval for this population parameter. Interpret this interval.

13.3   This problem uses the same small data set as that given in the third problem in Chapter 12, for rainfall, temperature, and yield of rye.

a)   Determine the simple correlations r_{X_1Y}, r_{X_2Y}, and $r_{X_1X_2}$. What do the values suggest about the bivariate relationships between the variables?

b)   Estimate $\rho_{Y|X_1X_2}$.

c)   Test the hypothesis $H_0 : \rho_{Y|X_1X_2} = 0$ (using $\alpha = 0.05$). What do you conclude from this test? What other test is equivalent to this one?

d)   Estimate $\rho_{X_2Y|X_1}$. Determine a 95% confidence interval for this population parameter. Interpret this interval.

e)   Test the hypothesis $H_0 : \rho_{X_2Y|X_1} = 0$. What do you conclude from this test? What other tests are equivalent to this one? Write out the corresponding null hypotheses.

13.4   Use the data given in Problem 12.4 for mean temperature, $X_1 =$ altitude, $X_2 =$ longitude and $X_3 =$ latitude of 16 cities to answer the following:

a)   Find $r_{X_2,Y}$, $R_{Y|X_2,X_3}$, and $R_{Y|X_1,X_2,X_3}$.

b)   Estimate the partial correlation $r_{X_2,Y|X_3}$. Determine a 95% confidence interval for $\rho_{X_2,Y|X_3}$.

REFERENCES

1. Cleveland, W.S. [1993]. *Visualizing Data*, Summit, NJ: Hobart Press, 181–272.

2. Cook, R.D. and Weisberg, S. [1999]. *Applied Regression Including Computing and Graphics*, New York: John Wiley & Sons.

3. Draper, N. R. and Smith, H. [1998]. *Applied Regression Analysis*, 3rd ed. New York: John Wiley & Sons.

4. Friendly, M. [2002]. Corrgrams: Exploratory Displays for Correlation Matrices, *The American Statistician*, 56, 316–324.

5. Looney, S.W. [1995]. How to Use Tests for Univariate Normality to Asses Multivariate Normality, *The American Statistician*, 49, 64–69.

6. Montgomery, D.C., Peck, E.A., and Vining, G.G. [2001]. *Introduction to Linear Regression*, 3rd ed. New York: John Wiley & Sons.

7. Ryan, T.P. [1996]. *Modern Regression Methods*, New York: John Wiley & Sons.

14

Miscellaneous Topics
in Regression

In this chapter, we briefly discuss four different topics that are relevant to multiple regression, but were not taken up in earlier chapters on regression. The first topic concerns the treatment of nominal independent variables. Since there is no ordering associated with the levels of these variables, it is not meaningful to fit a regression equation without making some modification to these types of X variables. The handling of nominal independent variables by the creation of dummy or indicator variables is discussed in Section 14.1.

The second topic concerns interactions between two independent variables. In Chapter 5, we discussed interaction in the context of two-way cross-classifications. An *interaction* was said to exist if the effect of one of the factors depended on the level of the second factor. Here, we describe how to incorporate interactions between independent variables in regression and how to interpret the results in Section 14.2.

The third topic concerns the inclusion of polynomial terms in a regression model. It may be that the relationship between the Y and an X variable is not linear but quadratic. In this case, adding X^2 as an independent variable may provide a better representation of the data. Addition of higher order terms, such as cubic (X^3) or quartic (X^4), also might provide better-fitting models. This topic is taken up in Section 14.3.

The final topic, variable selection, is applicable when investigators have collected information on many variables and they wish or need to identify a model which includes a smaller number of X variables. A variety of variable selection strategies are briefly introduced in Section 14.4. The entire chapter is summarized in Section 14.5.

14.1   MODELS WITH DUMMY VARIABLES

In earlier regression chapters, we assumed either a fixed X model, where differences between successive X values were accurately known, or the multivariate normal model. If neither of these models is appropriate, the X variable can be transformed to a set of variables called *dummy* or *indicator* variables. These new variables allow the researcher to investigate the more general question of whether or not there is any association between the two variables.

Before we describe what dummy variables are, let's first consider some situations in which an investigator would be interested in transforming an X variable to a set of dummy variables.

(1) The variable may be nominal, so there is no ordering associated with the levels; a regression analysis with such an independent variable would not be meaningful. Examples of such variables include sex, race, and religion.

(2) The variable may be ordinal. If it isn't appropriate to assume that there is close to an equal distance between levels of the categories, a regression analysis with such a variable would be difficult to interpret. Examples include degree of severity (low, medium, high).

Now, let's consider how dummy variables are created. There are a variety of ways that dummy variables can be defined; we illustrate a common method here, which is called *reference cell coding*. The simplest situation is one is which the X variable has two categories (for example, sex has two categories, male and female). With two categories, a single dummy variable, D_1, identifies the two by assigning different numerical values to them, say, 1 and 0.

Example. There are 111 males and 44 females in the cardiac rehabilitation data set. We can construct a single dummy variable for sex,

$$D_1 = \begin{cases} 1 & \text{if female,} \\ 0 & \text{if male.} \end{cases}$$

Regressing weight in pounds (Y) on sex (D_1), the following sample regression equation is obtained:

$$\hat{Y} = 190.8 - 37.3D_1,$$

so that for males $\hat{Y} = 190.8$ and, for females $\hat{Y} = 190.8 - 37.3 = 153.5$. These fitted values correspond to the mean weight (in pounds) for males and females. The slope, -37.3, is the difference in mean weight between men and women. The test that the slope is 0 is equivalent to the test that mean weight is the same for men and women; this test can be performed as a two-sample t test or as ANOVA F test (with $p < 0.0001$).

Dummy variables can also be used in conjunction with other variables in a regression equation. For example, suppose sex, age (in years) and hip measurement (in inches) are included in the same regression equation. For the data example, the expression for the sample regression plane is

$$\hat{Y} = -119 - 35 \times \text{sex} - 0.547 \times \text{age} + 8.16 \times \text{hip}$$

The Y intercept is different for men (-119) and women ($-154 = -119 - 35 \times 1$), but the estimated partial regression coefficients for age and hip are the same for both men and women. Another way of saying this is that the regression plane for males is parallel to the regression plane for females. The predicted weight is 175 pounds for a 60 year-old-man with hip measurement of 40; it is 140 pounds for a woman with the same age and hip measurement. The difference in the predicted values (women $-$ men), $140 - 175 = -35$, is the same at all age and hip determinations.

Suppose a categorical variable X assumes $a = 3$ levels. As an example, suppose subjects' smoking history is categorized into three groups as current smokers, former smokers, and never smokers. Two dummy variables, D_1 and D_2, could be created — for example,

Level	D_1	D_2
Current	1	0
Former	0	1
Never	0	0

Without any other independent variables in the regression model, the least squares equation has the following form:

$$\hat{Y} = a + b_1 D_1 + b_2 D_2,$$

or, more specifically,

Level	$\hat{Y}$
Current	$a + b_1$
Former	$a + b_2$
Never	a

The intercept, a, is the mean value of Y for the third level of the X variable (never smokers), $\bar{Y}_3$. The quantity b_1 is the difference in mean values of Y between the first and third levels (current smokers $-$ never smokers), or $\bar{Y}_1 - \bar{Y}_3$, and b_2 is the difference in mean values of Y between the second and third levels (former smokers $-$ never smokers), or $\bar{Y}_2 - \bar{Y}_3$. This gives us an idea of why this method of coding is referred as reference coding. When interpreting the partial regression coefficients, individual levels of X are compared with the *referent category* — the category to which all dummy variables are given the value of 0. In this example, dummy variables could have been defined in such a way that current smokers or former smokers could have been the referent group. The choice of the referent category should be based on what statements the investigators wish to make; never smokers is a reasonable selection if the investigators are particularly interested in highlighting comparisons between all types of smokers and never smokers.

More generally, if a categorical variable assumes a levels, it is possible to define $a - 1$ dummy variables. There are a variety of ways in which these variables can be defined; we continue to illustrate reference coding. For example,

$$D_1 = \begin{cases} 1 & \text{if level 1,} \\ 0 & \text{otherwise,} \end{cases}$$

$$D_2 = \begin{cases} 1 & \text{if level 2,} \\ 0 & \text{otherwise,} \end{cases}$$

$$\vdots$$

$$D_{a-1} = \begin{cases} 1 & \text{if level } a - 1, \\ 0 & \text{otherwise.} \end{cases}$$

Data analysts can create their own dummy variables, and some software packages will create them if requested. Either way, there are a few points to keep in mind. First, it's important to verify how dummy variables have been coded. Otherwise, analysts run the risk of interpreting their computer output incorrectly. With reference coding, the referent category must be chosen. Typically, analysts choose a category that would be most interesting to make comparisons with and has a comparatively large sample size. There are alternatives to the reference coding strategy discussed here [1, 6].

For hypothesis testing, analysts generally want to test that all partial regression coefficients associated with the set of dummy variables are simultaneously equal to zero. If the dummy variables are the only variables included in the model, then the test that all partial regression coefficients are equal to 0 is performed. This test is equivalent to the test of equality of means in the context of one-way ANOVA. If other independent variables are included in the regression model, then a test of a subset of partial regression coefficients must be made. This is usually done automatically when the software program has created the dummy variables. If the user has created the dummy variables, the software doesn't know that the set of partial regression coefficients should be treated as a group; the user has to request that this set be all 0.

When some dummy variables created from a particular category are included in a model but others are not, interpretation of the regression equation requires care. Consider the example of the three smoking categories. Suppose D_2, the dummy variable associated with former smokers, is found to be not statistically significant, so the analyst decides to include only D_1 in the model. Without D_2, D_1 is redefined so that the referent group becomes nonsmokers and former smokers. This may not be what the investigator intended. It is generally preferable to include all dummy variables created for a categorical variable.

If there are several categorical variables for which dummy variables are created, then it is possible to have a large number of predictor variables in the model. For example, suppose there are four categorical variables which an investigator wishes to include in a model as dummy variables. These are sex (two levels), smoking history (three levels), religion (four levels), and race (five levels). Then the regression equation has $(2-1) + (3-1) + (4-1) + (5-1) = 10$ predictors. Analysts would want to make sure they haven't created too many predictor variables for a particular sample size. Otherwise, the sample regression coefficients will have larger estimated standard errors and the resulting model likely won't be very good at predicting the outcome variable for another data set. If this situation occurs, the model is said to be *overfitted*.

14.2 MODELS WITH INTERACTION TERMS

When investigators think that the effects of two X variables (say, X_1 and X_2) are not strictly additive (as $\beta_1 X_1 + \beta_2 X_2$), then an interaction term can be included in predicting Y. A new independent variable, X_3, is created to take into account the lack of additivity. A common practice is to use the product $X_1 X_2 = X_3$ as the new variable.

It is easiest to illustrate and understand the concept of interaction when one of the variables is a single dummy variable and the other is a quantitative variable. (The same general principles apply for the interaction between two quantitative variables.)

If D_1 is a dummy variable which assumes values 1 and 0 and X_2 is the quantitative variable, then a regression equation with an interaction term,

$$\hat{Y} = a + b_1 D_1 + b_2 X_2 + b_3 (D_1 X_2),$$

can be fitted. In this case, for the referent group we have, with $D_1 = 0$,

$$\hat{Y} = a + b_2 X_2,$$

and when $D_1 = 1$, the equation is

$$\hat{Y} = (a + b_1) + (b_2 + b_3) X_2.$$

Here, by including the variable $D_1 X_2$, we have allowed the regression lines for the two categories to have different slopes and different intercepts; without the interaction variable, the regression slope coefficients are necessarily equal.

The a is interpreted as the Y intercept when $D_1 = 0$ and $X_2 = 0$, so its interpretation is the same, whether or not an interaction term is included.

However, the partial regression coefficients have different interpretations when an interaction term has been added. The coefficient b_1 can be interpreted as the change in the Y intercept when D_1 is changed from 0 to 1. Or it can be interpreted as the change in $\hat{Y}$ when D_1 is changed from 0 to 1 and X_2 is 0. The coefficient b_2 is the change in $\hat{Y}$ for a one unit change in X_2 when D_1 is 0. That is, the two sample partial regression coefficients are interpreted with a second X variable set equal to 0. Recall that for additive regression models, the sample partial regression coefficients are interpreted with the linear effects of a second variable removed. The coefficient b_3 represents the change in slope when X_2 is changed by one unit and D_1 equals 1. If other variables, $X_4, \ldots, X_k$, were also included in the model, b_1 would be interpreted as the change in $\hat{Y}$ when D_1 is changed from 0 to 1, $X_2 = 0$, and $X_3, \ldots, X_k$ are held constant.

A common way to assess whether an interaction term should be included in a regression model is through hypothesis testing. The null hypotheses is

$$H_0 : Y = \alpha + \beta_1 D_1 + \beta_2 X_2 + \varepsilon,$$

and the alternative is specified as

$$H_1 : Y = \alpha + \beta_1 D_1 + \beta_2 X_2 + \beta_3 D_1 X_2 + \varepsilon.$$

In addition to reporting the results of the hypothesis test, it can also be helpful to summarize the fit of the model in terms of the increased R^2 when an interaction term is introduced into the model.

It is also important to check that the multiple regression assumptions are satisfied. Outliers can be responsible for significant interactions among variables. Further details about regression models with interaction terms can be found in [1, 9, 10].

14.3   MODELS WITH POLYNOMIAL TERMS

We turn now to the regression of Y on a single X variable, with a brief discussion of fitting a polynomial.

Sometimes a polynomial is fitted because there are theoretical reasons for believing that the population regression curve is a polynomial of a certain degree. On the other hand, often it is fitted without any theoretical reason but simply because a straight line appears not to give a good fit to the data. Looking at a scatter plot of the data to get an idea of the relationship between the X and the Y variable is a good way to start.

Fitting a polynomial curve would be appropriate for the data which were used in Problem 4.1 of Chapter 4. A plant scientist was interested in investigating the relationship between the percentage of fungal spores that germinate and temperature. He selected $a = 4$ temperatures (15, 20, 25, and 30 degrees Celsius) and incubated $b = 4$ microscopic slides at each of the four temperatures. A scatter diagram showed that the percentage of spores germinated was lower at the lowest and highest temperatures and higher at the middle temperatures. Assuming a linear relationship between temperature and percentage of spores that germinate would not provide a good representation of the data. (Problem 14.2 at the end of this chapter uses polynomial regression to model the relationship between the two variables.)

It is possible to approximate any regression curve as closely as is desired by using a polynomial of sufficiently high degree. However, in fitting a polynomial to a set of data, we are not just interested in obtaining a curve that lies very close to the sample data points. Rather, we are attempting to obtain a curve that approximates the population regression curve (curve of population means). If our primary interest *were* in fitting the curve to the data points, we could actually fit a polynomial of such high degree that it would pass *exactly* through every data point. A straight line (polynomial of degree 1) can be passed through any two points; a quadratic (degree 2) can be passed through any three points; a cubic (degree 3) can be passed through any four points; and so on. Usually, k, the degree of the fitted polynomial, is chosen to be 2 or 3; certainly k should be quite small compared with n, the sample size.

The polynomial of degree k can be written

$$Y^{(k)} = a + b_1 X + b_2 X^2 + \cdots + b_k X^k. \qquad (14.1)$$

We now seek the curve of this form that minimizes the sum of squared vertical deviations $\sum_{i=1}^{n}(Y_i - \hat{Y}_i)^2$. Polynomial regression can be considered as a special case of multiple regression by simply defining $X_1 = X$, $X_2 = X^2$, ..., $X_k = X^k$. Equation 14.1 becomes

$$Y^{(k)} = a + b_1 X_1 + b_2 X_2 + \cdots + b_k X_k. \qquad (14.2)$$

Note first that it is permissible to change X^2 to a new variable X_2. Here X_2 is merely a characteristic measured on each individual or object; it can perfectly well be X^2 measured on each individual. The value of a is still the ordinate at $X = 0$. It is clear that, by setting $X^i = X_i$, $i = 1, \ldots, k$, any multiple regression program can be used to find the least squares Equation 14.1 and perform the analyses; thus in one sense there is nothing new about polynomial regression. Indeed, polynomial regression is regarded as a special case of regression in most software packages.

Scatter plots of Y versus X are useful for deciding on the degree of the polynomial.

It is also possible to fit a second degree polynomial for one predictor variable along with others that are linear. Increasing the value of one X variable may cause an increase and then a decrease in Y, suggesting a second degree polynomial, while increasing the values of other X variables will result in an increase in Y, suggesting linear terms.

14.3.1 Polynomial Model

The model underlying polynomial regression is that for each value of X, there is a population of Y's, and:

(1) The Y populations are normally distributed.

(2) Their means are on a polynomial in X of known degree k.

(3) Their variances are equal.

The data consist of n independent observations from these populations and so can be expressed in the form

$$Y_i^k = \alpha + \beta_1 X_i + \beta_2 X_i^2 + \cdots + \beta_k X_i^k + \varepsilon_i, \qquad (14.3)$$

where $\varepsilon_i \sim \text{IND}(0, \sigma^2)$, $i = 1, \ldots, n$.

With $X = X_1$, $X^2 = X_2, \ldots, X_k = X^k$, Equation 14.3 is the same as the multiple regression model discussed in Chapter 12. Therefore, we can make an ANOVA table, find confidence intervals, and test hypotheses, exactly as in multiple regression. In the multiple regression problems, we were able to assume that $E(Y|X_1, \ldots, X_k) = \alpha + \beta_1 X_1 + \cdots + \beta_k X_k$ and then make confidence intervals for the β_i and to test $H_0 : \beta_i = 0$. In polynomial regression, since the value of X_i is determined by the value of X, $E(Y|X, X^2, \ldots, X^k) = E(Y|X)$. The tests usually made are that the highest degree term can be omitted; that is, we assume $E(Y|X) = \alpha + \beta_1 X + \cdots + \beta_k X^k$ and test $\beta_k = 0$. If we do not reject the null hypothesis, we may assume that $E(Y|X) = \alpha + \beta_1 X + \cdots + \beta_{k-1} X^{k-1}$ and test $H_0 : \beta_{k-1} = 0$. Note that polynomial regression modeling can be done for fixed X's or for random X's.

Most software packages consider polynomial regression as a special case of multiple regression. Many of those that are menu-driven allow analysts to request that quadratic (or higher order) terms be included when specifying the model. Otherwise, analysts need to create new variables before a model is requested. For example, if a quadratic term were desired, a new variable, a transformation of the measured variable, must be made, such as $X_2 = X \cdot X$.

14.4 VARIABLE SELECTION

Often in regression analysis with the joint distribution model, data are obtained on a large (sometimes extremely large) number of possible X variables, and the investigator needs to decide which to use in the analysis. Such is often the case in exploratory situations when little is known about relations among the variables. In the fixed X situation, the values of only a few independent variables are fixed, and these are of course selected before the data are gathered; it is then comparatively easy for the investigator to decide on the X's to be used in the final regression equation. Thus the methods of variable selection discussed in this section are usually applied only to the joint distribution model.

When we wish to predict Y from a small set of X's, the situation is comparatively simple. Adding more variables to predict Y always gives a new regression equation that fits the points at least as well as did the original equation. However, the sample regression plane may also describe characteristics which are unique to that random sample. If the equation were used to predict Y for another random sample, its fit might be poor. Thus if two equations predict the Y values of the data equally well, we generally choose the one with the smaller set of X variables. Also, if a larger set appears to predict Y just slightly better than a smaller set, we may still choose the smaller set. As a general rule, if more variables do not improve the fit appreciably over a smaller set in a regression equation, the larger set will predict less well in a new setting.

Before we get into some of the specific techniques of variable selection, we emphasize that it is also good to look at scatter diagrams, check for outliers, and consider possible transformations — that is, to do initial data screening as described in Chapter 1 and previous regression chapters. Furthermore, we stress that variable selection can require the fitting and refitting of regression equations; whether or not the data fit the specified model needs to be checked repeatedly. Fortunately, software programs are available to help us with this task.

In seeking the *important* variables (the variables which, in combination, account for a sizable percentage of the variation in Y), the situation is more difficult. If investigators start with, say, 25 X variables and find that four of them in combination predict Y quite well, they cannot claim that these four are *the* important variables for predicting Y — that the remaining 21 variables are unimportant in predicting Y. They should look at many different regressions before drawing any conclusions.

For either purpose, investigators need criteria for evaluating and comparing subsets of the X variables as well as methods for identifying subsets of the available X's to include in the regression. We first describe four criteria that can be used in variable selection and then discuss four methods for generating models, which will be compared.

14.4.1 Criteria for Evaluating and Comparing Models

We now consider four criteria that have been suggested for comparing different models. Many other criteria have been proposed, but we are focusing on these four because they are among the most widely used.

We are assuming that there are k possible X variables, but the following statistics are computed for a model fit with p X variables, where $p \leq k$.

The criterion that is probably most familiar is R^2, as described in Chapters 11 and 13. For each model fit, this statistic is calculated as

$$R^2 = \frac{\text{SS}_{reg}}{\text{SS}_t} = 1 - \frac{\text{SS}_r}{\text{SS}_t}. \tag{14.4}$$

Here SS_r is the residual sum of squares obtained from the regression of Y on $X_1, \ldots, X_p$, and SS_t is the total sum of squares of Y. This statistic is routinely printed out from most regression programs, and because it has a definite range from 0 to 1, a lot of analysts feel they can interpret it. However, as the number of variables, p, is increased, the residual sum of squares decreases and R^2 increases. If researchers were deciding to choose a model with the highest R^2, they would always select the model with all the variables. Consequently, the selected model is the most complex one and there is the possibility that the model is overfitted. Instead, an investigator may want to select the model where the increase in R^2 starts to become small; but it may be difficult to decide what is small.

To get around this limitation of the increasing R^2, statisticians looked for alternative measures which would balance the advantages of more X variables (i.e., reducing the residual sum of squares) with its disadvantages (i.e., overfitting).

One solution, the second criterion, is the adjusted R^2. This is is calculated as

$$\text{adjusted } R^2 = 1 - \frac{\text{MS}_r}{s_Y^2}. \tag{14.5}$$

Here, MS_r is calculated as the ratio of the residual sum of squares obtained when Y is regressed on $X_1, \ldots, X_p$ to $n - p - 1$, and s_Y^2 is $\text{SS}_t/(n-1)$. Like R^2, it is routinely printed out from many regression programs. Examining Equation 14.5 reveals several characteristics of it. First, it is a ratio of sums of squares to numbers of degrees of freedom, so that its value depends on the number of X variables in the equation (p) and the sample size (n). It can never be larger than R^2. When the sample size is large relative to k, the adjusted R^2 is close to R^2; when the number of variables included is nearly as large as the sample size, the adjusted R^2 is appreciably smaller than R^2. The adjusted R^2 can even be negative if R^2 is very small or if k is large relative to n. As more variables are added to a model, the adjusted R^2 increases but then decreases when the additional variables have a small effect on R^2. A regression model with the highest adjusted R^2 won't necessarily be the most complex one. (If all variables $Y, X_1, \ldots, X_k$ are jointly normally distributed, R^2 is a biased estimate of $\rho_{Y|X_1,\ldots,X_k}^2$, tending to overestimate the square of the population correlation; the adjusted R^2 is more nearly unbiased than R^2 [11]. This is another advantage of adjusted R^2 over R^2.) Analysts using this criterion to compare models would select models with higher adjusted R^2.

A third criterion is Mallow's C_p. This statistic can be calculated as

$$C_p = \frac{\text{SS}_r(X_1, \ldots, X_p)}{\text{MS}_r(X_1, \ldots, X_k)} - n + 2(p+1). \tag{14.6}$$

In this equation, $SS_r(X_1, \ldots, X_p)$ is the residual sum of squares obtained from the regression of Y on $X_1, \ldots, X_p$ and MS_r refers to the residual mean square obtained from the regression of Y on all X variables, $X_1, \ldots, X_k$. (Note that we have altered the notation for residual sums of squares to clarify how many variables are used in determining a particular sum of squares.) This definition of Mallow's C_p is the one that most software programs use in the computations. However, some packages make use of alternative definitions.

Examining the equation for Mallow's C_p gives us an idea of some of its properties. Note that $SS_r(X_1, \ldots, X_p)$ is always $\geq SS_r(X_1, \ldots, X_k)$, so that the ratio of the residual sums of squares in the numerator to the mean square residual in the denominator is $\geq n - k - 1$. At its minimum, the ratio is equal to $n - k - 1$, so that $C_p \geq 2p + 1 - k$. When $p = k$, C_p assumes its minimum value, $p + 1$. When comparing models, analysts using this criterion would select models with low values of C_p.

A fourth criterion for comparing models is the Akaike information criterion, generally denoted by AIC. There are a variety of ways of calculating it, and different software packages use different definitions, but for multiple regression models, it may be calculated (excluding a constant term) as

$$\text{AIC} = n\log\frac{SS_r(X_1, \ldots, X_p)}{n} + 2(p + 1). \tag{14.7}$$

An advantage of AIC is that it can be computed for a more general class of models than those that we have been considering in this book: its application is not restricted to normally distributed Y variables. (R^2, the adjusted R^2, and Mallow's C_p are limited to the models that we have been discussing in this book.) The development of AIC was based on the assumption that there is no one "true" model [3].

When models with the same Y and same number of X variables are compared, selecting the model with the highest R^2 is equivalent to selecting the model with the highest F value or lowest p value for testing that all partial regression coefficients are 0. Furthermore, in this case, the ordering of the models from best fitting to poorest fitting in terms of R^2 (highest to lowest) is the same as that for the other measures: adjusted R^2 (highest to lowest), Mallows's C_p (lowest to highest) and AIC (lowest to highest). The ordering won't necessarily be the same when comparing models with different numbers of X variables.

In summary, when comparing the models obtained using these criteria, analysts select those that have comparatively high R^2, high adjusted R^2, low C_p, and low AIC. Our statements regarding criteria for selection of variables are intentionally a bit vague. Certainly, an analyst can follow a specific rule for a given criterion, such as selecting the model with the highest R^2, highest adjusted R^2, lowest C_p, or lowest AIC. But flexibility is often used in variable selection. If there is only minimal difference in values for a particular criterion, analysts may wish to use a simpler model, or to indicate that they cannot distinguish between the models, or to use a more complex model if they believe some variables should be retained for theoretical reasons. This decision is usually left to the investigator, although some guidelines are available. For example, for nested models (one is a special case of another) it has been suggested that models should not be distinguished when differences in their AIC values are between 0 and 2 but that they should be when they are greater than approximately 10 [3].

14.4.2   Methods for Variable Selection

Here we discuss five different methods for identifying "better" combinations of variables: all possible subsets, best subsets, forward selection, backward elimination, and forward stepwise procedures. What the best models are can depend on which of the criteria are used for comparing the different models. For each of the methods of variable selection given here, we could use the four criteria given above to select variables.

All Possible Subsets. It seems most straightforward to determine the criteria given above for all possible subsets of the variables. For example, suppose there are three X's being considered for possible inclusion in a model: X_1, X_2, and X_3. There are seven possible subsets: X_1; X_2; X_3; X_1 and X_2; X_1 and X_3; X_2 and X_3; X_1, X_2, and X_3. A researcher can then compare the results for the seven models and choose the ones that are best (for example, with the lowest AIC score). The advantage to using this procedure is that it considers all possible models, so that the preferred models can readily be identified. The disadvantage is that a very large number of models have to be considered as k becomes large. Even with $k = 5$, there are 31. The software that is available for applying this method is limited (particularly for large numbers of X variables), so analysts may have to generate many of the possible models using the standard regression procedures.

Best Subsets. To reduce the number of models, a method called *best subsets* can also be considered. A common application is to find the subset of models with a given number of X variables that are best. Suppose there are five X's. The best models with one X, two X's, three X's, four X's, and five X's are selected, according to some criterion. When applying this procedure, it is possible for analysts to force some X variables to be in the regression model. This is advantageous if the investigator wants to make use of knowledge that particular X variables are related to the Y.

An alternative to selecting best subsets for a given number of variables is to select the best subsets in terms of a given criterion. For example, we may wish to compare models with the highest adjusted R^2's or lowest C_p, without regard to the number of variables selected.

The main advantage to the best subsets procedure is that it is less overwhelming than looking at all possible subsets. The disadvantage is that some models that are quite similar to the chosen ones could be missed.

Forward Selection. One selection method commonly used is called *forward selection*. This procedure starts with no X variables in the model and adds variables one at a time until a stopping rule is satisfied. For most software packages, the criterion for comparing models is based on R^2.

The first variable selected is the one whose simple correlation with Y is the largest in magnitude (i.e. $|r_{X_iY}|$). We may denote this variable by X_1. This X variable also has the largest calculated F value or smallest p value for testing $H_0 : \beta_i = 0$ under the assumption that $E(Y|X_i) = \alpha + \beta_i X_i$. If there are k variables for possible inclusion in the model, there are k simple correlations, F values, or p values that are compared when selecting this first variable.

The forward selection procedure next selects as X_2, the second variable to be entered, the variable which, with X_1, yields the largest $R^2_{Y|X_1,X_i}$. (There are a variety of ways for stating the same thing. In terms of statistics, we could say that X_2 is the variable whose partial correlation with Y given X_1 is largest in magnitude, that is, that has the largest $|r_{X_iY|X_1}|$. In terms of hypothesis testing, we could say that the selected variable is the one with the largest calculated F value or smallest p value for testing $H_0 : \beta_2 = 0$ or $H_0 : \rho_{X_2Y|X_1} = 0$ or $H_0 : \rho_{Y|X_1X_2} = \rho_{Y|X_1}$ under the assumption that $E(Y|X_1X_2) = \alpha + \beta_1 X_1 + \beta_2 X_2$.) With this choice, any variable highly correlated with X_1 is unlikely to enter. For this second step, there are $k-1$ variables for possible entry into the model, so $k-1$ multiple correlations, partial correlations, or p values are compared when selecting this second variable.

Variables are added, one at a time, until a stopping rule is satisfied. One common stopping rule is to stop entering more variables whenever the p values for all tests performed for selecting the next variable are greater than a specified cutpoint. For example, suppose two variables out of k have already been selected. To select a third variable, at least one of the $k-3$ tests must give a p value less than the cutpoint. If none of the $k-1$ p values satisfy this criterion, the procedure stops; it has selected a model with two variables out of k.

We are used to seeing significance levels for hypothesis tests set at $\alpha = 0.05$. But the usual values do not apply for forward selection procedures. At each step, the variable with the *largest* calculated F is selected. Simulation studies have shown that the distribution of the largest calculated F's does not follow an F distribution when the tested partial regression coefficient is 0. Because the appropriate distributions are not easily determined, statisticians have looked for approximations.

Most statistical packages allow the user to specify a cutpoint, which may be referred to as "significance level for entry" or as an F value for entry. A recommended choice for the significance level is a value of 0.15 [2]. With the cutpoint 0.15, the variable with the smallest associated p value is entered into the regression model if the p value is less than 0.15. If the variable with the smallest p value is greater than 0.15, the forward selection procedure stops. Forward selection doesn't necessarily give the "best" model according to any criterion.

One variation on forward selection is to force some variables to be included in the model. This is useful if prior investigations or knowledge of the subject matter indicate that certain variables are predictive of the Y variable. When a set of dummy variables has been created for a categorical data, it is recommended that the set be tested simultaneously for entry [4].

Backward Elimination. The backward elimination procedure starts with all k of the X variables in the regression equation and then removes or eliminates the variables one at a time until a stopping rule is satisfied. The variable that is removed first, X_k, is the one with the largest p value for testing $H_0 : \beta_k = 0$ under the assumption that $E(Y|X_1, \ldots, X_k) = \alpha + \beta_1 X_1 + \cdots + \beta_k X_k$. The variable that is removed is considered the least useful: the R^2 is decreased the least, and the partial correlation between it and Y when the remaining $k-1$ variables are included is smallest. This process is then repeated with the $k - 1$ remaining variables. It continues deleting variables until the smallest p value for the compared tests is less than the specified cutpoint. That is, all remaining variables contribute to the fit of the model. The same problems with determining a reasonable cutpoint encountered with forward selection are also found in backward elimination. A recommended choice for the cutoff is a p value of 0.25 [1].

Because it starts with all the X variables in the equation, it allows inclusion of variables that need one or more other variables to form a good predictive set. This is its main advantage, particularly when compared with forward selection.

Stepwise Procedure. The forward stepwise procedure combines features from forward selection and backward elimination. In this method, *step* refers to the addition of a variable to the regression equation. Like forward selection, it begins with no X variables in the model. At step 1, the variable with the smallest p value for the test $H_0 : \beta_i = 0$ assuming the model $E(Y|X_i) = \alpha + \beta_i X_i$ is entered, provided it is below the specified significance level for entry. At step 2, the second variable is entered as in forward selection. After the second variable is entered, however, an F test is made for each of the two X variables to determine whether it can be removed. If either the first or second variable entered has a p value greater than the specified significance level for removal, that variable is removed. The procedure continues to add variables one at a time and to check after each entry whether any of the variables already entered can now be removed. The process stops when no variables can either be added or eliminated according to the specified cutpoints for entry and removal.

Data analysts specify the cutpoints for entry and removal of variables. The p value for entry must be smaller than the p value for removal (or the F value for entry must be larger than the F value for removal). Otherwise, the same variable is entered and removed repeatedly. If the p value for removal is much smaller than the p value for entry (0 at the extreme), the resulting equation is the same as in forward selection, because no variables are removed.

14.4.3   General Comments on Variable Selection

Automated variable selection schemes are controversial. They tend to ignore any knowledge of the subject matter. This is why these techniques are considered most appropriate for exploratory analyses. Once a field has progressed far enough that relationships among some variables are known and understood, this knowledge should be used in fitting equations to data.

Simulation studies have found problems with these procedures, such as selecting noise rather than authentic variables, obtaining highly inflated R^2's and adjusted R^2's, too narrow confidence intervals (coverage rates smaller than the specified one) for partial regression coefficients in the selected models, and so on [5, 8, 13]. When variable selection methods are used, multiple tests are performed and the best variables are picked. Since a great many models are considered, the p values are not to be trusted. See [12] for a review of problems encountered with these variable selection techniques.

With all selection methods, and especially the best subset method, the resulting models and regression equations are highly dependent on the particular sample being used; they should be viewed as exploratory results.

It is particularly important that analysts pay attention to their sample size when different groups of variables are considered in variable selection. Even when each variable does not have many missing data, if what is missing varies from case to case, it is not unusual to end up identifying models which are based on a small percentage of the data; variable selection procedures use complete cases only.

As results can be so data dependent, and an equation developed from one sample may not provide a good fit to another sample, a simple option is to randomly divide the data set into two parts and to determine regression equations for each part separately. If the two equations are similar, this suggests that the model provides a good representation of the data. If they are not similar, application of the diagnostic measures discussed in Chapters 10 and 11 is recommended. Presence of outliers could account for dissimilar results.

Investigators tend to use these methods to report one "best" model. In fact, various models can be nearly comparable. It seems appropriate to report these alternatives. The objective of variable selection may not be to find a single model but to find sets of regression equations that are comparable. An alternative approach to model selection, which takes this view, is described in [3]. This approach makes use of differences in AIC between models and is based on information theory. It can easily be implemented with standard statistical software.

Example. We wish to identify variables for inclusion in a model to predict weight (in pounds) from age (in years), height (in inches), waist (in inches) and hip (in inches) for women in the cardiac rehabilitation data set.

A preliminary look at the data reveals that waist and hip measurements are missing for three women. The original sample size was 43, and we are basing our analysis on the 40 women who had complete data. We are assuming that these data are missing at random, and we are deleting these cases. Initial data screening indicated that age is skewed to the left, but the other variables are each approximately normally distributed and there are no outlying observations. Summary statistics for the five variables are given in Table 14.1.

The simple correlations among the variables can be summarized in a 5 by 5 correlation matrix, with rows and columns ordered as weight, age, height, waist, and hip:

$$
\begin{pmatrix}
1.00 & -0.23 & 0.33 & 0.84 & 0.93 \\
-0.23 & 1.00 & -0.06 & -0.07 & -0.20 \\
0.33 & -0.06 & 1.00 & 0.03 & 0.10 \\
0.84 & -0.07 & 0.03 & 1.00 & 0.92 \\
0.93 & -0.20 & 0.10 & 0.92 & 1.00
\end{pmatrix}.
$$

Weight is most strongly correlated with waist and hip measurements and less correlated with age. Among the four predictors, waist and hip are highly correlated, but the correlations among the other pairs of predictors are small. These correlations are consistent with what we would expect, as women who weigh more should be taller and have larger waists and hips. (This example is not a realistic application of the use of variable selection, as we do have some knowledge of the subject matter. However, it is a straightforward illustration of variable selection criteria and methods.)

We first illustrate best subsets. Table 14.2 identifies the four models that have the lowest values of C_p. The lowest value of C_p was found when weight was regressed on age, height, and hip. Note that there isn't much difference in the R^2's, adjusted R^2's, C_p's or AIC's. Also, note how similar the R^2's and adjusted R^2's are; this reflects the small number of variables relative to the sample size.

The same four models were selected when adjusted R^2 was used as the criterion. The only difference was that rows 2 and 3 of Table 14.2 are reversed. On the basis of any of the criteria used, we can't distinguish between any of

Table 14.1 Summary Statistics for Example Variables

Statistic	Weight	Age	Variable Height	Waist	Hip
Sample size	43	43	43	40	40
Minimum	99.75	36	59	27	34.5
Mean	153.5	64	63.4	35.1	42.0
Standard deviation	30.0	10.0	2.3	4.9	4.2
Maximum	242.25	81	68	45.75	52.0

these four models. In this case, we would select height and hip, as this would provide the simplest model.

If we were using this method to select a model, we would likely select two variables for inclusion in the model: height and hip. While this model isn't the one with the absolute lowest C_p, it is the simplest one. We could also argue that we are unable to distinguish among these four, since there are essentially no differences in the R^2's, adjusted R^2's, or AIC's.

Alternatively, the best subsets for a given number of variables in the regression equation may be reported. A greater number of sets of selected variables are summarized in Table 14.3. One variable is selected in the first four rows, two variables are selected in the next four rows, three variables are selected in the next four rows, and all four variables are included in the last row. Table 14.3 provides a broader range of values for each of the four criteria; while R^2 and adjusted R^2 cannot exceed 1, C_p and AIC can become quite large. Note that for a given number of variables, the R^2's and adjusted R^2's are ordered from largest to smallest, while the C_p and AIC are ordered from largest to smallest.

Age, height, and hip are found to be the best combination of variables when this method is used, although this set doesn't really seem appreciably better than just height and hip.

Finally, the results of the forward selection procedure are presented in Table 14.4. We selected 0.15 as our significance level for entry of the variables into the regression model. The first variable entered is hip; hip has the highest simple correlation with weight. The second variable entered is height; hip and height produced the highest R^2 among all sets containing hip and one other variable. (Or, after adjustment for hip, height had the highest partial correlation with weight.) The next variable that would have been entered is age. However, the p value associated with the test that the multiple correlation between weight and hip, height, and age (three variables) is greater than the multiple correlation between weight and hip and height (two variables) is 0.16, which does not quite satisfy the selection cutpoint of 0.15. Thus, if we were using forward variable selection, only hip and height would been selected.

Table 14.2 Best Model Selection on the Basis of C_p

Selected Variables	R^2	Adjusted R^2	C_p	AIC
Age, height, hip	0.93	0.92	3.05	176
Height, hip	0.92	0.92	3.08	177
Age, height, waist, hip	0.93	0.92	5.00	178
Height, waist, hip	0.92	0.92	5.04	179

Table 14.3 Best Model Selection on the Basis of R^2

Selected Variables	R^2	Adjusted R^2	C_p	AIC
Hip	0.87	0.87	24.9	194.4
Waist	0.70	0.69	105.8	228.2
Height	0.10	0.08	388.2	272.0
Age	0.06	0.04	406.1	273.7
Height, hip	0.92	0.92	3.1	176.6
Age, hip	0.88	0.87	24.6	194.9
Waist, hip	0.87	0.87	26.0	195.8
Height, waist	0.79	0.77	67.2	216.7
Age, height, hip	0.93	0.92	3.0	176.3
Height, waist, hip	0.92	0.92	5.0	178.5
Age, waist, hip	0.88	0.87	26.3	196.7
Age, height, waist	0.82	0.81	52.6	211.6
Age, height, waist, hip	0.93	0.92	5.0	178.3

Table 14.4 Summary of Forward Selection Method

Step	Variable Entered	R^2	C_p
1	Hip	0.87	24.9
2	Height	0.92	3.1

In this particular example, for all the methods and criteria used, we select the same two variables: hip and height. (Examples can be found when the different methods select different combinations of variables.)

The results make sense when we go back and examine the correlation matrix above. Weight, hip and height are all highly correlated. The correlation between weight and hip ($r = 0.93$) is greater than the correlation between weight and waist ($r = 0.84$). The correlation between waist and hip is $r = 0.92$. This suggests there is little gain by including both hip and waist in the same regression equation. The other predictor variables (height and age) are essentially uncorrelated with waist and hip. This suggests that the variation in weight explained by these variables would not be greatly affected by waist or hip; these are picking up different sources of variation. Height has a moderate correlation with weight ($r = 0.33$), while age has a smaller correlation with weight ($r = -0.23$). Thus, it is not surprising that hip and height were selected by the methods selected.

The regression model that is selected is

$$\text{weight} = \alpha + \beta_1 \times \text{hip} + \beta_2 \times \text{height} + \varepsilon,$$

and the sample regression plane is

$$\widehat{\text{weight}} = -310.23 + 6.65 \times \text{hip} + 2.92 \times \text{height}.$$

Graphic checks that the data fit the model were made by examining the histogram of the residuals, the normal quantile plot of the residuals, and plots of residuals versus fitted values, hip, and height. These are not shown here; no violations of the assumptions were apparent.

14.5 SUMMARY

In earlier regression and correlation chapters (Chapters 10 – 13) we described general concepts and analyses. Here, we discussed four more specific topics. The first topic concerned how to deal with nominal or ordinal independent variables in the context of regression; we focused on dummy variables using reference coding.

The second topic concerned interaction of independent variables in regression. Interaction between two X variables could be introduced into a regression model by the creation of a new variable which is a product of the two original variables. We focused on the interpretation of the regression coefficients and how the interpretation changes when interactions are and are not included in the regression equation.

The third topic was polynomial regression, an option to consider when a curve gives a better representation of the relationship between the Y and X variables than a straight line.

Finally, we addressed variable selection techniques to identify a reasonable subset of X variables for inclusion in a regression model. We considered four criteria (R^2, adjusted R^2, Mallow's C_p, and AIC) and several variable selection methods: forward, backward, stepwise, best subsets, and all possible subsets. We described these different criteria and methods and used them to illustrate variable selection for a particular example. We indicated that these techniques are controversial and are most appropriate for exploratory data analyses. When knowledge of the subject matter is available, this should be incorporated into the variable selection process.

Problems

14.1   Using the data from the example in Chapter 2, perform a regression analysis using dummy variables for the factor smoking.

   a)   If nonsmoker is the reference category, define the dummy variables.

   b)   Compare and contrast the computer output from ANOVA and from regression.

   c)   What do you see as advantages and disadvantages of regression versus ANOVA for this example?

14.2   A plant scientist is interested in investigating the relationship between the percentage of fungal spores that germinate (Y) and temperature (X). He selects $a = 4$ temperatures (15, 20, 25, and 30 degrees Celsius) and incubates $b = 4$ microscopic slides at each of the four temperatures. The data are as follows:

Slide	Temp, degrees Celsius			
	15	20	25	30
1	33.1	52.8	61.8	6.0
2	31.3	52.3	47.5	3.8
3	25.6	63.2	43.7	3.1
4	27.9	65.0	55.5	10.1

   a)   Draw a scatter diagram of the percentage of fungal spores that germinate versus temperature. Does the relationship between the two variables appear linear? What degree of polynomial looks like it might fit?

   b)   Specify the model which corresponds to a polynomial of degree 2 (a quadratic function).

   c)   Estimate the quadratic regression curve, and plot it on the scatter diagram.

   d)   Check whether the data fit the model, by looking at histograms or normal probability plots of the residuals, residuals versus fitted values, residuals versus temperature, and residuals versus the square of temperature.

   e)   Transform the percentage of fungal spores germinated using the square root transformation, and refit the model. Repeat the four subproblems above.

   f)   Would you recommend that the nontransformed outcome or square root transformed outcome be used in the analysis? Why?

14.3   This problem makes use of the rye yield, yearly rainfall, and temperature data given in Problem 11.4. Create two new variables: the square of rainfall (rainfall $\times$ rainfall and the interaction between rainfall and temperature (rainfall $\times$ temperature.

a)   Regress yield on rainfall, the square of rainfall and temperature. Construct a normal plot of residuals and plot residuals versus rainfall and residuals versus temperature. Do the assumptions of the multiple regression model appear to be satisfied?

b)   Regress yield on rainfall, temperature, and the interaction between rainfall and temperature. Construct a normal plot of residuals and plot residuals versus rainfall and residuals versus temperature. Do the assumptions of the multiple regression model appear to be satisfied?

c)   Compare the fit of these models with those fit in Problem 11.4 and in Problem 12.3. Which of the models provides the best representation of the data? Justify your answer.

14.4   In the text, we performed variable selection using the subset of 43 women. In this problem, we look at the subset of men. (Data are available from the Wiley ftp site.)

a)   Create the correlation matrix of weight, age, height, waist, and hip for men. What does the matrix suggest about the bivariate relationships among the variables? How many subjects have missing data, and which variables are missing?

b)   Perform variable selection using the best subset method and minimum C_p as the criterion. Which model(s) do you recommend? Why?

c)   Perform variable selection using the forward selection procedure, with R^2 as the criterion and significance level for variable entry of 0.15. Which model(s) do you recommend? Why?

d)   Compare your findings with what was found in the text for women. Does your comparison suggest that there may be some interaction between sex and weight? Explain.

14.5   Use the data given in Problem 12.4 on the altitude, longitude, latitude, and mean temperature of 16 cities to answer the following:

a)   Using forward selection, with significance level for variable entry set at $\alpha = 0.15$, which combination of variables (altitude, longitude, and/or latitude) would you recommend be selected to predict temperature?

b)   Using best subsets (sets of one variable, two variables, three variables), rank the models in terms of R^2 and adjusted R^2. Which combination of variables (altitude, longitude and/or latitude) would you recommend be selected to predict temperature? Compare your results with what you found in Problems 12.4 and 13.4 and the forward selection procedure.

14.6   This problem deals with measurements obtained from adult males and females. They are a subsample from a study of the effects of air pollution on lung function. The variables measured are sex (coded as $1 =$ male and $2 =$ female), age (in years), height (in inches), weight (in pounds), FEV1 (in liters), and FVC (in liters). FEV1 is the volume of air expelled during the first second when a participant has been told to breathe in deeply and then expel as much air as possible. FVC (forced vital capacity) is the total volume of air which an individual can expel regardless of how long it takes. The data for these 39 individuals are available on the Wiley ftp site.

a)   Using FVC as the Y variable, perform a best subsets selection using age, height, and weight for males only.

b)   Using FVC as the Y variable, perform a best subsets selection for females only using age, height, and weight. Compare the results with what you found for males only.

c)   Using FVC as the Y variable, perform a best subsets selection using sex, age, height, and weight. Use a dummy variable for sex (i.e., recode to 0 and 1). Compare the results with what you found for males only and females only.

d)   Using FEV1 as the Y variable, perform backward elimination using age, height, and weight for males only.

e)   Using FEV1 as the Y variable, perform backward selection using age, height, and weight for females only. Compare the results with what you found for males only.

f)   Using FEV1 as the Y variable, perform backward elimination using sex, age, height, and weight. Use a dummy variable for sex (i.e., recode to 0 and 1). Compare the results with what you found for males only and females only.

REFERENCES

1. Afifi, A.A., Clark, V.A., and May, S.J. [2003]. *Computer-Aided Multivariate Analysis*, 4th ed., Boca Raton, FL: Chapman and Hall.

2. Bendel, R.B. and Afifi, A.A. [1977.] Comparison of Stopping Rules in Forward Stepwise Regression, *Journal of the American Statistical Association*, 72, 46–53.

3. Burnam, K.P. and Anderson, D. R. [2002]. *Model Selection and Inference: A Practical Information-Theoretic Approach*, 2nd ed., New York: Springer-Verlag.

4. Cohen, A. [1991]. Dummy Variables in Stepwise Regression, *The American Statistician*, 45, 226–228.

5. Flack, V.F. and Chang, P.C. [1987]. Frequency of Selecting Noise Variables in a Subset Regression Analysis: A Simulation Study, *The American Statistician*, 41, 84–86.

6. Hardy. [1994]. *Regression with Dummy Variables,* Sage University Paper Series on Quantitative Applications in the Social Sciences, 07-093, Thousand Oaks, CA: Sage.

7. Hocking, R.R. [1976]. The Analysis and Selection of Variables in Linear Regression, *Biometrics, 32,* 1–50.

8. Hurvich, C.M. and Tsai, C-L. [1990]. The Impact of Model Selection on Inference in Linear Regression, *The American Statistician, 44,* 214–217.

9. Jaccard, J., Turrisi, R., and Wan, C.K. [1990]. *Interaction Effects in Multiple Regression,* Sage University Paper Series on Quantitative Applications in the Social Sciences, 07-072, Newbury Park, CA: Sage.

10. Judd, C.M. and McClelland, G.H. [1989]. *Data Analysis: A Model Comparison Approach,* San Diego, CA: Harcourt, Brace Jovanovich, 247–252.

11. Kendall, M.G. and Stuart, A. [1977]. *The Advanced Theory of Statistics, Volume 1: Distribution Theory,* 4th ed., London: Charles Griffin & Company Limited, 417–418.

12. Miller, A.J. [1984]. Selection of Subsets of Regression Variables (with discussion), *Journal of the Royal Statistical Society, Series A, 147,* 389–425.

13. Rencher, A.C. and Pun, F.C. [1980]. Inflation of R^2 in Best Subset Regression, *Technometrics, 22,* 49–53.

15

Analysis of Covariance

In the ANOVA designs in earlier chapters, we compared various linear combinations of sample means. In Chapters 10 through 14, we used regression techniques to study the relation of a response variable Y to one or more independent variables $X_1, \ldots, X_k$. A combination of these two techniques is known as *analysis of covariance* or ANCOVA.

There are a variety of ways of looking at ANCOVA, but we focus here on it as a technique for assessing equality of population means, while removing the linear effects of X variables, referred to as *covariates*. The covariates, if ignored, may have two undesirable effects on comparisons of means. First, variation that can be explained by the linear relations between the outcome and the covariate ends up as part of the residual variation. Second, if the distributions of the covariate (X) differ across the populations, failure to control for it may introduce bias into the comparison of means. It can be unclear whether mean responses (Y) of several populations differ (or don't differ) because the covariate distributions are unequal or because of the factors which define the populations.

As with other procedures discussed in this book, ANCOVA can be applied in either experimental or nonexperimental settings, but its advantages are not the same for both. In the experimental setting, in which units are randomly assigned to treatment groups, the main objective of ANCOVA is reduction of the residual error term that is used in making inferences. Covariance analysis can result in shorter confidence intervals, more powerful tests, or smaller required sample sizes than with ANOVA. The residual variation can be reduced because part of it can be explained by the linear relations between the Y variable and the covariates (X variables). There is less concern about covariate distributions being unequal; we expect them to be approximately the same because of randomization.

In the nonexperimental setting, there is greater potential for covariates to be unequally distributed across the treatment groups. The second objective, of removing the effect of the covariates on population means, is of greater concern in observational studies. Comparisons among population means are made at the same levels of the covariates.

In this chapter, we confine ourselves mainly to the simplest type of covariance problem — namely, a combination of a one-way ANOVA with linear regression on a single X variable. An example is introduced in Section 15.1. The ANCOVA model and its interpretation are presented in Section 15.2. Estimation of model parameters is described in Section 15.3. This is followed by a discussion of hypothesis testing in Section 15.4. Estimation of adjusted means, their estimated standard errors, and confidence intervals are discussed in Section 15.5. How to tell if the data fit the ANCOVA model is considered in Section 15.6, and what to do they they don't is addressed in Section 15.7. The advantages and limitations of ANCOVA in nonexperimental studies are reviewed in Section 15.8. Desirable characteristics for covariates are summarized in Section 15.9, and some comments about measurement error, which can occur in both response variables and covariates, are presented in Section 15.10. ANCOVA is compared and contrasted with other methods of covariate adjustment in Section 15.11. Some comments about available statistical software for performing ANCOVA are given in Section 15.12. The chapter is summarized in Section 15.13.

15.1   EXAMPLE

As an example of a covariance analysis, we use some data on language scores Y for students taught by three different methods. Measurements on IQ (X) taken before the language instruction are also available. The data are given in Table 15.1. Altogether, 30 students were randomly assigned to treatment group, which in this example is teaching method. Ten students were allocated to each method.

The main question that we wish to ask is whether the mean language score is the same for the three teaching methods. Just from looking at the mean language scores for each of the three teaching methods given in Table 15.1, we see that the highest value is obtained from method 2 (81.40), and the lowest from method 3 (73.70); the sample mean language score associated with method 1 is between the other two (78.70). As we've seen in Chapter 2, we could make inferences by one-way ANOVA, as in Table 15.2. Teaching method is not significant at $\alpha = 0.05$; $p = 0.11$. [For convenience, we use $\phi(\alpha) = \sum_{i=1}^{a} (\alpha_i - \bar{\alpha})^2 / (a - 1)$ in the EMS column of Table 15.2.]

A possible limitation on the above analysis is related to the fact that IQ score was ignored. The residual variation may be higher than it needs to

EXAMPLE   377

Table 15.1 Data on Language Scores (Y) Using Three Teaching Methods and IQ Scores (X)

	Method 1		Method 2		Method 3	
	Language	IQ	Language	IQ	Language	IQ
	72	87	85	110	71	95
	75	119	93	128	77	120
	85	121	68	117	79	125
	70	112	83	94	83	107
	73	100	78	107	71	85
	86	133	85	125	73	98
	92	135	93	111	70	100
	68	109	76	80	82	138
	91	139	79	123	71	112
	75	105	74	95	60	90
Mean	78.70	116.00	81.40	109.00	73.70	107.00
SD	8.92	16.65	8.02	15.44	6.82	16.75

be. Any effect of the linear relation between language and IQ score would be included in the residual variation; if we were to control for the linear relation between the two, we would expect the residual variation to be lowered.

To get an idea of the relation between language score and IQ, let's look at a scatter diagram of language score versus IQ score, in Figure 15.1. On this graph, we have identified the different teaching methods by different symbols (a circle for method 1, a triangle for method 2, and a square for method 3). It seems from the plot that there is a tendency for language score to be positively related to IQ score.

Table 15.2 Analysis of Variance Table for Language Score For Three Teaching Methods

Source of Variation	SS	df	MS	EMS	Computed F	p Value
Method	305.27	2	152.63	$\sigma^2 + 10\phi(\alpha)$	2.41	0.11
Residual	1712.60	27	63.43	σ^2		
Total	2017.87	29				

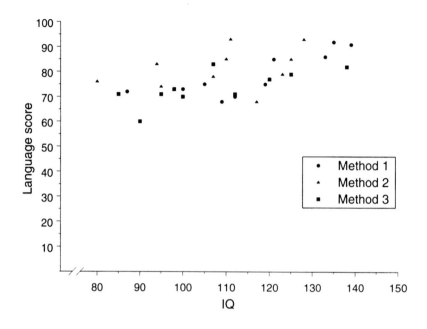

Fig. 15.1   Language score versus IQ score, by teaching method.

15.2   THE ANCOVA MODEL

Underlying the analysis of covariance, we make certain assumptions. For each treatment and any fixed value of the covariate X, the distribution of the outcome Y is normal. For each treatment, the means of these populations lie on a specified type of regression curve (here, a straight line); the variances are all equal.

The underlying ANCOVA model can be expressed in such a way that its regression aspects or its ANOVA aspects are emphasized. With emphasis on regression, the more common representation, each observation is expressed as

$$Y_{ij} = \alpha_{0i} + \beta X_{ij} + \varepsilon_{ij}, \qquad i = 1, \ldots, a, \quad j = 1, \ldots, n_i, \qquad (15.1)$$

where $\varepsilon_{ij} \sim \text{IND}(0, \sigma^2)$. In Equation 15.1, Y_{ij} and X_{ij} denote the Y and X values for the jth individual on the ith treatment. The number of treatments is a, and the number of individuals in the ith sample is n_i.

In this form, the $\alpha_{0i} + \beta X_{ij}$ represent a parallel population regression lines; each line has a different Y intercept α_{0i} but the same slope β.

An alternative statement of the underlying model that exhibits the ANOVA aspect of ANCOVA is

$$Y_{ij} = \mu + \alpha_i + \beta(X_{ij} - \bar{X}_{..}) + \varepsilon_{ij}, \qquad i = 1, \ldots, a, \quad j = 1, \ldots, n_i, \quad (15.2)$$

with $\sum_{i=1}^{a} \alpha_i = 0$, $\varepsilon_{ij} \sim \text{IND}(0, \sigma^2)$, and X_{ij} and β just as in Equation 15.2. (Note that $\bar{X}_{..} = \sum_{i=1}^{a} \sum_{j=1}^{n_{ij}} X_{ij}/N$, where $N = \sum_{i=1}^{a} n_i$.)

In this form, because the X_{ij} are all from the same population of X's when units are randomly assigned to treatment group, the population mean of $X_{ij} - \bar{X}_{..}$ is zero. We therefore have $E(Y_{ij}) = \mu + \alpha_i$ as the population mean of the Y's on the ith treatment. Just as in one-way ANOVA, μ is the average of the a population means, and α_i is the effect of the ith treatment.

Example. For our example of language scores, teaching method, and IQ scores, the model can expressed as

$$Y_{ij} = \alpha_{0i} + \beta X_{ij} + \varepsilon_{ij}, \qquad i = 1, \ldots 3, \quad j = 1, \ldots, 10.$$

In particular, there are $a = 3$ teaching methods and $n_1 = n_2 = n_3 = 10$ students who are taught by each teaching method.

The assumptions implied by the model are:

(1) For any fixed IQ score, language scores for a given teaching method are normally distributed.

(2) The means of the language scores for fixed IQ scores have means lying on a straight line. The population regression lines are $E(Y_{ij}) = \alpha_{0i} + \beta X_{ij}$. The three regression lines are parallel.

(3) For any fixed IQ score, the distributions of language scores have equal variances σ^2.

Figure 15.2 illustrates the ANCOVA model as we defined it. Here, there are three parallel population regression lines. The slopes (β) are the same, but the Y intercepts (α_{0i}) are different. The mean language score depends on IQ as well as on teaching method. Because the slope is positive, there is a positive relationship between language score and IQ. For a one unit increase in IQ, the mean language score changes by β units. The different Y intercepts reflect the effect of teaching method. With parallel regression lines, the difference in mean language score between, say, teaching methods 1 and 3 is simply $\alpha_{01} - \alpha_{03}$ (the difference of the intercepts) at *every* value of IQ.

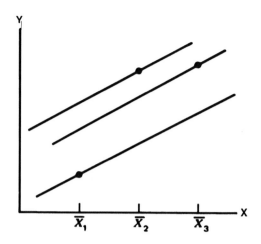

Fig. 15.2 Population regression lines for the ANCOVA model.

15.3 ESTIMATION OF MODEL PARAMETERS

The estimation of the α_{0i}'s, β, and σ^2 is based on the same procedures that we have discussed throughout the book.

We saw in Section 15.2 that ANCOVA has aspects of ANOVA as well as regression; the model includes both a factor and a continuous covariate. Therefore, it is probably easiest to obtain parameter estimates through use of a general linear model procedure; with this, models with factors only (as in ANOVA) or more general X variables (as in regression) or some combination of the two (as in ANCOVA) can be fitted.

Alternatively, regression procedures can be used. However, an a level factor (where $a \geq 3$) may need to be transformed to $a - 1$ dummy variables (see Chapter 14).

The estimate of each α_{0i} is equal to $\bar{Y}_{i.} - b\bar{X}_{i.}$. The sample regression line for the ith factor level goes through the point $(\bar{X}_{i.}, \bar{Y}_{i.})$.

Example. When we fit the ANCOVA model with parallel population regression lines, we obtain three parallel sample regression lines. For the three teaching methods (factors), these lines are:

$$
\begin{aligned}
\hat{Y}_1 &= 42.104 + 0.315X, \\
\hat{Y}_2 &= 47.013 + 0.315X, \\
\hat{Y}_3 &= 39.944 + 0.315X.
\end{aligned}
$$

To estimate these sample regression lines with the same slope, we fit a model with the factor (teaching method) and covariate (IQ score) — a usual AN-COVA model. In the program we used (SAS proc glm), we needed to request that estimates be printed out, using the solution command.

15.4 HYPOTHESIS TESTS

We describe two different hypothesis tests here. Each is straightforward and is based on exactly the same assumptions as in a linear regression: independent observations, normal distributions of Y at particular values of X, equal variances, and, for each treatment, population means on a straight line.

The hypothesis that we are most interested in testing is whether the regression lines are the same for the a different treatments. For the null model, not only are the regression lines parallel, but they overlap, as illustrated in Figure 15.3a. The slopes are all equal and the Y intercepts are all equal. For our example, this suggests that teaching method has no effect on mean language score, but that a student's IQ score does.

The null and alternative hypotheses can be written as

$$H_0 : E(Y_{ij}) = \alpha_0 + \beta X_{ij},$$

$$H_1 : E(Y_{ij}) = \alpha_{0i} + \beta X_{ij}. \tag{15.3}$$

Note that this null model is a regression model, as described in Chapter 11. There is a single X variable, and the factor is completely ignored.

Of less interest is testing whether the parallel regression lines have a slope of zero. We expect them to have a nonzero slope. Otherwise, knowledge of the covariate's value contributes nothing to the prediction of Y, so there is no gain in doing ANCOVA with this covariate. The main reason for doing this test is to verify that a reasonable covariate has been selected. For the null model, there are a parallel regression lines, each with slope 0, as illustrated in Figure 15.3b. The null and alternative hypotheses can be expressed as

$$H_0 : E(Y_{ij}) = \alpha_{0i},$$

$$H_1 : E(Y_{ij}) = \alpha_{0i} + \beta X_{ij}. \tag{15.4}$$

Note that this null model is a one-way ANOVA model, as described in Chapter 2. (Each α_{0i} can be reexpressed as $\mu + \alpha_i$ or μ_i.) There is one factor, and the covariate is completely ignored. In terms of our example, the null model suggests that knowledge of IQ score does not provide information about language score.

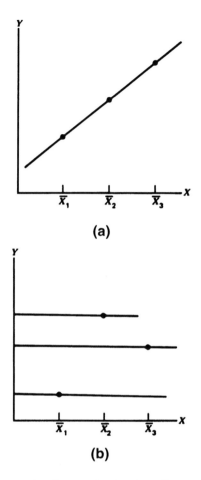

(a)

(b)

Fig. 15.3 Population regression lines under two hypotheses: (a) $E(Y_{ij}) = \alpha_0 + \beta X$ and (b) $E(Y_{ij}) = \alpha_{0i}$.

These two null hypotheses can be tested from the same ANOVA table, which is given in Table 15.3. In this table, three sources of variation are identified: variation due to the factor (after adjustment has been made for the covariate), variation due to the covariate (after adjustment has been made for the factor), and residual variation.

The SS_a denotes the adjusted or Type III sums of squares for the factor; a is to the number of levels of the treatment factor, so $a - 1$ is the associated number of degrees of freedom. The SS_X denotes the adjusted or Type III sums of squares for the covariate, X. In this model, there is only one covariate, so there is one degree of freedom associated with this source of variation. To test for no effect of the treatment factor, as in Equation 15.4, the F statistic

Table 15.3 Analysis of Covariance Table for Testing Effects of Factor and Covariate)

Source of Variation	Adjusted SS	df	MS	F
Factor	SS_a	$a - 1$	MS_a	MS_a/MS_r
Covariate	SS_X	1	MS_X	MS_X/MS_r
Residual	SS_r	$N - a - 1$	MS_r	
Total	SS_t	$N - 1$		

is the ratio of the factor mean square to the residual mean square, that is, MS_a/MS_r. Similarly, to test for no effect of the covariate, as in Equation 15.5 the F statistic is the ratio of the covariate mean square to the residual mean square, that is, MS_X/MS_r.

The two adjusted sums of squares plus the residual sum of squares do not add up to the total sum of squares in ANCOVA. However, if SS_a and SS_r are summed, as well as their numbers of degrees of freedom $(a - 1 + N - a - 1 = N - 2)$, an ANOVA table for simple linear regression is obtained. (There are two sources of variation: regression and residual. The resulting ANOVA table would be produced by fitting the null model given in Equation 15.4 to the data; the factor is ignored.) Also, if SS_X and SS_r are summed, as well as their numbers of degrees of freedom $(1 + N - a - 1 = N - a)$, a one-way ANOVA table is obtained. (There are two sources of variation: factor and residual. The resulting ANOVA table would be generated by fitting the null model given in Equation 15.5; the covariate X is ignored.)

However, since ANCOVA involves both classification variables or factors and continuous X variables or covariates, it is easiest to perform the analyses using software that allows both types of variables to be specified in a model. These procedures are generally referred to as *general linear modeling* procedures and are more general than those that deal exclusively with ANOVA or with regression. (See Chapter 8 for an overview of different types of models.) Many of the standard statistical packages have a general linear model program (e.g., the glm procedure in SAS, or the general linear model option as a special case of ANOVA in Minitab.) Since these are general procedures, analysts need to know how to apply them in special cases. Both on-line documentation and manuals can be quite helpful in this regard, as they frequently give specific examples.

Example. The two hypothesis tests for our example are summarized in Table 15.4. (Note that the sums of squares do not add up to the total; we are reporting adjusted, or Type III, sums of squares. The sum of squares for method is determined with linear effects of IQ removed. The sum of squares for IQ score is calculated with effects of teaching method removed.)

As an aside, before looking at the F tests, we note some characteristics of the sums of squares. Recall from Chapter 12 that there are multiple ways to break apart or combine sums of squares. Addition of the covariate (after factor) sum of squares to the residual sum of squares yields $713.618 + 998.982 = 1712.6$, the residual sum of squares in Table 15.2 for the one-way ANOVA. Similarly, we can verify that $262.439 + 998.982 = 1261.421$, the residual sum of squares for a simple linear regression model. (This is not shown here.)

The calculated F statistic for testing the hypothesis given in Equation 15.4 is $F = 3.42$, and $p = 0.048$. From this, we reject the null hypothesis that there is no effect of teaching method when we adjust for IQ. In the context of regression, the three population regression lines are parallel, but not overlapping.

We also conclude that there is an effect of IQ score on mean language score, when we adjust for teaching method, since $F = 18.57$ and $p = 0.0002$. In terms of regression, the three parallel population regression lines do not have slope 0.

What was the advantage of using ANCOVA in this example? The gain can be seen by comparing the residual sum of squares for the one-way ANOVA when IQ score was ignored (Table 15.2, $SS_r = 1712.60$) with the residual sum of squares for the ANCOVA (Table 15.4, $SS_r = 998.98$). In this example, this represents a reduction of $(1712.60 - 998.98)/1712.60$, or 42%. Thus, 42% of the residual variation from the one-way ANOVA can be explained by the linear relation between language score and IQ score. In terms of residual mean squares, we see $MS_r = 63.43$ when IQ score was ignored (Table 15.2), compared with $MS_r = 38.42$ when adjustment was made for IQ score (Table 15.4). Confidence intervals (as described in Section 15.5.2) are also shorter, because they make use of the square root of the residual mean square. The length of a confidence interval is $\sqrt{38.42/63.43} = 0.78$ times as long with IQ specified as the covariate. Thus, from the point of view of reduction in variability, using IQ score as a covariate was a good choice. The reduction in residual variability translates into increased power to detect differences in mean language score and narrower confidence intervals. This is consistent with the main objective of using ANCOVA in experiments.

We also note that the mean square for method (after IQ score), 131.219, is somewhat smaller than the sum of squares for method, 153.63, from the one-way ANOVA in Table 15.2. When adjustment is made for IQ score, the mean square in the numerator is also smaller. In experimental settings such as this one, we don't expect a large reduction in the mean square for the factor (method), because we rely on the randomization to equalize effects of the covariate (IQ score) across the groups (teaching method). A smaller mean square in the numerator could have the effect of decreasing the F statistic, but the greater reduction in the residual mean square in this example increases the F statistic.

Table 15.4   Analysis of Covariance Table for Language Scores (Y) on IQ Scores (X)

Source of Variation	Adjusted SS	df	MS	Computed F	p
Method	262.44	2	131.22	3.42	0.048
IQ Score	713.62	1	713.62	18.57	0.0002
Residual	998.98	26	38.42		
Total	2017.87	29			

15.5   ADJUSTED MEANS

15.5.1   Estimation of Adjusted Means and Standard Errors

When investigators wish to compare the mean response in the a different populations, it is generally not appropriate to rely exclusively on the sample means $\bar{Y}_{1.}, \bar{Y}_{2.}, \ldots, \bar{Y}_{a.}$ when it is known that a covariate X is related to the response Y. If the distribution of the X values differs across the different populations, then some of the difference in mean response could be attributable to differences in the levels of the covariates. For population i, the population mean depends on X as

$$E(\bar{Y}_{i.}|X) = \alpha_{0i} + \beta X,$$

and the corresponding sample mean at a specified level of X is

$$\begin{aligned}
\hat{Y}_i &= a_i + bX \\
&= \bar{Y}_{i.} + b(X - \bar{X}_{i.}),
\end{aligned}$$

where a_i is the Y intercept and b is the slope of the sample regression line.

One way to address the effect of the differing distributions of X across the populations is to determine the mean at the same value of X. Typically, the value of X that is selected is the overall mean, $\bar{X}_{..}$ (or in the case of unequal sample sizes, the mean of the group-specific means, $\sum_{i=1}^{a} \bar{X}_{i.}/a$). These are referred to as *adjusted means* or as *least square means*. The population adjusted mean, which we denote by $\bar{\mu}_{i.}$ is estimated by

$$\begin{aligned}
\text{adj } \bar{Y}_{i.} &= a_i + b\bar{X}_{..} \\
&= \bar{Y}_{i.} + b(\bar{X}_{..} - \bar{X}_{i.}). \quad (15.5)
\end{aligned}$$

From this equation, we can see that if the mean covariate value is the same across the a samples, no adjustment is made. If the sample slope is positive and the mean value of the covariate for a particular population is less than the overall mean, then the sample mean response, $\bar{Y}_{i.}$, is increased to what it is predicted to be when $X = \bar{X}_{..}$.

Since adj $\bar{Y}_{i.}$ is a linear combination, it is straightforward to estimate its variance and standard error. The same procedures were used in Chapter 10 for simple linear regression:

$$\text{Var adj } \bar{Y}_{i.} = \text{Var}(\bar{Y}_{i.} + b(\bar{X}_{..} - \bar{X}_{i.})) \tag{15.6}$$

$$= \left[\frac{1}{n_i} + \frac{(\bar{X}_{..} - \bar{X}_{i.})^2}{\sum_{i=1}^{a} \sum_{j=1}^{n_i}(X_{ij} - \bar{X}_{i.})^2} \right] \sigma^2. \tag{15.7}$$

As in simple linear regression, we see that the variance is smaller when sample sizes (n_i) are larger and when the covariate mean is close to the overall mean, that is, $\bar{X}_{i.} - \bar{X}_{..}$ is small. The estimated variance is obtained by substituting σ^2 by its estimate, the residual mean square MS_r as specified in Table 15.3. The estimated standard error is the square root of the estimated variance.

Example. Ignoring IQ score, the sample means for the three different teaching methods are $\bar{Y}_1 = 78.7$, $\bar{Y}_2 = 81.4$, and $\bar{Y}_3 = 73.7$. The sample mean IQ scores for the three groups are $\bar{X}_1 = 116.0$, $\bar{X}_2 = 109.0$, and $\bar{X}_3 = 107.0$. The overall mean IQ score is $\bar{X}_{..} = 110.67$. Note that — as expected in an experimental study such as this one, in which students were randomized to teaching method — the sample mean IQ scores are approximately equal in the three groups. Therefore, we expect little difference between the mean language score and the adjusted mean language score. However, because of the linear relationship between language score and IQ score, we expect the estimated standard errors to be lower for the adjusted means.

Substituting the value of $X = \bar{X}_{..} = 110.67$, we obtain the adjusted means. The estimated standard errors can be found by replacing σ^2 with its estimate (38.44) and specifying the sample covariate means and sample sizes in Equation 15.7. The (unadjusted) means and their estimated standard errors (estimated using methods described in Chapter 2 and substituting $\text{MS}_r = 63.43$) are summarized in Table 15.5.

Since there was little difference in the mean IQ score for the three groups, we see little difference in the sample means and the adjusted means. For teaching method 1, the adjusted mean is slightly lower than the mean, because the mean IQ was slightly higher than the overall mean IQ. The mean language score is determined at IQ $= 110.67$ rather than at 116. For methods 2 and 3, the adjusted means are higher; these reflect mean IQ scores below the overall mean for methods 2 and 3.

Also as expected, the estimated standard errors for the adjusted means are all lower than those for the means. The sample sizes in this example were all equal, so differences in estimated standard errors reflect only differences between the mean IQ score for each group and the overall mean. The estimated standard error is smallest for teaching method 2, since its mean IQ score, $\bar{X}_{2.} = 109.0$, is closest to the overall mean of 110.67. Similarly, the estimated standard error is largest for teaching method 1, since its mean IQ score, $\bar{X}_{1.} = 116.0$, is farthest from the overall mean.

Sometimes adjusted means are computed to enable investigators to report mean values for the outcome variable that has been adjusted for a well-known value of the covariate. For our example, the investigator may wish to report language scores that have been adjusted to an IQ score of 100.

15.5.2 Confidence Intervals for Adjusted Means

Probably the most useful confidence intervals in ANCOVA are those for differences in population adjusted mean response. These will allow us to identify differences in the population adjusted means as well as to obtain an interval estimate for how disparate population adjusted means are.

The expression for the $100(1-\alpha)\%$ confidence interval for the difference in population adjusted means of populations i and i', $(\bar{\mu}_{i.|X=\bar{X}_{..}}) - (\bar{\mu}_{i'.|X=\bar{X}_{..}})$, is

$$\text{adj } \bar{Y}_{i.} - \text{adj } \bar{Y}_{i'.} \pm t_{[1-\alpha/2, N-a-1]} \, \text{se}(\text{adj } \bar{Y}_{i.} - \text{adj } \bar{Y}_{i'.}), \qquad (15.8)$$

where the estimated standard error is

$$\sqrt{\left[\frac{1}{n_i} + \frac{1}{n_{i'}} + \frac{(\bar{X}_{i.} - \bar{X}_{i'.})^2}{\sum_{i=1}^{a} \sum_{j=1}^{n_i} (X_{ij} - \bar{X}_{i.})^2}\right] \text{MS}_r}. \qquad (15.9)$$

The number of degrees of freedom associated with the t distribution is the same as that used in calculation of the residual mean square, MS_r.

Example. The 95% confidence intervals for the three possible pairwise differences in the population adjusted means and in the population means are given in Table 15.6. The three paired differences compare the adjusted mean

Table 15.5 Comparisons of Adjusted Mean and Mean Language Scores and Their Estimated Standard Errors

Teaching Method	Adjusted Means		Means	
	Estimate	Standard Error	Estimate	Standard Error
1	77.02	2.00	78.70	2.52
2	81.93	1.96	81.40	2.52
3	74.86	1.98	73.70	2.52

language score (adjusted to the overall mean IQ score of $\bar{X}_{..} = 110.67$). The lengths of the intervals are smaller for the differences in the population adjusted means; this can be attributed to the smaller residual mean square that is used in the calculations.

The three confidence intervals for the differences in population adjusted mean language scores suggest that the population adjusted means for teaching methods 2 and 3 are unequal; this confidence interval for $\bar{\mu}_{2.|X=110.67} - \bar{\mu}_{3.|X=110.67}$ was the only one of the three that did not cover 0. On the basis of these intervals, we conclude that, for students with an IQ score of 110.67, the three teaching methods may be equal. For the population means, all three confidence intervals include 0; we have no evidence that the three population means are unequal.

In summary, Table 15.4 suggests that when adjustment is made for IQ, there is a difference in mean language score for the three methods. The calculated p value was 0.048, which is quite close to a cutpoint of 0.05. For students with an IQ score of 110.67, when adjustment is made for multiple comparisons, we don't have evidence that mean language scores are unequal. Without adjustment for multiple comparisons, we do find a difference for teaching methods 2 and 3. These findings are not entirely consistent, and different analysts might not agree in how to interpret the results. We would likely say that there is only marginal evidence that the adjusted means are unequal and would conclude that, when adjustment is made for IQ score, there may not be a difference in mean language score.

15.6 CHECKING IF THE DATA FIT THE ANCOVA MODEL

Since all of the inferences that are made are based on the assumption that the model is appropriate, it is important to investigate whether the underlying assumptions are correct. Most of the assumptions — normal distributions, equal variances, straight line regressions, and independence of observations — can be evaluated as discussed in Chapter 10.

It's always important to identify the extent of missing data; many programs which perform ANCOVA use only cases with complete data for the variables included in the analysis. This can become a problem, particularly when ANCOVA is generalized to include multiple covariates.

Since multiple regression lines, with parallel slopes, are a new concept in this chapter, this assumption is now discussed in greater detail.

If the regression lines are not parallel, they may be pictured as in Figure 15.4. We have three population regression lines, each with a different Y intercept (α_{0i}) and a different slope (β_i). In terms of our example, this suggests that there is interaction between teaching method and IQ score on mean language score. In this situation, it would not be possible to make simple statements about differences in population mean language scores between the teaching methods, since the difference depends on the value of a student's

Table 15.6   95% Confidence Intervals for Differences in Mean Language Score

Confidence Interval Based On	
Adjusted Means	Means
$-10.70 \leq \bar{\mu}_{1.\|X=110.67} - \bar{\mu}_{2.\|X=110.67} \leq 0.89$	$-11.53 \leq E(\bar{Y}_{1.} - \bar{Y}_{2.}) \leq 6.13$
$-3.70 \leq \bar{\mu}_{1.\|X=110.67} - \bar{\mu}_{3.\|X=110.67} \leq 8.02$	$-3.83 \leq E(\bar{Y}_{1.} - \bar{Y}_{3.}) \leq 13.83$
$1.36 \leq \bar{\mu}_{2.\|X=110.67} - \bar{\mu}_{3.\|X=110.67} \leq 12.78$	$-1.13 \leq E(\bar{Y}_{2.} - \bar{Y}_{3.}) \leq 16.53$

IQ score. Similarly, it would not be possible to make simple statements about the slopes of the regression lines, since they depend on the teaching method. In this case, the equation for the underlying model can be expressed as

$$Y_{ij} = \alpha_{0i} + \beta_i X_{ij} + \varepsilon_{ij}, \qquad i = 1, \ldots, a, \quad j = 1, \ldots, n_i. \qquad (15.10)$$

As with all other methods of data screening, it helps to look at scatter diagrams and to calculate summary statistics. In this case, graphs of outcome versus covariate, with the sample regression line for each treatment separately, provide an indication of equality of slopes. Comparison of slopes — both point estimates and confidence intervals — for each treatment can also provide an initial summary.

Finally, a hypothesis test can be performed to investigate whether or not the regression lines are parallel. The null and alternative hypothesis can be expressed as

$$H_0 : Y_{ij} = \alpha_{0i} + \beta X_{ij} + \varepsilon_{ij},$$

$$\qquad (15.11)$$

$$H_1 : Y_{ij} = \alpha_{0i} + \beta_i X_{ij} + \varepsilon_{ij}.$$

The alternative hypothesis can be viewed as a model that involves main effects of the factor and covariate as well as the interaction between the two variables; there is no interaction between the two in the null model. Thus, this is a test of no interaction between the factor and the covariate.

The test is performed using ANOVA. In Table 15.7, we see that four sources of variation are identified: the factor, the covariate, the factor by covariate interaction, and the residual. The table reflects a single factor with a levels and a single covariate X. The sums of squares are adjusted (or type III). The only rows of the table that are needed for the test for parallel slopes are the factor by covariate interaction and the residual.

The F statistic is determined as the ratio of the factor by covariate interaction mean square to the residual mean square, MS_{aX}/MS_r. When the slopes of the population regression lines are equal, the F statistic follows an

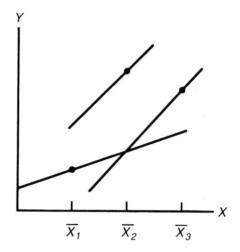

Fig. 15.4 Population regression lines when $E(Y_{ij}) = \alpha_{0i} + \beta_i X_{ij}$.

Table 15.7 Analysis of Covariance Table for Test of Parallel Slopes

Source of Variation	Adjusted SS	df	MS	F
Factor	SS_a	$a - 1$	MS_a	MS_a/MS_r
Covariate	SS_X	1	MS_X	MS_X/MS_r
Factor by covariate interaction	SS_{aX}	$a - 1$	MS_{aX}	MS_{aX}/MS_r
Residual	SS_r	$N - 2a$	MS_r	
Total	SS_t	$N - 1$		

F distribution with $\nu_1 = a - 1$ and $\nu_2 = N - 2a$. [The number of degrees of freedom associated with the interaction mean square is the product of the number of degrees of freedom associated with the factor and the covariate, here $(a - 1) \times 1$.]

Analysts should be aware of a possible limitation on basing their conclusions about whether the slopes are parallel on this test. If the hypothesis is not rejected, there is always the possibility that a Type II, or β, error has been made, that is, that the population regression lines have unequal slopes but the hypothesis test fails to detect it. A way to decrease the chance of making this error is to increase the chance of making a Type I, or α, error, by increasing the level of significance α. However, it isn't clear what the appropriate level of significance is. Therefore, many statisticians prefer to make a decision on the basis of scatter plots and overlap of confidence intervals for the separate population slopes.

Example. Scatter diagrams for language score versus IQ score are shown in Figure 15.5 for each teaching method separately. A sample regression line for each treatment group is also included. Comparison of these graphs gives the impression that the three lines are more or less parallel. At least, for each teaching method there appears to be an increasing relation between language score and IQ score; all slope estimates are positive and approximately equal.

We can get an idea of how similar the slopes are by estimating 95% confidence intervals for each slope. First, we regress language score on IQ score for each of the three teaching methods separately. The fitted regression lines for the three teaching methods are

$$\hat{Y}_1 = 26.84 + 0.45 \text{ IQ},$$
$$\hat{Y}_2 = 60.75 + 0.19 \text{ IQ},$$
$$\hat{Y}_3 = 42.40 + 0.29 \text{ IQ},$$

where $\hat{Y}_1$, $\hat{Y}_2$, and $\hat{Y}_3$ denote the predicted value of language score when teaching methods 1, 2, and 3 are used. It is difficult to assess whether the popu-

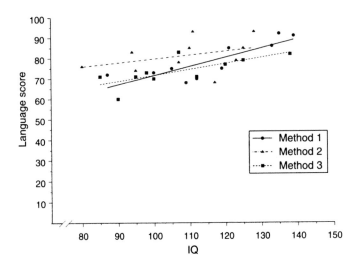

Fig. 15.5 Language score versus IQ score by teaching method.

lation regression lines are equal from the point estimates of the slopes alone; the estimated standard errors for the slope estimates for methods 1, 2, and 3 are 0.10, 0.17, and 0.10, respectively.

Next, we can use the point estimates and estimated standard errors to construct confidence intervals for β_1, β_2, and β_3, the slopes of the population regression lines for methods 1, 2, and 3. The 95% confidence intervals are

$$0.21 \leq \beta_1 \leq 0.69,$$
$$-0.20 \leq \beta_2 \leq 0.58,$$
$$0.06 \leq \beta_3 \leq 0.52.$$

There is quite a bit of overlap for these three confidence intervals. As discussed in Chapter 3, overlapping confidence intervals are suggestive that the population parameters are the same (but it is recommended that conclusions be based on formal hypothesis tests) [9].

For completeness, we also present the ANOVA table which is constructed to test whether or not there is interaction between teaching method and IQ score; see Table 15.8. (Again, note that the sums of squares are adjusted and so do not add up to the total.) Here, the calculated $F = 1.03$ and $p = 0.37$, so we conclude that the three regression lines may be parallel.

15.7 WHAT TO DO IF THE DATA DON'T FIT THE MODEL

If the ANCOVA assumptions are violated, transformations of the variables are considered. In many applications, a transformation may obviate violations of more than one assumption.

We have assumed here that there is a linear relation between the Y and the X variable. If this is found not to be the case, either a transformation of the X variable or a change in the regression curve (for example, polynomial regression, as described in Chapter 14.)

If it is difficult or impossible to find transformations which will remove interaction between the covariate and the factor, one possibility is to perform multiple analyses, each one restricted to a different range, with a different width, of the covariate values.

15.8 ANCOVA IN OBSERVATIONAL STUDIES

When the assignment of individuals to a different groups has not been made randomly, a covariance analysis can be carried out in precisely the same manner as under random assignment; all the formulas hold. ANCOVA with non-random assignment to groups, as in observational studies or surveys, has both

Table 15.8   Test for Parallel Regression Lines

Source of Variation	Adjusted SS	df	MS	Computed F	p
Method	103.59	2	51.79	1.35	0.28
IQ Score	684.05	1	684.05	17.84	0.0003
Method by IQ Interaction	78.68	2	39.34	1.03	0.37
Residual	920.30	24	38.35		
Total	2017.87	29			

a major advantage and a major disadvantage. The advantage is that investigators may be able to reduce the effect of a variable that tends to obscure the true picture of the mean differences. (In contrast, in experimental studies, we rely on randomization to equalize distributions of covariates.) The disadvantage is that the interpretation of the results may be difficult. How difficult it is depends on the nature of the covariate. The characteristics of a good covariate are discussed in Section 15.9 below.

We can see the role that ANCOVA can play in bias reduction by re-examining the model, as given in Equation 15.2. For convenience, this model is repeated here.

$$Y_{ij} = \mu + \alpha_i + \beta(X_{ij} - \bar{X}_{..}) + \varepsilon_{ij}, \qquad i = 1, \ldots, a, \quad j = 1, \ldots, n_i,$$

The mean of Y for the ith population is

$$E(\bar{Y}_{i.}) = \mu + \alpha_i + \beta(\bar{X}_{i.} - \bar{X}_{..}),$$

and the mean of Y for the i'th population is

$$E(\bar{Y}_{i'.}) = \mu + \alpha_{i'} + \beta(\bar{X}_{i'.} - \bar{X}_{..}),$$

so that the difference in means is

$$E(\bar{Y}_{i.}) - E(\bar{Y}_{i'.}) = (\alpha_i - \alpha_{i'}) + \beta(\bar{X}_{i.} - \bar{X}_{i'.}).$$

The $\beta(\bar{X}_{i.} - \bar{X}_{i'.})$ is the bias in the difference in means. If the covariate means are the same in the populations, there is no bias. So when the adjusted means are determined as

$$\begin{aligned} \bar{\mu}_{i.} &= \alpha_{0i} + \beta\bar{X}_{..} \\ \bar{\mu}_{i'.} &= \alpha_{0i'} + \beta\bar{X}_{..} \end{aligned}$$

their difference is

$$\bar{\mu}_{i.} - \bar{\mu}_{i'.} = \alpha_{0i} - \alpha_{0i'},$$

and the bias is removed.

While reduction in bias is probably the main reason analysts would apply ANCOVA, it can also be used to reduce residual variation. Thus, as with experimental studies, hypothesis tests may be more powerful and confidence intervals narrower.

15.9   WHAT MAKES A GOOD COVARIATE

An important characteristic of good covariates is that they are highly correlated with the dependent variable. As in regression with random X's, the covariates should be measurable on an interval scale. Often, investigators decide whether or not to perform a covariance analysis with X as a covariate by examining r_{XY}, the correlation calculated from their data between the response variable Y and X. Or they may make the decision on whether to measure X by estimating ρ, the population correlation coefficient of Y and X, from previous analyses or from the literature. Recall from Chapter 11 that the conditional variance of Y when X is fixed is $\sigma^2 = \sigma_Y^2(1-\rho^2)$ and that r_{XY}^2, the squared correlation between Y and X is the proportion of the variance of Y that is removed by the regression of Y on X. Thus if the correlation is small, the small reduction in variance may not make the more complex covariance analysis worthwhile. For example, if $\rho = 0.3$, then $\rho^2 = 0.09$, and so with the sample r_{XY}^2 somewhere in the neighborhood of 0.09, a very small reduction is achieved. Alternatively, if a covariate can be found with $\rho = 0.7$, then r_{XY}^2 estimates $\rho^2 = 0.49$. A substantial reduction can then be expected; for a given sample size, confidence intervals will be shorter and F tests more sensitive. ANCOVA is often not considered to be worthwhile when the estimate of ρ is less than 0.3.

One word of caution should be given about the calculation of r_{XY} using data collected from several populations. It is potentially misleading to calculate the correlation by pooling the data from the multiple samples; the correlation will include the effects of the classification factor. One way to get around this problem is to calculate the sample correlation for each level of the factor separately. Alternatively, the analyst can remove the effect of the factor. To do this, the usual ANOVA model is fitted and the residuals computed. The simple correlation between the residuals and the covariate can be computed; this is the correlation between Y and X when adjustment has been made for the factor. Ideally, the covariate should have the same correlation with the outcome across the levels of the factor.

In experimental studies, it is important that a covariate is not affected by treatment. Otherwise, when adjustment is made for its effect in the analysis, some of the treatment effect is removed as well. One way to ensure that the covariate is not affected by the treatment is to measure it before treatment is applied. Often, the covariate is chosen to be the pretreatment value of the outcome. Here again is a demonstration of the importance of knowledge of the subject matter. The more the investigators know about how variables interrelate and whether there are any causal relationships among them, the better the study can be designed and analyzed. (In our chapter example, a student's assignment to treatment is not likely to affect IQ score.)

Another desirable characteristic of good covariates is that their distributions do not differ widely between groups. As discussed in Section 15.4, in experimental studies, large differences among the sample means are less likely to occur because of the randomization; this can be more problematic for observational studies. When there are sizable differences in covariate values across the a populations, the interpretation of the adjusted means may be suspect. These are computed at the estimated overall mean, $\bar{X}_{..}$. If the value of $\bar{X}_{..}$ is not a reasonable value for the X to assume, the adjusted mean might be meaningless. (As an analogy, recall that, in regression analyses in Chapters 10, 11, and 12, inferences about the intercept α were not made if X values near 0 were meaningless or if there were no data for values of X close 0.) If no measurements of Y were made near the overall sample mean, the adjusted mean would be determined by extrapolating the sample regression line to a region where there is no evidence that the linear relation holds. The estimated standard errors are unstable, and this is reflected in wide confidence intervals. It may then be difficult to detect significant differences in the adjusted means. The correct conclusion would not be that the adjusted means may be equal, but that these comparisons are suspect.

During the planning phase of a study, the investigators should be aware of possible covariates, so that appropriate measurements are taken. This is important for both experimental and observational studies. Otherwise, the analysts can't make use of the advantages provided by ANCOVA. It might turn out that the most important covariate is one that is unknown or not measured. This is particularly problematic in observational studies, because a source of bias is not removed.

Further discussion concerning identification of covariates and their impact on ANCOVA is provided in [2, 3, 5, 7].

15.10 MEASUREMENT ERROR

In our presentation of regression and covariance analysis, we have tacitly assumed that the observations on X and Y are precisely correct. Mistakes in the data set can arise from a variety of causes, and of course must be eliminated insofar as possible. Even with such mistakes eliminated, however, the observations are not exact except for discrete variables, such as teaching method. For a continuous variable, measurements can never be said to be exact. Weight, for example, may be recorded correct to the nearest kilogram, or correct to the nearest gram or even to the nearest milligram, but never exactly correctly. This inherent inaccuracy in measurement data causes little difficulty provided the measurements are made with reasonable accuracy. It is present, however, whenever variables are continuous, and should be kept as small as possible.

We shall now assume that other errors have been eliminated and that there remain just the unavoidable measurement errors; these can reasonably be assumed to be symmetrically distributed with zero means. We now distinguish three cases in a covariance analysis in which sizable measurement errors may be a concern.

(1) In either a random experiment or a survey, Y values are subject to sizable measurement error. In this case, measurement errors do not bias either estimates of the adjusted means or of the regression coefficient b; these estimates obtained are, on the average, correct. However, the variability of the estimates in increased because the measurement errors increase the residual sum of squares.

(2) In a randomized experiment, if X is subject to measurement error, the observed X data are more variable than the true X values. A flatter regression line is fitted, so less of the covariate effect is removed. Since the calculated sum of squared deviations about the mean is *larger* than it would be if it could be calculated from true values of X, and since it is in the denominator of the equation for computing b, the calculated regression coefficient tends to be *smaller* than the population regression coefficient.

(3) In surveys, X is measured with error. As in the randomized experiment, that means β tends to be underestimated. Now, however, there may be large difference among the groups in X values (e.g., men tend to weigh more than women). With a lower value of b than would have been calculated if exact X values had been available, the linear effect of the covariate is removed to a lesser extent. There is thus a tendency to underadjust for differences among groups. Failure to make sufficient adjustment for differences in the covariate may result in incorrect interpretation of the data.

15.11   ANCOVA VERSUS OTHER METHODS OF ADJUSTMENT

In Chapter 6 we studied blocking, another method for reducing residual mean square error by removing some of the effect of an unwanted variable. The objectives of blocking are comparable to those of ANCOVA.

A critical difference between ANCOVA and the randomized complete block is in the method of assigning subjects to treatment; thus the choice between the two designs must be made at the beginning of the study. In the experiment discussed in this chapter, students were randomly assigned to teaching method, regardless of their IQ score. The linear effect of IQ score on language score was taken care of in the data analysis through ANCOVA. In contrast, if the blocked design had been implemented, categories of IQ scores would have been defined (e.g. 80–99, 100–119, 120–139). Students within each IQ category would have been randomized to one of the three teaching methods. The data analysis would have reflected the design.

The randomized block design is often favored when the variable whose effect is to be eliminated is a categorical variable with no underlying scale. When the variable whose effect the investigator wishes to remove is continuous, the randomized block design can still be used by creating groups with specified cutpoints. By categorizing rather than using the actual X values, some information would be lost, so ANCOVA would be the preferable strategy, unless the relationship between the Y and X variables were nonlinear; no specific relation between the two variables needs to be assumed when blocking is used.

Another method for covariate adjustment is *restriction*, in which only a subset of the possible values of a variable are included in an analysis. This is particularly useful when the investigator wishes to make statements about subgroups of a more general population (such as men or women, or subjects in different age groups) or when there is interaction between variables that cannot be removed by transformation. Restriction can be used either in the design phase of the study or in the analysis phase.

Analyzing differences is another method to adjust for covariates. This is particularly appropriate when the Y and X are the same variable, only measured at two points in times. Researchers may choose to calculate change and use it in the analysis. For example, suppose a study is designed to investigate weight loss and subjects are randomly assigned to one of two treatments. X is their pretreatment weight, and Y is their posttreatment weight. In this context, change in weight is the outcome variable, and the factor is treatment [1]. Alternatively, researchers may divide the final weight by the pretreatment weight and multiply this ratio by 100 to obtain a ratio of final weight to initial weight, in percent. Or they may divide the difference of the final and initial weights by the initial weight and multiple this ratio by 100 to obtain a relative change in weight, in percent. The choice between these methods would depend upon the characteristics of the data set and the conclusions the researchers wish to make. For a discussion of why covariance analysis is often preferred to measuring change, see [6].

ANCOVA can be generalized by increasing the numbers of factors and/or number of covariates.

15.12   COMMENTS ON STATISTICAL SOFTWARE

Most statistical software allows the fitting of ANCOVA models through general linear modeling procedures. Locations vary in the different packages. For example, the general linear model is an option of the ANOVA procedures in

Minitab, it is a separate procedure in SAS, and it is a special case of regression in S-PLUS. In each case, analysts identify factors as well as covariates.

15.13   SUMMARY

We introduced ANCOVA as an analysis procedure which is useful when independent variables include both classification variables and interval-scaled covariates. It can be used to investigate two types of questions: (1) is the mean response across the different levels of the factor the same when adjustment is made for the covariates? and (2) what is the relationship between the response and the covariates for different levels of the factor? Obtaining numerical results tends to be more complex than in some other statistical procedures, since analysts must use more general programs, such as general linear model procedures. Since both factors and covariates are used in AN-COVA, procedures which combine characteristics of ANOVA and regression must be applied.

We indicated ANCOVA can be applied in both experimental and nonexperimental studies, and compared and contrasted its objectives for the two types of studies. In experimental studies, its objective is to decrease the lengths of confidence intervals or increase the power of hypothesis tests; this is accomplished by reducing residual variance through removing that portion which can be explained by the linear relation between X and Y. In nonexperimental studies, there is an additional objective: to adjust for the effects of unequal covariate distributions on mean response across the different factor levels.

The interpretation of ANCOVA is tends to be more difficult in nonexperimental studies especially if the covariates differ appreciably in their mean value among the groups being studied. Data should be graphed and examined carefully.

We defined the ANCOVA model and described its special cases. We described relevant hypothesis tests and discussed the estimation of adjusted mean outcomes — the mean response at each factor level, determined at the overall mean covariate value. We described characteristics of a good covariate.

We discussed the importance of checking that the ANCOVA model does indeed hold and focused on the assumption that the population regression lines are parallel across the levels of the factor.

We compared and contrast ANCOVA with blocking, another method for achieving similar objectives in experimental and nonexperimental investigations.

Problems

15.1   In an agricultural experiment comparing yields Y of three varieties of corn (bushels/acre), rainfall X was measured (inches). Assume that the three

varieties have been randomly assigned to the plots of land. The data are as
follows:

Variety I		Variety II		Variety III	
X	Y	X	Y	X	Y
14	68.5	30	81.5	15	70.0
36	83.0	33	85.2	11	84.0
31	83.0	39	87.1	42	75.2
27	66.5	26	69.3	14	67.5
15	58.1	43	73.5	15	66.0
17	82.4	31	65.5	42	79.1
		18	73.4	26	75.5
		14	56.1		

a)   Plot yield versus rainfall for the three varieties of corn on a single
graph. Do the relationships between yield and rainfall appear linear?

b)   For each variety of corn, determine the sample regression line and
draw the three lines on the plot constructed in part a.

c)   Use one-way ANOVA to test for equality of mean yield for the three
varieties of corn.

d)   Under the assumption that the population regression lines are parallel, test whether there are differences in mean yield among the three varieties
of corn.

e)   Determine 1) the (unadjusted) means and 2) the adjusted means.
Is it reasonable that the means and adjusted means are similar or dissimilar?
Explain.

f)   Estimate 1) the variance in yield, when no adjustment is made
for rainfall and 2) the variance in yield when adjustment has been for the
linear relationship between yield and rainfall. Is it reasonable that these two
variance estimates are similar or dissimilar? Explain.

15.2   In studying intelligence of children with heart disease, two groups of
patients were considered: those who underwent surgery and those who did not.
The children were not randomly assigned to surgery. Investigators measured
IQ at the beginning of the study (X) and IQ at the end of the study (Y) for
24 children who had surgery and for 24 children who did not. The following
data were obtained:

Nonsurgery				Surgery			
Y	X	Y	X	Y	X	Y	X
127	124	82	95	86	78	99	90
124	127	111	125	99	87	106	114
100	90	89	100	119	100	90	81
104	93	96	92	102	103	114	108
130	115	100	96	113	114	107	107
94	100	94	85	99	97	88	98
121	111	100	112	105	113	83	95
100	97	90	98	111	111	88	88
101	109	105	109	119	104	100	105
110	95	105	99	102	92	87	85
104	110	112	115	113	107	107	72
88	117	100	88	103	118	109	100

a) Test that IQ at the beginning of the study was equal in the two groups.

b) Plot IQ at the end of the study versus IQ at the beginning of the study for each group of children on the same graph.

c) Determine the sample regression lines for each group separately and draw them on a scatter diagram obtained in part a.

d) Determine the sample regression lines when the population regression lines are assumed to be parallel, and draw them on a scatter diagram obtained in part a.

e) Assuming parallel regression lines, estimate the population mean final IQ for children who undergo surgery and have an initial IQ of 100. Determine a 95% confidence interval.

f) Determine 1) the (unadjusted) means and 2) the adjusted means. Is it reasonable that the means and adjusted means are similar or dissimilar? Explain.

g) Estimate 1) the variance in final IQ, when no adjustment is made for initial IQ and 2) the variance in final IQ when adjustment has been for the linear relationship between final and initial IQ. Is it reasonable that these two variance estimates are similar or dissimilar? Explain.

REFERENCES

1. Brogan, D. and Kutner, M.H. [1980]. Comparative Analysis of Pre-test Post-test Research Designs, *The American Statistician*, 34, 229–232.

2. Cochran, W.G. [1957]. Analysis of Covariance: Its Nature and Uses, *Biometrics*, 13, 261–281.

3. Cox, D.R. and McCullagh, P. [1982]. Some Aspects of Analysis of Covariance (with discussion), *Biometrics,* 38, 541–561.

4. Dean, A. and Voss, D. [1999]. *Design and Analysis of Experiments,* New York: Springer-Verlag, 277–291.

5. Egger, M.J., Coleman, M.L., Ward, J.R., Reading, J.C., and Williams, H.J. [1985]. Uses and Abuses of Analysis of Covariance in Clinical Trials, *Controlled Clinical Trials,* 6, 12–24.

6. Fleiss, J. L. [1986]. *The Design and Analysis of Clinical Experiments,* New York: John Wiley & Sons, 187–194.

7. Lord, F.M. [1967]. A Paradox in the Interpretation of Group Comparisons, *Psychological Bulletin,* 68, 304–305.

8. Milliken, G.A. and Johnson, D.E. [2002]. *Analysis of Messy Data, Volume III: Analysis of Covariance,* Boca Raton, FL: Chapman and Hall / CRC.

9. Schenker, N. and Gentleman, J. [2001]. On Judging the Significance of Differences by Examining the Overlap between Confidence Intervals, *The American Statistician,* 55, 182–186.

10. Wildt, A.R. and Ahtola, O.T. [1978]. *Analysis of Covariance,* Sage University Paper Number 12, Thousand Oaks, CA: Sage Publications.

11. Winer, B.J. [1971]. *Statistical Principles in Experimental Design,* New York: McGraw-Hill Company, 752–812.

16

Summaries, Extensions, and Communication

We have two objectives for this final chapter. First, we want to summarize and suggest extensions of the models we have described in this book. This is done in Section 16.1. Second, we want to put the methods we have discussed in the broader context of the role of statistics in research. An important part of this concerns the communication of the statistical methods and the data analyses. This is described in Section 16.2.

16.1 SUMMARIES AND EXTENSIONS OF MODELS

In this book, we have discussed specific models: the one-way ANOVA with fixed effects, multiple regression, and so forth. They all assume that there is a single Y variable that is normally distributed. The material in this book covers two classes of models: general linear models and mixed models.

A general linear model is defined to be of the form

$$Y = \alpha + \beta_1 X_1 + \cdots + \beta_k X_k + \varepsilon,$$

where

$$Y | X_1, \ldots, X_k \sim \mathrm{ND}(0, \sigma^2)$$

or

$$\varepsilon \sim \mathrm{IND}(0, \sigma^2).$$

The X variables can be classification variables (factors) and/or continuous variables. All of the parameters $(\alpha, \beta_1, \ldots, \beta_k)$ are fixed, and we are interested in making inferences concerning these parameters.

In contrast, a mixed model has both fixed and random effects. Two of the examples we considered are the two-way ANOVA with one random and one fixed factor, and repeated measures. In our applications of the mixed models, we assumed that each of the random effects was independent and normally distributed, and that assumption determined the variance and covariance of the Y's. It is possible to consider other variance and covariance structures, and there is software available to do this.

Actually, the general linear model can be regarded as a special case of the mixed model, with the constraint that the only random part of the model is ε.

Alternatively, the general linear model and the mixed model can be thought of as specific cases of more general models. Both the *generalized linear model* [2] and the *general mixed model* relax the assumption that the outcome variable Y is normally distributed. This allows the modeling of outcomes that are binary (as in logistic regression) or as counts (as in Poisson regression), and so forth. The more complex models do not use the method of least squares for estimation and inferences, but rely for these purposes on other methods such as maximum likelihood or restricted maximum likelihood. While the details are different, the objectives are largely the same — estimation of summary statistics, statistical inference in terms of hypothesis tests and confidence intervals, and the general investigation of how variables are interrelated. A good source of information about and illustrations of these more complex models is the documentation that accompanies the software that performs these sorts of analyses [3, 4, 5, 6]. Not all software packages implement these procedures.

In summary, there are a large number of models that could be fit for a set of data. In this book, we have considered some in detail, have made reference to others, and have not mentioned still others. We recommend that analysts pay particularly close attention to the models which they assume and make some checks that they are appropriate.

16.2   COMMUNICATION OF STATISTICS IN THE CONTEXT OF A RESEARCH PROJECT

We began this book with a brief overview of the central role that statistics plays in the planning and execution of a research study. Now, in this final chapter, we want to come back to this topic and summarize how the statistical methods that we have been discussing are put into the larger context of a research project. Since a study usually ends with dissemination of the work, it seems appropriate for us to conclude this book with some further guidelines for communicating statistical aspects of a study.

One form of communication is through the written word; examples include a thesis or dissertation, poster, report, or published manuscript. The work may be available on paper or electronically. An alternative means of communication is the spoken word; examples include oral defense of a thesis or dissertation, or presentation of the material to a class, at a seminar, or at a professional meeting. Frequently, these oral presentations are illustrated with material created with software such as Power Point.

Statistics plays a role in all aspects of a research study. In the design phase, application of statistical concepts helps ensure that the study is designed so that its data can be analyzed appropriately with respect to the investigator's research hypotheses and so that it is as efficient as possible in making use of available time, money, and other scarce resources.

During the data collection phase of a study, statistical practices can assist in monitoring of data quality and completeness.

While we have described some study designs and mentioned a little about data collection, we have mainly focused on the data analysis and interpretation phases in this book.

An important part of data analysis and interpretation involves communicating the research findings to others. A good way to get an understanding of how to present such portions of a paper is to take a look at some of the articles you have been reading in your field and try outlining them.

Either a written or an oral presentation of scientific work is generally divided into sections: abstract, introduction, methods, results, discussion, and references. An abstract is an overall summary of the work. The introduction provides motivation for the study and states the study objectives. The methods section describes what was done: from identifying the study design, to study execution, to data collection (including detailed laboratory techniques, if applicable). The results section contains a presentation of study findings. The discussion section includes conclusions, comparisons of the study findings with other work, limitations of the study, and suggestions of what might be done next. The reference section identifies all sources that were cited in the work.

Statistical issues may or may not be relevant to an introduction or a discussion, but they are almost always presented in the methods and results sections.

We provide here some of our broad recommendations concerning what should be presented and how. We focus on the methods and results portions of a written report, but the recommendations apply equally well to an oral presentation. There are always items specific to a particular research study, so our discussion certainly is not complete.

From a statistics perspective, some of the items that are appropriate to put in a methods section include:

- how variables were defined and measured,

- which variables were transformed and how this was done,

- what was the study design,

- how subjects were randomized to treatment or selected for inclusion in the study,

- how the sample size was selected,

- what statistical procedures were used, including those for multiple comparisons or variable selection,

- what other procedures were used but not reported because comparable results were found (e.g., nonparametric analyses or transformed data),

- what rules were followed to declare something statistically significant (e.g., $\alpha = 0.05$),

- what methods were used to check whether the assumptions were satisfied,

- how missing data were handled, and

- which software packages and procedures were used.

When summarizing results, it's a good idea to construct the tables and figures which tell the story you want to tell. This also helps you confirm what your main findings are. Writing the results section is much easier if these are available and appropriately labeled. In some cases, the writing of the results can be as simple as describing what is given in the tables and figures.

There is a great deal of software available that can be used to prepare creative tables and graphical displays. Ideally, a reader should be able to look at the tables and figures and grasp the main findings of the work. Thus, these should be easy to read, with captions that succinctly describe what their contents are. Some have suggested that a caption should begin with a statement of what is in the body of the table (for example, means, standard deviations, etc.) For graphs, the axes should be labeled, with units of measurement identified.

The results section should focus on your main findings, which should reflect the objectives and main research hypotheses for your work. Lesser findings or supporting work should come after your main findings. From a statistics perspective, some of the items you want to present in a results section include:

- Graphical summarizations of data (histograms, boxplots, plots of sample means with error bars, scatter plots), and/or

- Numerical summaries of data: for continuous variables that are approximately normally distributed, means and standard deviations; for continuous variables that are skewed, medians and interquartile ranges or ranges; for categorical variables, the frequencies and percentages. These may be presented by group (e.g., by treatment group). They should be presented as the original, nontransformed variables, unless some other practice is standard in the investigator's field. The sample size should always be given.

- Statistics and their estimated standard errors (means, adjusted means, sample regression coefficients, sample regression lines, correlation coefficients, coefficients of determination, etc.).

- Inferences, preferably expressed in terms of confidence intervals, with lower and upper levels, or as calculated test statistics (such as t or F with degrees of freedom) and p values.

When transformations have been used to satisfy the assumptions for the statistical methods, it is advisable to back-transform point and interval estimates, so that they are presented in terms of the original scales. For example, suppose a variable has been $\log_{10}$ transformed and a confidence interval for the $\log_{10}$ of the population mean has been computed. The lower and upper limits of the confidence interval for the population mean can then be obtained by back-transforming, that is, raising 10 to the power of the lower and upper values of the confidence interval for the $\log_{10}$ population mean.

Another point to keep in mind concerns the accuracy of the measurements. Many statistics packages give large numbers of digits to the right of a decimal point. This is appropriate for computations, particularly when you wish to confirm by hand how something is computed. However, it isn't a good idea to report so many digits; it is difficult for a reader to absorb all of them, and it can give a misleading picture of the accuracy to which some quantity has been measured. Some statisticians like to report estimates of standard deviations and standard errors with one extra digit. This way, readers can calculate or verify confidence intervals without sacrificing accuracy.

Some statisticians recommend that p values contain two significant digits [1]. Note that zeros before other numbers are not counted as significant digits but that zeros after other numbers are. So, for example, p values of 0.80 and 0.025 both have two significant digits. When reporting a p value, it is better to give the value rather than just indicate whether or not a result was statistically significant. Findings associated with a p value of 0.051 would likely be interpreted differently than those with a p value of 0.91.

A researcher giving an oral presentation or a poster may want to omit some of the details suggested above, particularly when time or space is limited. (However, it is good to have these details available, so that the presenter can respond to questions.) In these settings, one of the best recommendations is to limit the amount of material that is presented. There should be no more than three or four points made on each slide. Graphical displays tend to be more effective than numerical displays for communicating information, particularly in these settings.

Regardless of the form of the presentation, careful communication of the statistical aspects of a study is beneficial, as it helps others evaluate the work. It adds credibility to a study that was well designed and analyzed, and it can help others be aware of the strengths and limitations of the research project. It can provide information that will allow others to decide whether or not it is appropriate to compare the investigation with earlier ones and can assist future investigators in the planning of their own studies (for example, by providing estimates of population parameters for sample size calculations). The process of producing a summary that is complete and clear also helps the investigators themselves be more precise in their thinking about their own work.

REFERENCES

1. Lang, T.A. and Secic, M. [1997]. *How to Report Statistics in Medicine,* Philadelphia: American College of Physicians, 39–40, 76.

2. McCullagh, P. and Nelder, J.A. [1989]. *Generalized Linear Models,* 2nd ed., London: Chapman and Hall.

3. http://www.sas.com

4. http://www.spss.com

5. http://www.mathsoft.com/splus

6. http://www.stata.com

7. Venables, W.N. and Ripley, B.D. [1999]. *Modern Applied Statistics with S-Plus,* 3rd ed., New York: Springer-Verlag.

Appendix A

A.1 EXPECTED VALUES AND PARAMETERS

The *expected value* of any quantity is its value averaged over the entire population. The symbol E denotes expected value.

The *population mean* for a variable Y is defined as the expected value of Y. It is usually denoted by μ:

$$\mu = E(Y). \tag{A.1}$$

The *population variance* is defined as the expected value of the quantity $(Y - \mu)^2$. It is usually denoted by σ^2. In symbols, we have

$$
\begin{aligned}
\sigma^2 &= E[(Y - \mu)^2] &\text{(A.2)}\\
&= E[(Y - \mu)(Y - \mu)] \\
&= E(Y^2) - 2\mu E(Y) + \mu^2 \\
&= E(Y^2) - [E(Y)]^2. &\text{(A.3)}
\end{aligned}
$$

The population variance is a measure of the variability of the population; a large value of σ^2 occurs when the population is widely spread about the mean. The *population standard deviation* is the square root of the population variance and is denoted by σ.

The *population covariance* of two variables X and Y is defined as the expected value of the quantity $(X - \mu_X)(Y - \mu_Y)$. It is usually denoted by σ_{XY}:

$$\sigma_{XY} = E[(X - \mu_X)(Y - \mu_Y)]. \qquad (A.4)$$

The population covariance is positive when large values of X tend to correspond to large values of Y and small values to small values; it is negative when large values of one variable correspond to small values of the other variable.

The *population correlation coefficient* between X and Y is defined as the covariance of X and Y divided by the product of their standard deviations. It is denoted by ρ. In symbols,

$$\rho = \frac{\sigma_{XY}}{\sigma_X \sigma_Y}. \qquad (A.5)$$

Throughout the book, we make repeated use of several rules about expected values. For simplicity, we state these for two variables, X and Y; they can be generalized to any number of variables.

(1) The expected value of a constant times a variable is the constant times the expected value of the variable:

$$E(aY) = aE(Y). \qquad (A.6)$$

(2) The expected value of a sum of variables is the sum of the expected values of the variables:

$$E(X + Y) = E(X) + E(Y). \qquad (A.7)$$

(3) If variables are independent, then the expectation of their product is the product of their expectations:

$$E(XY) = E(X)E(Y). \qquad (A.8)$$

A.2   LINEAR COMBINATIONS OF VARIABLES AND THEIR PARAMETERS

Often, it is desirable to form new variables by combining several variables. In particular, linear combinations of variables occur frequently. Linear combinations are weighted sums. The population means, variances, and covariances of such linear combinations are obtained easily in terms of the parameters of the original variables.

We first consider two small examples, where we work through the details of getting means, variances, and covariances of linear combinations.

Example. Consider a simple example where there are two variables, Y_1 and Y_2. We want the mean and variance of the linear combination $V = Y_1 + 3Y_2 + 10$. The following parameters are given: $E(Y_1) = 10$, $E(Y_2) = 12$, $\text{Var}(Y_1) = 11$, $\text{Var}(Y_2) = 12$, and $\text{Cov}(X, Y) = 2$.

The mean of V can be obtained by applying Equations A.6 and A.7:

$$
\begin{aligned}
E(V) &= E(Y_1 + 3Y_2 + 10) \\
&= E(Y_1) + 3E(Y_2) + 10 \\
&= 10 + 36 + 10 \\
&= 56.
\end{aligned}
$$

To obtain the variance of V, we must also apply Equations A.2 and A.8:

$$
\begin{aligned}
\text{Var}(V) &= E[(Y_1 + 3Y_2 + 10) - E(Y_1 + 3Y_2 + 10)]^2 \\
&= E\{[Y_1 - E(Y_1)] + [3Y_2 - 3E(Y_2)]\}^2 \\
&= E\{[Y_1 - E(Y_1)]^2 + [3Y_2 - 3E(Y_2)]^2 \\
&\quad + 2[Y_1 - E(Y_1)][3Y_2 - 3E(Y_2)]\} \\
&= \text{Var}(Y_1) + 9\,\text{Var}(Y_2) + 6\,\text{Cov}(Y_1, Y_2) \\
&= 11 + 108 + 12 \\
&= 131.
\end{aligned}
$$

Example. Consider two linear combinations, $U = 0.4X_1 + 0.6X_2$ and $V = 0.3Y_1 + 0.3Y_2 + 0.4Y_3$. The variance of U is 108.4, and the variance of V is 98.9. The covariances between the X's and the Y's are

$$\text{Cov}(X_1, Y_1) = 40, \quad \text{Cov}(X_1, Y_2) = 20, \quad \text{Cov}(X_1, Y_3) = 60,$$

$$\text{Cov}(X_2, Y_1) = 50, \quad \text{Cov}(X_2, Y_2) = 10, \quad \text{Cov}(X_2, Y_3) = 50.$$

The covariance between U and V can be determined from the definition of the covariance (Equation A.4):

$$
\begin{aligned}
\text{Cov}(U, V) &= E\{[U - E(U)][V - E(V)]\} \\
&= E\{[0.4X_1 + 0.6X_2 - 0.4E(X_1) - 0.6E(X_2)] \\
&\quad \times [0.3Y_1 + 0.3Y_2 + 0.4Y_3 - 0.3E(Y_1) - 0.3E(Y_2) - 0.4E(Y_3)]\}
\end{aligned}
$$

$$
\begin{aligned}
&= E\{0.4[X_1 - E(X_1)] + 0.6[X_2 - E(X_2)]\} \times \\
&\quad \times \{0.3[Y_1 - E(Y_1)] + 0.3[Y_2 - E(Y_2)] + 0.4[Y_3 - E(Y_3)]\} \\
&= (0.4)(0.3)E\{[X_1 - E(X_1)][Y_1 - E(Y_1)]\} \\
&\quad + (0.4)(0.3)E\{[X_1 - E(X_1)][Y_2 - E(Y_2)]\} \\
&\quad + (0.4)(0.4)E\{[X_1 - E(X_1)][Y_3 - E(Y_3)]\} \\
&\quad + (0.6)(0.3)E\{[X_2 - E(X_2)][Y_1 - E(Y_1)]\} \\
&\quad + (0.6)(0.3)E\{[X_2 - E(X_2)][Y_2 - E(Y_2)]\} \\
&\quad + (0.6)(0.4)E\{[X_2 - E(X_2)][Y_3 - E(Y_3)]\} \\
&= 0.12\,\mathrm{Cov}(X_1, Y_1) + 0.12\,\mathrm{Cov}(X_1, Y_2) + 0.16\,\mathrm{Cov}(X_1, Y_3) \\
&\quad + 0.18\,\mathrm{Cov}(X_2, Y_1) + 0.18\,\mathrm{Cov}(X_2, Y_2) + 0.24\,\mathrm{Cov}(X_2, Y_3) \\
&= 0.12(40) + 0.12(20) + 0.16(60) \\
&\quad + 0.18(50) + 0.18(10) + 0.24(50) \\
&= 39.60.
\end{aligned}
$$

The two combinations U and V happen to have no variables in common, but it is perfectly possible to have two linear combinations containing some common variables. In this case, we would need to know the variances of the common variables. With no variables in common, we only need the covariances among the X's and Y's.

To find the correlation coefficient of U and V, we calculate their standard deviations. The standard deviation of U equals $\sqrt{108.4}$, or 10.4; the standard deviation of V equals $\sqrt{98.9}$, or 9.94. Applying Equation A.5, the correlation coefficient between U and V is 39.60 / $[(10.4)(9.94)]$, or 0.38.

A more practical illustration of expected values is in the determination of $E(\bar{Y})$ and $\mathrm{Var}(\bar{Y})$. If a simple random sample of size n is drawn from a population with mean μ and variance σ^2. There are n variables, $Y_1, Y_2, \ldots, Y_n$, each with mean μ and variance σ^2, and each of these variables is independent of the others. (Because independence is assumed, the covariance between any two variables, say the ith and jth, is $\sigma_{ij} = 0$, and their correlation $\rho_{ij} = 0$.)

Consider the sample mean $\bar{Y}$, a linear combination of the variables with weights all equal to $1/n$. Assuming simple random sampling, the n variables are independent:

$$
\bar{Y} = \frac{Y_1 + Y_2 + \cdots + Y_n}{n}. \tag{A.9}
$$

The expected value of $\bar{Y}$ is

$$
\begin{aligned}
E(\bar{Y}) &= E\left(\frac{Y_1 + Y_2 + \cdots + Y_n}{n}\right) \\
&= n\frac{\mu}{n} \\
&= \mu.
\end{aligned}
$$

By definition, the variance of $\bar{Y}$ is

$$
\begin{aligned}
\sigma_{\bar{Y}}^2 &= E(\bar{Y} - \mu)^2 \\
&= E\left(\frac{Y_1 + Y_2 + \cdots + Y_n}{n} - \frac{n\mu}{n}\right)^2 \\
&= E\left[\left(\frac{Y_1}{n} - \frac{\mu}{n}\right) + \left(\frac{Y_2}{n} - \frac{\mu}{n}\right) + \cdots + \left(\frac{Y_n}{n} - \frac{\mu}{n}\right)\right]^2 \\
&= E\left[\frac{(Y_1 - \mu)^2}{n^2} + \frac{(Y_1 - \mu)(Y_2 - \mu)}{n^2} + \cdots \right. \\
&\qquad + \frac{(Y_1 - \mu)(Y_n - \mu)}{n^2} + \frac{(Y_2 - \mu)^2}{n^2} + \cdots \\
&\qquad \left. + \frac{(Y_{n-1} - \mu)(Y_n - \mu)}{n^2} + \frac{(Y_n - \mu)^2}{n^2}\right] \\
&= (\sigma^2 + 0 + \cdots + 0 \\
&\qquad + 0 + \sigma^2 + \cdots + 0 \\
&\qquad + \cdots \\
&\qquad + 0 + 0 + \cdots + \sigma^2)/n^2 \\
&= \sigma^2/n.
\end{aligned}
$$

The following are rules for finding means, variances, and covariances of linear combinations. These rules can all be verified through repeated application of the rules for expected values given above.

(1) A rule for finding the mean of the linear combination $a_1 Y_1 + a_2 Y_2 + \cdots + a_n Y_n$ is

$$
E\left(\sum_{i=1}^{m} a_i Y_i\right) = \sum_{i=1}^{m} a_i E(Y_i). \tag{A.10}
$$

(2) A rule for finding the variance of the linear combination $a_1 Y_1 + a_2 Y_2 + \cdots + a_n Y_n$ is

$$
\operatorname{Var}\left(\sum_{i=1}^{m} a_i Y_i\right) = \sum_{i=1}^{m} a_i^2 \operatorname{Var}(Y_i) + \sum_{i=1}^{m}\sum_{j=1}^{m} a_i a_j \operatorname{Cov}(Y_i, Y_j), \tag{A.11}
$$

where $i \neq j$.

(3) A rule for finding the covariance of two linear combinations $a_1 Y_1 + a_2 Y_2 + \cdots + a_m Y_m$ and $b_1 Y_1 + b_2 Y_2 + \cdots + b_n Y_m$ is

$$\text{Cov}\left(\sum_{i=1}^{m} a_i Y_i, \sum_{j=1}^{m} b_j Y_j\right) = \sum_{i=1}^{m} a_i b_i \text{ Var}(Y_i) + \sum_{i=1}^{m}\sum_{j=1}^{m} a_i b_j \text{ Cov}(Y_i, Y_j),$$

(A.12)

where $i \neq j$.

In these expressions, $Y_1, Y_2, \ldots, Y_m$ denote any m variables, and $a_1, \ldots, a_m$, $b_1, \ldots, b_m$ denote any constants. Since some of the constants may be zero, the two linear combinations may or may not contain the same variables, and they also may or may not contain the same number of variables. Often the Y_i and Y_j are independent. In this case, $\text{Cov}(Y_i, Y_j)$ equals zero and the formula simplify to

$$\text{Var}\left(\sum_{i=1}^{m} a_i Y_i\right) = \sum_{i=1}^{m} a_i^2 \text{ Var}(Y_i) \qquad \text{(A.13)}$$

$$\text{Cov}\left(\sum_{i=1}^{m} a_i Y_i, \sum_{j=1}^{m} b_j Y_j\right) = \sum_{i=1}^{m} a_i b_i \text{ Var}(Y_i). \qquad \text{(A.14)}$$

Most of the remaining material in this appendix is selected applications of these rules for finding means, variances, and covariances of linear combinations which we make use of in the book.

A.3 BALANCED ONE-WAY ANOVA, EXPECTED MEAN SQUARES

A.3.1 To show $E(MS_a) = \sigma^2 + n \sum_{i=1}^{a} \alpha_i^2/(a-1)$

First, let's consider only the sum of squares, SS_a. In this derivation, we make use of Equation A.3 to express $E(Y^2) = \text{Var}(Y) + [E(Y)]^2$. Then

$$E \sum_{i=1}^{a}\sum_{j=1}^{n}(\bar{Y}_{i.} - \bar{Y}_{..})^2 = \sum_{i=1}^{a}\sum_{j=1}^{n} E(\bar{Y}_{i.} - \bar{Y}_{..})^2$$

$$= \sum_{i=1}^{a}\sum_{j=1}^{n} \text{Var}(\bar{Y}_{i.} - \bar{Y}_{..}) + [E(\bar{Y}_{i.} - \bar{Y}_{..})]^2.$$

Next, consider $\text{Var}(\bar{Y}_{i.} - \bar{Y}_{..})$. Note that $\bar{Y}_{..}$ is a linear combination of a $\bar{Y}$'s. On the right hand side of the first line in the following set of equations, $\bar{Y}_{i.}$ is included in the first term and not in the second term; the second term includes $\bar{Y}_{1.} + \cdots + \bar{Y}_{i-1.} + \bar{Y}_{i+1.} + \cdots + \bar{Y}_{a.}$, that is, $a-1$ sample means.

$$\mathrm{Var}(\bar{Y}_{i.} - \bar{Y}_{..}) = \mathrm{Var}\left[\left(\frac{a-1}{a}\right)\bar{Y}_{i.} - \frac{\bar{Y}_{1.} + \cdots + \bar{Y}_{a.}}{a}\right]$$

$$= \left(\frac{a-1}{a}\right)^2 \frac{\sigma^2}{n} + \frac{a-1}{a^2}\frac{\sigma^2}{n}$$

$$= \frac{(a-1)\sigma^2}{an}.$$

This is a constant, so that when it is summed over i and j, we get

$$\sum_{i=1}^{a}\sum_{j=1}^{n}\mathrm{Var}(\bar{Y}_{i.} - \bar{Y}_{..}) = (a-1)\sigma^2.$$

Next, consider

$$[E(\bar{Y}_{i.} - \bar{Y}_{..})]^2 = [(\mu + \alpha_i) - \mu]^2$$

$$= \alpha_i^2.$$

This depends only on i, so that when it is summed over i and j, it equals

$$n\sum_{i=1}^{a}\alpha_i^2.$$

Thus, $E\sum_{i=1}^{a}\sum_{j=1}^{n}(\bar{Y}_{i.} - \bar{Y}_{..})^2 = (a-1)\sigma^2 + n\sum_{i=1}^{a}\alpha_i^2$. Dividing both terms by $a-1$, we obtain

$$E(\mathrm{MS}_a) = \sigma^2 + n\frac{\sum_{i=1}^{a}\alpha_i^2}{a-1}.$$

A.3.2 To Show $E(\mathrm{MS}_r) = \sigma^2$

First, let's consider only the sums of squares. Again, we make use of Equation A.3:

$$E\sum_{i=1}^{a}\sum_{j=1}^{n}(Y_{ij} - \bar{Y}_{i.})^2 = \sum_{i=1}^{a}\sum_{j=1}^{n}E(Y_{ij} - \bar{Y}_{i.})^2$$

$$= \sum_{i=1}^{a}\sum_{j=1}^{n}\mathrm{Var}(Y_{ij} - \bar{Y}_{i.}) + [E(Y_{ij} - \bar{Y}_{i.})]^2.$$

Next, consider $\mathrm{Var}(Y_{ij} - \bar{Y}_{i.})$. Note that $\bar{Y}_{i.}$ is a linear combination of n Y's. On the right-hand side of the first line in the following set of equations, Y_{ij} is included in the first term and not in the second term; the second term includes $Y_{i1} + \cdots + Y_{i,j-1} + Y_{i,j+1} + \cdots + Y_{in}$, that is, $n-1$ of the individual Y's:

$$
\begin{aligned}
\mathrm{Var}(Y_{ij} - \bar{Y}_{i.}) &= \mathrm{Var}\left[\left(\frac{n-1}{n}\right)Y_{ij} - \frac{Y_{i1} + \cdots + Y_{in}}{n}\right]\\
&= \left(\frac{n-1}{n}\right)^2 \frac{\sigma^2}{n} + \frac{n-1}{n}\frac{\sigma^2}{n^2}\\
&= \frac{(n-1)\sigma^2}{n}.
\end{aligned}
$$

This is a constant, so that when it is summed over i and j, we get

$$
\sum_{i=1}^{a}\sum_{j=1}^{n}\mathrm{Var}(Y_{ij} - \bar{Y}_{i.}) = a(n-1)\sigma^2.
$$

Next, consider

$$
\begin{aligned}
[E(Y_{ij} - \bar{Y}_{i.})]^2 &= [(\mu + \alpha_i) - (\mu + \alpha_i)]^2\\
&= 0.
\end{aligned}
$$

Thus, $E\sum_{i=1}^{a}\sum_{j=1}^{n}(Y_{ij} - \bar{Y}_{i.})^2 = a(n-1)\sigma^2$. Dividing this by $a(n-1)$, we obtain

$$
E(\mathrm{MS}_r) = \sigma^2.
$$

A.4   BALANCED ONE-WAY ANOVA, RANDOM EFFECTS

The model is $Y_{ij} = \mu + \alpha_i + \varepsilon_{ij}$, with $i = 1, \ldots, a$, $j = 1, \ldots, n$, and where $\alpha_i \sim \mathrm{IND}(0, \sigma_a^2)$, $\varepsilon_{ij} \sim \mathrm{IND}(0, \sigma^2)$, and α_i and ε_{ij} are independent. The variance of Y_{ij} is equal to

$$
\begin{aligned}
\mathrm{Var}(Y_{ij}) &= \mathrm{Var}(\mu + \alpha_i + \varepsilon_{ij})\\
&= \sigma_a^2 + \sigma^2.
\end{aligned}
$$

Since μ is a constant, there is no variance associated with it. The covariance between Y_{ij} and $Y_{ij'}$, where $j \neq j'$ is

$$
\begin{aligned}
\mathrm{Cov}(Y_{ij}, Y_{ij'}) &= \mathrm{Cov}(\mu + \alpha_i + \varepsilon_{ij}, \mu + \alpha_i + \varepsilon_{ij'})\\
&= \sigma_a^2,
\end{aligned}
$$

so that the correlation between Y_{ij} and $Y_{ij'}$ where $j \neq j'$ is

$$\rho = \frac{\mathrm{Cov}(Y_{ij}, Y_{ij'})}{\sqrt{\mathrm{Var}(Y_{ij})}\sqrt{\mathrm{Var}(Y_{ij'})}}$$

$$= \frac{\sigma_a^2}{\sigma_a^2 + \sigma^2}.$$

This correlation ρ is called the *intraclass* correlation.

A.5   BALANCED NESTED MODEL

The nested model, as we defined it, is $Y_{ijk} = \mu + \alpha_i + \beta_{i(j)} + \varepsilon_{ijk}$, where $\sum_{i=1}^a \alpha_i = 0$, $\beta_{i(j)} \sim \mathrm{IND}(0, \sigma_b^2)$, and $\varepsilon_{ijk} \sim \mathrm{IND}(0, \sigma^2)$; the $\beta_{i(j)}$ and ε_{ijk} are independent.

The variance of Y_{ijk} is the variance of a linear combination of μ, α_i, $\beta_{i(j)}$, and ε_{ijk}. This is a combination of two constants, μ and α_i, together with the two terms which have variability associated with them, $\beta_{i(j)}$ and ε_{ijk}. So

$$\mathrm{Var}(Y_{ijk}) = \sigma_b^2 + \sigma^2. \tag{A.15}$$

The variance of $(\bar{Y}_{i..})$ can also be computed as the variance of a linear combination:

$$\mathrm{Var}(\bar{Y}_{i..}) = \mathrm{Var}\left(\frac{\sum_{j=1}^n \sum_{k=1}^n Y_{ijk}}{bn}\right)$$

$$= \mathrm{Var}\left(\frac{(Y_{i11} + \cdots + Y_{i1n}) + \cdots + (Y_{ib1} + \cdots + Y_{ibn})}{bn}\right).$$

The variables Y_{ijk} that have the same subscript j have covariances associated with them, for example, $\mathrm{Cov}(Y_{i11}, Y_{i1k}) = \sigma_b^2$. Using Equation A.2, we can determine

$$\mathrm{Var}(\bar{Y}_{i..}) = \frac{bn\,\mathrm{Var}(Y_{ijk})}{(bn)^2} + \frac{bn(n-1)\,\mathrm{Cov}(Y_{ijk}, Y_{ijk'})}{(bn)^2}$$

$$= \frac{\sigma_b^2 + \sigma^2}{bn} + \frac{(n-1)\sigma_b^2}{bn}$$

$$= \frac{\sigma_b^2}{b} + \frac{\sigma^2}{bn}. \tag{A.16}$$

The variance of the difference of two means, $\mathrm{Var}(\bar{Y}_{i..} - \bar{Y}_{i'..})$, where $i \neq i'$, is equal to the sum of the variances of all the means as in Equation A.13, because the Y's from different treatment groups are assumed to be independent. That is,

$$\begin{aligned}
\mathrm{Var}(\bar{Y}_{i..} - \bar{Y}_{i'..}) &= \mathrm{Var}(Y_{i..}) + \mathrm{Var}(Y_{i'..}) \\
&= 2\left(\frac{\sigma_b^2}{b} + \frac{\sigma^2}{bn}\right).
\end{aligned} \tag{A.17}$$

A.6   MIXED MODEL

The mixed effects model can be expressed as $Y_{ijk} = \mu + \alpha_i + \beta_j + \alpha\beta_{ij} + \varepsilon_{ijk}$, where $\sum_{i=1}^{a} \alpha_i = 0$ (i.e., this factor has fixed effects), $\beta_j \sim \mathrm{IND}(0, \sigma_b^2)$ (i.e., this factor has random effects), $\alpha\beta_{ij} \sim \mathrm{IND}(0, \sigma_{ab}^2)$ (i.e., the interaction between the fixed and random factors is considered random), and $\varepsilon_{ijk} \sim \mathrm{IND}(0, \sigma^2)$. The β_j, $\alpha\beta_{ij}$, and ε_{ijk} are independent.

A.6.1   Variances and Covariances of Y_{ijk}

First, we present variances and covariances of the Y_{ijk}; these follow directly from the assumptions of the mixed model and properties of linear combinations.

$$\begin{aligned}
\mathrm{Var}(Y_{ijk}) &= \mathrm{Var}(\mu + \alpha_i + \beta_j + \alpha\beta_{ij} + \varepsilon_{ijk}) \\
&= \sigma_b^2 + \sigma_{ab}^2 + \sigma^2,
\end{aligned}$$

$$\begin{aligned}
\mathrm{Cov}(Y_{ijk}, Y_{ijk'}) &= \mathrm{Cov}(\mu + \alpha_i + \beta_j + \alpha\beta_{ij} + \varepsilon_{ijk}, \\
&\qquad \mu + \alpha_i + \beta_j + \alpha\beta_{ij} + \varepsilon_{ijk'}) \\
&= \sigma_b^2 + \sigma_{ab}^2,
\end{aligned}$$

$$\begin{aligned}
\mathrm{Cov}(Y_{ijk}, Y_{i'jk'}) &= \mathrm{Cov}(\mu + \alpha_i + \beta_j + \alpha\beta_{ij} + \varepsilon_{ijk}, \\
&\qquad \mu + \alpha_{i'} + \beta_j + \alpha\beta_{i'j} + \varepsilon_{i'jk'}) \\
&= \sigma_b^2.
\end{aligned}$$

All other covariances are equal to 0.

A.6.2   Variance of $\bar{Y}_{i..}$

The variance of $\bar{Y}_{i..}$ is a linear combination of variables, the Y_{ijk}, not all of which are independent. The covariance of the Y's that have the same second subscript, j, needs to be taken into account.

$$\mathrm{Var}(\bar{Y}_{i..}) = \mathrm{Var}\left[\frac{(Y_{i11} + \cdots + Y_{i1n}) + \cdots + (Y_{ib1} + \cdots + Y_{ibn})}{bn}\right]$$

$$= \text{Var}\left(\frac{Y_{i11} + \cdots + Y_{i1n}}{bn}\right)$$

$$+ \text{Var}\left(\frac{Y_{i21} + \cdots + Y_{i2n}}{bn}\right)$$

$$+ \cdots$$

$$+ \text{Var}\left(\frac{Y_{ib1} + \cdots + Y_{ibn}}{bn}\right).$$

For each of the b levels of the random factor, there are n Y's that have the same value of j. Applying Equation A.2 for these n Y's, we obtain

$$\begin{aligned} \text{Var}(Y_{ij1} + \cdots + Y_{ijn}) &= n\,\text{Var}(Y_{ijk}) + n(n-1)\,\text{Cov}(Y_{ijk}, Y_{ijk'}) \\ &= n(\sigma_b^2 + \sigma_{ab}^2 + \sigma^2) + n(n-1)(\sigma_b^2 + \sigma_{ab}^2). \end{aligned}$$

The variance of $\bar{Y}_{i..}$ is then

$$\begin{aligned} \text{Var}(\bar{Y}_{i..}) &= \frac{b[n(\sigma_b^2 + \sigma_{ab}^2 + \sigma^2) + n(n-1)(\sigma_b^2 + \sigma_{ab}^2)]}{(bn)^2} \\ &= \frac{\sigma_b^2}{b} + \frac{\sigma_{ab}^2}{b} + \frac{\sigma^2}{bn}. \end{aligned} \tag{A.18}$$

A.6.3 Variance of $\bar{Y}_{i..} - \bar{Y}_{i'..}$

To compute the variance of $\bar{Y}_{i..} - \bar{Y}_{i'..}$, we must make use of Equation A.2, since

$$\text{Var}(\bar{Y}_{i..} - \bar{Y}_{i'..}) = \text{Var}(\bar{Y}_{i..}) + \text{Var}(\bar{Y}_{i'..}) - 2\,\text{Cov}(\bar{Y}_{i..}, \bar{Y}_{i'..}).$$

In Section A.6.2 we determined that the variance of $\bar{Y}_{i..}$ is equal to the variance of $\bar{Y}_{i'..}$. Here, we focus on the covariance.

$$\text{Cov}(\bar{Y}_{i..}, \bar{Y}_{i'..}) = \text{Cov}\left(\frac{Y_{i11} + \cdots + Y_{i1n} + \cdots + Y_{ib1} + \cdots + Y_{ibn}}{bn},\right.$$

$$\left.\frac{Y_{i'11} + \cdots + Y_{i'1n} + \cdots + Y_{i'b1} + \cdots + Y_{i'bn}}{bn}\right).$$

There are b levels of the random factor, and for each one, there are n^2 covariances between the Y's. For example, for level j,

$$\text{Cov}(Y_{ij1} + \cdots + Y_{ijn}, Y_{i'j1} + \cdots + Y_{i'jn}) = n^2 \sigma_b^2,$$

so the covariance between $\bar{Y}_{i..}$ and $\bar{Y}_{i'..}$ is

$$\text{Cov}(\bar{Y}_{i..}, \bar{Y}_{i'..}) = \frac{bn^2\sigma_b^2}{(bn)^2}$$

$$= \frac{\sigma_b^2}{b}. \tag{A.19}$$

Thus, the variance is equal to

$$\text{Var}(\bar{Y}_{i..} - \bar{Y}_{i'..}) = \text{Var}(\bar{Y}_{i..}) + \text{Var}(\bar{Y}_{i'..}) - 2\,\text{Cov}(\bar{Y}_{i..}, \bar{Y}_{i'..})$$

$$= 2\left(\frac{\sigma_b^2}{b} + \frac{\sigma_{ab}^2}{b} + \frac{\sigma^2}{bn}\right) - 2\frac{\sigma_b^2}{b}$$

$$= 2\left(\frac{\sigma_{ab}^2}{b} + \frac{\sigma^2}{bn}\right). \tag{A.20}$$

A.7   SIMPLE LINEAR REGRESSION — DERIVATION OF LEAST SQUARES ESTIMATORS

For the simple linear regression model, with $Y|X \sim N(\alpha + \beta X, \sigma^2)$, we wish to obtain the least squares estimators of α and β. That is, we minimize the sum of squared vertical deviations of Y_i from its expected value, $E(Y_i|X_i)$, which is:

$$Q = \sum_{i=1}^{n}(Y_i - \alpha - \beta X_i)^2.$$

We minimize Q by taking the partial derivatives $\partial Q/\partial \alpha$ and $\partial Q/\partial \beta$, setting them equal to 0, and solving for the least squares estimators, a and b:

$$\frac{\partial Q}{\partial \alpha} = 2\sum_{i=1}^{n}(Y_i - a - bX_i)(-1) = 0,$$

$$\sum_{i=1}^{n}Y_i = \sum_{i=1}^{n}(a + bX_i)$$

$$= na + b\sum_{i=1}^{n}X_i,$$

$$a = \bar{Y} - b\bar{X};$$

$$\frac{\partial Q}{\partial \beta} = 2\sum_{i=1}^{n}(Y_i - a - bX_i)(-X_i) = 0,$$

$$\sum_{i=1}^{n} X_i Y_i = a \sum_{i=1}^{n} X_i + b \sum_{i=1}^{n} X_i^2$$

$$= (\bar{Y} - b\bar{X}) \sum_{i=1}^{n} X_i + b \sum_{i=1}^{n} X_i^2$$

$$= n\bar{Y}\bar{X} - b \frac{(\sum_{i=1}^{n} X_i)^2}{n} + b \sum_{i=1}^{n} X_i^2,$$

$$\sum_{i=1}^{n} X_i Y_i - n\bar{Y}\bar{X} = b \left(\sum_{i=1}^{n} X_i^2 - \frac{(\sum_{i=1}^{n} X_i)^2}{n} \right)$$

$$b = \frac{\sum_{i=1}^{n} X_i Y_i - n\bar{Y}\bar{X}}{\sum_{i=1}^{n} X_i^2 - n\bar{X}^2}$$

$$= \frac{\sum_{i=1}^{n} (X_i - \bar{X})(Y_i - \bar{Y})}{\sum_{i=1}^{n} (X_i - \bar{X})^2};$$

$$\sum_{i=1}^{n} Y_i = n\bar{Y},$$

$$\sum_{i=1}^{n} (Y_i - \bar{Y})^2 = \sum_{i=1}^{n} Y_i^2 - 2\bar{Y}Y_i + n\bar{Y}^2$$

$$= \sum_{i=1}^{n} Y_i^2 - \frac{(\sum_{i=1}^{n} Y_i)^2}{n}$$

$$= \sum_{i=1}^{n} Y_i^2 - n\bar{Y}^2.$$

A.8   DERIVATION OF VARIANCE ESTIMATES FROM SIMPLE LINEAR REGRESSION

In deriving the variance estimates of the statistics obtained from simple linear regression, the values of Y, $Y_1, Y_2, \ldots, Y_n$ are regarded as random while the X's are fixed.

The statistics $\bar{Y}$ (the height of the line at $X = \bar{X}$) and b are simply linear combinations of the n independent observations $Y_1, Y_2, \ldots, Y_n$. We have

$$\bar{Y} = \frac{Y_1 + Y_2 + \cdots + Y_n}{n}.$$

The variance for the linear combination is

$$\text{Var}(\bar{Y}) = \left(\frac{1}{n}\right)^2 \text{Var}(Y_1) + \left(\frac{1}{n}\right)^2 \text{Var}(Y_2) + \cdots + \left(\frac{1}{n}\right)^2 \text{Var}(Y_n)$$

$$= \left(\frac{1}{n}\right)^2 (n\sigma^2)$$

$$= \frac{\sigma^2}{n}.$$

Since $b = \sum_{i=1}^{n}(Y_i - \bar{Y})(X_i - \bar{X}) / \sum_{i=1}^{n}(X_i - \bar{X})^2$, and, since $\sum_{i=1}^{n}(Y_i - \bar{Y})(X_i - \bar{X})$ can be expressed as $\sum_{i=1}^{n} Y_i(X_i - \bar{X})$, b can also be written as a linear combination of the Y's:

$$b = \frac{Y_1(X_1 - \bar{X}) + Y_2(X_2 - \bar{X}) + \cdots + Y_n(X_n - \bar{X})^2}{\sum_{i=1}^{n}(X_i - \bar{X})^2}.$$

Thus the variance of b is

$$\text{Var}(b) = \frac{[(X_1 - \bar{X})^2 + (X_2 - \bar{X})^2 + \cdots + (X_n - \bar{X})^2]\sigma^2}{[\sum_{i=1}^{n}(X_i - \bar{X})^2]^2}$$

$$= \frac{\sigma^2}{\sum_{i=1}^{n}(X_i - \bar{X})^2}.$$

To find the variance of $a + bX^*$, we first express it as $\bar{Y} + b(X^* - \bar{X})$:

$$\text{Var}[\bar{Y} + b(X^* - \bar{X})] = \text{Var}(\bar{Y}) + (X^* - \bar{X})^2 \text{Var}(b) + 2(X^* - \bar{X}) \text{Cov}(\bar{Y}, b).$$

Here $\text{Cov}(\bar{Y}, b)$ is the covariance of two different linear combinations of Y_1, Y_2, ..., Y_n. Using the rule for determining the covariance of two linear combinations, we obtain

$$\text{Cov}(\bar{Y}, b) = \frac{[(X_1 - \bar{X}) + (X_2 - \bar{X}) + \cdots + (X_n - \bar{X})]\sigma^2}{n \sum_{i=1}^{n}(X_i - \bar{X})^2}$$

$$= 0,$$

because $\sum_{i=1}^{n}(X_i - \bar{X}) = 0$. Then $\text{Var}(a + bX^*)$ is

$$\text{Var}(a + bX^*) = \text{Var}(\bar{Y}) + (X^* - \bar{X})^2 \text{Var}(b)$$

$$= \sigma^2 \left(\frac{1}{n} + \frac{(X^* - \bar{X})^2}{\sum_{i=1}^{n}(X_i - \bar{X})^2}\right).$$

This variance is used in a confidence interval for $E(Y|X^*)$, the mean of the Y population at $X = X^*$.

The variance of the difference between an observed and predicted Y is used in obtaining $\text{Var}(Y^*)$. When Y^* is a new observation, not used in the calculation of the least squares line,

$$
\begin{aligned}
\text{Var}[Y^* - \bar{Y} - b(X^* - \bar{X})] &= \text{Var}(Y^*) + \text{Var}(\bar{Y}) \\
&\quad + (X^* - \bar{X})^2 \, \text{Var}(b) \\
&= \sigma^2 \left(1 + \frac{1}{n} + \frac{(X^* - \bar{X})^2}{\sum_{i=1}^{n}(X_i - \bar{X})^2} \right),
\end{aligned}
$$

because the observation Y^* is independent of the n observations.

Alternatively, if we wanted the variance of the ith residual $Y_i - \bar{Y} - b(X_i - \bar{X})$, we would need to take into account $\text{Cov}(Y_i, \bar{Y}) = \sigma^2/n$ and $\text{Cov}(Y_i, (X_i - \bar{X})b) = \sigma^2(X_i - \bar{X})/\sum_{i=1}^{n}(X_i - \bar{X})^2$. That is,

$$
\begin{aligned}
\text{Var}[Y_i - \bar{Y} - b(X_i - \bar{X})] &= \text{Var}(Y_i) + \text{Var}(\bar{Y}) + (X_i - \bar{X})^2 \, \text{Var}(b) \\
&\quad - 2 \, \text{Cov}(Y_i, \bar{Y}) - 2 \, \text{Cov}[Y_i, b(X_i - \bar{X})] \\
&= \sigma^2 \left(1 - \frac{1}{n} - \frac{(X_i - \bar{X})^2}{\sum_{i=1}^{n}(X_i - \bar{X})^2} \right).
\end{aligned}
$$

Thus, the variance of the residuals is not constant but depends on the values of X.

Appendix B

Table B.1   The Standard Normal Distribution*

$z[\lambda]$	λ	$z[\lambda]$	λ	$z[\lambda]$	λ	$z[\lambda]$	λ
0.00	.5000						
0.01	.5040	0.51	.6950	1.01	.8438	1.51	.9345
0.02	.5080	0.52	.6985	1.02	.8461	1.52	.9357
0.03	.5120	0.53	.7019	1.03	.8485	1.53	.9370
0.04	.5160	0.54	.7054	1.04	.8508	1.54	.9382
0.05	.5199	0.55	.7088	1.05	.8531	1.55	.9394
0.06	.5239	0.56	.7123	1.06	.8554	1.56	.9406
0.07	.5279	0.57	.7157	1.07	.8577	1.57	.9418
0.08	.5319	0.58	.7190	1.08	.8599	1.58	.9229
0.09	.5359	0.59	.7224	1.09	.8621	1.59	.9441
0.10	.5398	0.60	.7257	1.10	.8643	1.60	.9452
0.11	.5438	0.61	.7291	1.11	.8665	1.61	.9463
0.12	.5478	0.62	.7324	1.12	.8686	1.62	.9474
0.13	.5517	0.63	.7357	1.13	.8708	1.63	.9484
0.14	.5557	0.64	.7389	1.14	.8729	1.64	.9495
0.15	.5596	0.65	.7422	1.15	.8749	1.65	.9505
0.16	.5636	0.66	.7454	1.16	.8770	1.66	.9515
0.17	.5675	0.67	.7486	1.17	.8790	1.67	.9525
0.18	.5714	0.68	.7517	1.18	.8810	1.68	.9535
0.19	.5753	0.69	.7549	1.19	.8830	1.69	.9545
0.20	.5793	0.70	.7580	1.20	.8849	1.70	.9554
0.21	.5832	0.71	.7611	1.21	.8869	1.71	.9564
0.22	.5871	0.72	.7642	1.22	.8888	1.72	.9573
0.23	.5910	0.73	.7673	1.23	.8907	1.73	.9582
0.24	.5948	0.74	.7704	1.24	.8925	1.74	.9591
0.25	.5987	0.75	.7734	1.25	.8944	1.75	.9599
0.26	.6026	0.76	.7764	1.26	.8962	1.76	.9608
0.27	.6064	0.77	.7794	1.27	.8980	1.77	.9616
0.28	.6103	0.78	.7823	1.28	.8997	1.78	.9625
0.29	.6141	0.79	.7852	1.29	.9015	1.79	.9633
0.30	.6179	0.80	.7881	1.30	.9032	1.80	.9641
0.31	.6217	0.81	.7910	1.31	.9049	1.81	.9649
0.32	.6255	0.82	.7939	1.32	.9066	1.82	.9656
0.33	.6293	0.83	.7967	1.33	.9082	1.83	.9664
0.34	.6331	0.84	.7995	1.34	.9099	1.84	.9671
0.35	.6368	0.85	.8023	1.35	.9115	1.85	.9678
0.36	.6406	0.86	.8051	1.36	.9131	1.86	.9686
0.37	.6443	0.87	.8078	1.37	.9147	1.87	.9693
0.38	.6480	0.88	.8106	1.38	.9162	1.88	.9699
0.39	.6517	0.89	.8133	1.39	.9177	1.89	.9706
0.40	.6554	0.90	.8159	1.40	.9192	1.90	.9713
0.41	.6591	0.91	.8186	1.41	.9207	1.91	.9719
0.42	.6628	0.92	.8212	1.42	.9222	1.92	.9726
0.43	.6664	0.93	.8238	1.43	.9236	1.93	.9732
0.44	.6700	0.94	.8264	1.44	.9251	1.94	.9738
0.45	.6736	0.95	.8289	1.45	.9265	1.95	.9744
0.46	.6772	0.96	.8315	1.46	.9279	1.96	.9750
0.47	.6808	0.97	.8340	1.47	.9292	1.97	.9756
0.48	.6844	0.98	.8365	1.48	.9306	1.98	.9761
0.49	.6879	0.99	.8389	1.49	.9319	1.99	.9767
0.50	.6915	1.00	.8413	1.50	.9332	2.00	.9772

Table B.1   (*Continued*)

z[λ]	λ	z[λ]	λ	z[λ]	λ	z[λ]	λ
2.01	0.9778	2.51	.9940	3.01	.9987	3.51	.9998
2.02	.9783	2.52	.9941	3.02	.9987	3.52	.9998
2.03	.9788	2.53	.9943	3.03	.9988	3.53	.9998
2.04	.9793	2.54	.9945	3.04	.9988	3.54	.9998
2.05	.9798	2.55	.9946	3.05	.9989	3.55	.9998
2.06	.9803	2.56	.9948	3.06	.9989	3.56	.9998
2.07	.9808	2.57	.9949	3.07	.9989	3.57	.9998
2.08	.9812	2.58	.9951	3.08	.9990	3.58	.9998
2.09	.9817	2.59	.9952	3.09	.9990	3.59	.9998
2.10	.9821	2.60	.9953	3.10	.9990	3.60	.9998
2.11	.9826	2.61	.9955	3.11	.9991	3.61	.9998
2.12	.9830	2.62	.9956	3.12	.9991	3.62	.9999
2.13	.9834	2.63	.9957	3.13	.9991	3.63	.9999
2.14	.9838	2.64	.9959	3.14	.9992	3.64	.9999
2.15	.9842	2.65	.9960	3.15	.9992	3.65	.9999
2.16	.9846	2.66	.9961	3.16	.9992	3.66	.9999
2.17	.9850	2.67	.9962	3.17	.9992	3.67	.9999
2.18	.9854	2.68	.9963	3.18	.9993	3.68	.9999
2.19	.9857	2.69	.9964	3.19	.9993	3.69	.9999
2.20	.9861	2.70	.9965	3.20	.9993	3.70	.9999
2.21	.9864	2.71	.9966	3.21	.9993	3.71	.9999
2.22	.9868	2.72	.9967	3.22	.9994	3.72	.9999
2.23	.9871	2.73	.9968	3.23	.9994	3.73	.9999
2.24	.9875	2.74	.9969	3.24	.9994	3.74	.9999
2.25	.9878	2.75	.9970	3.25	.9994	3.75	.9999
2.26	.9881	2.76	.9971	3.26	.9994	3.76	.9999
2.27	.9884	2.77	.9972	3.27	.9995	3.77	.9999
2.28	.9887	2.78	.9973	3.28	.9995	3.78	.9999
2.29	.9890	2.79	.9974	3.29	.9995	3.79	.9999
2.30	.9893	2.80	.9974	3.30	.9995	3.80	.9999
2.31	.9896	2.81	.9975	3.31	.9995	3.81	.9999
2.32	.9898	2.82	.9976	3.32	.9996	3.82	.9999
2.33	.9901	2.83	.9977	3.33	.9996	3.83	.9999
2.34	.9904	2.84	.9977	3.34	.9996	3.84	.9999
2.35	.9906	2.85	.9978	3.35	.9996	3.85	.9999
2.36	.9909	2.86	.9979	3.36	.9996	3.86	.9999
2.37	.9911	2.87	.9979	3.37	.9996	3.87	.9999
2.38	.9913	2.88	.9980	3.38	.9996	3.88	.9999
2.39	.9916	2.89	.9981	3.39	.9997	3.89	1.0000
2.40	.9918	2.90	.9981	3.40	.9997	3.90	1.0000
2.41	.9920	2.91	.9982	3.41	.9997	3.91	1.0000
2.42	.9922	2.92	.9982	3.42	.9997	3.92	1.0000
2.43	.9925	2.93	.9983	3.43	.9997	3.93	1.0000
2.44	.9927	2.94	.9984	3.44	.9997	3.94	1.0000
2.45	.9929	2.95	.9984	3.45	.9997	3.95	1.0000
2.46	.9931	2.96	.9985	3.46	.9997	3.96	1.0000
2.47	.9932	2.97	.9985	3.47	.9997	3.97	1.0000
2.48	.9934	2.98	.9986	3.48	.9997	3.98	1.0000
2.49	.9936	2.99	.9986	3.49	.9998	3.99	1.0000
2.50	.9938	3.00	.9986	3.50	.9998		

Footnotes to Table B.1

$*\lambda$ = Area under curve from $-\infty$ to $z[\lambda]$:

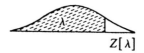

$$z[\lambda]$$

$z(0.50) = 0$, and for values of λ less than 0.50, $z(\lambda)$ is found by symmetry: $z(\lambda) = -z(1 - \lambda)$.

Data in the table are extracted from Owen, D. B. [1962] *Handbook of Statistical Tables* Reading, MA: Addison-Wesley, and are reprinted with permission.

Table B.2   Percentage Points $t[\lambda; \nu]$ of Student's t Distribution*

ν	$\lambda = 0.75$	0.90	0.95	0.975	0.99	0.995	0.9975	0.999
1	1.000	3.078	6.314	12.706	31.821	63.657	127.321	318.309
2	0.816	1.886	2.920	4.303	6.965	9.925	14.089	22.327
3	0.765	1.638	2.353	3.182	4.541	5.841	7.453	10.214
4	0.741	1.533	2.132	2.776	3.747	4.604	5.598	7.173
5	0.727	1.476	2.015	2.571	3.365	4.032	4.773	5.893
6	0.718	1.440	1.943	2.447	3.143	3.707	4.317	5.208
7	0.711	1.415	1.895	2.365	2.998	3.499	4.029	4.785
8	0.706	1.397	1.860	2.306	2.896	3.355	3.833	4.501
9	0.703	1.383	1.833	2.262	2.821	3.250	3.690	4.297
10	0.700	1.372	1.812	2.228	2.764	3.169	3.581	4.144
11	0.697	1.363	1.796	2.201	2.718	3.106	3.497	4.025
12	0.695	1.356	1.782	2.179	2.681	3.055	3.428	3.930
13	0.694	1.350	1.771	2.160	2.650	3.012	3.372	3.852
14	0.692	1.345	1.761	2.145	2.624	2.977	3.326	3.787
15	0.691	1.341	1.753	2.131	2.602	2.947	3.286	3.733
16	0.690	1.337	1.746	2.120	2.583	2.921	3.252	3.686
17	0.689	1.333	1.740	2.110	2.567	2.898	3.223	3.646
18	0.688	1.330	1.734	2.101	2.552	2.878	3.197	3.610
19	0.688	1.328	1.729	2.093	2.539	2.861	3.174	3.579
20	0.687	1.325	1.725	2.086	2.528	2.845	3.153	3.552
21	0.686	1.323	1.721	2.080	2.518	2.831	3.135	3.527
22	0.686	1.321	1.717	2.074	2.508	2.819	3.119	3.505
23	0.685	1.319	1.714	2.069	2.500	2.807	3.104	3.485
24	0.685	1.318	1.711	2.064	2.492	2.797	3.090	3.467
25	0.684	1.316	1.708	2.060	2.485	2.787	3.078	3.450
26	0.684	1.315	1.706	2.056	2.479	2.779	3.067	3.435
27	0.684	1.314	1.703	2.052	2.473	2.771	3.057	3.421
28	0.683	1.313	1.701	2.048	2.467	2.763	3.047	3.408
29	0.683	1.311	1.699	2.045	2.462	2.756	3.038	3.396
30	0.683	1.310	1.697	2.042	2.457	2.750	3.030	3.385
35	0.682	1.306	1.690	2.030	2.438	2.724	2.996	3.340
40	0.681	1.303	1.684	2.021	2.423	2.704	2.971	3.307
45	0.680	1.301	1.679	2.014	2.412	2.690	2.952	3.281
50	0.679	1.299	1.676	2.009	2.403	2.678	2.937	3.261
55	0.679	1.297	1.673	2.004	2.396	2.668	2.925	3.245
60	0.679	1.296	1.671	2.000	2.390	2.660	2.915	3.232
70	0.678	1.294	1.667	1.994	2.381	2.648	2.899	3.211
80	0.678	1.292	1.664	1.990	2.374	2.639	2.887	3.195
90	0.677	1.291	1.662	1.987	2.368	2.632	2.878	3.183
100	0.677	1.290	1.660	1.984	2.364	2.626	2.871	3.174
120	0.677	1.289	1.657	1.980	2.351	2.618	2.860	3.153
200	0.676	1.286	1.652	1.972	2.345	2.601	2.838	3.131
500	0.675	1.283	1.648	1.965	2.334	2.586	2.820	3.107
∞	0.674	1.282	1.645	1.960	2.326	2.576	2.807	3.090

Table B.2   (*Continued*)

ν	$\lambda = 0.9995$	0.99975	0.9999	0.99995	0.999975	0.99999
			$t[\lambda; \nu]$			
1	636.619	1.273.239	3.183.099	6.366.198	12.732.395	31.830.989
2	31.598	44.705	70.700	99.992	141.416	223.603
3	12.924	16.326	22.204	28.000	35.298	47.928
4	8.610	10.306	13.034	15.544	18.522	23.332
5	6.869	7.976	9.678	11.178	12.893	15.547
6	5.959	6.788	8.025	9.082	10.261	12.032
7	5.408	6.082	7.063	7.885	8.782	10.103
8	5.041	5.618	6.442	7.120	7.851	8.907
9	4.781	5.291	6.010	6.594	7.215	8.102
10	4.587	5.049	5.694	6.211	6.757	7.527
11	4.437	4.863	5.453	5.921	6.412	7.098
12	4.318	4.716	5.263	5.694	6.143	6.756
13	4.221	4.597	5.111	5.513	5.928	6.501
14	4.140	4.499	4.985	5.363	5.753	6.287
15	4.073	4.417	4.880	5.239	5.607	6.109
16	4.015	4.346	4.791	5.134	5.484	5.960
17	3.965	4.286	4.714	5.044	5.379	5.832
18	3.922	4.233	4.648	4.966	5.288	5.722
19	3.883	4.187	4.590	4.897	5.209	5.627
20	3.850	4.146	4.539	4.837	5.139	5.543
21	3.819	4.110	4.493	4.784	5.077	5.469
22	3.792	4.077	4.452	4.736	5.022	5.402
23	3.768	4.048	4.415	4.693	4.972	5.343
24	3.745	4.021	4.382	4.654	4.927	5.290
25	3.725	3.997	4.352	4.619	4.887	5.241
26	3.707	3.974	4.324	4.587	4.850	5.197
27	3.690	3.954	4.299	4.558	4.816	5.157
28	3.674	3.935	4.275	4.530	4.784	5.120
29	3.659	3.918	4.254	4.506	4.756	5.086
30	3.646	3.902	4.234	4.482	4.729	5.054
35	3.591	3.836	4.153	4.389	4.622	4.927
40	3.551	3.788	4.094	4.321	4.544	4.835
45	3.520	3.752	4.049	4.269	4.485	4.766
50	3.496	3.723	4.014	4.228	4.438	4.711
55	3.476	3.700	3.986	4.196	4.401	4.667
60	3.460	3.681	3.962	4.169	4.370	4.631
70	3.435	3.651	3.926	4.127	4.323	4.576
80	3.416	3.629	3.899	4.096	4.288	4.535
90	3.402	3.612	3.878	4.072	4.261	4.503
100	3.390	3.598	3.862	4.053	4.240	4.478
120	3.373	3.579	3.838	4.025	4.209	4.442
200	3.340	3.539	3.789	3.970	4.146	4.369
500	3.310	3.504	3.747	3.922	4.091	4.306
∞	3.291	3.481	3.719	3.891	4.056	4.265

Footnotes to Table B.2

$^*\lambda$ = area under curve from $-\infty$ to $t[\lambda; \nu]$.

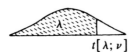

$t[\lambda; \nu]$

$t[0.50; \nu] = 0$, and for values of λ less than 0.50, $t[\lambda; \nu]$ is found by symmetry: $t[\lambda; \nu] = -t[1 - \lambda; \nu]$. Note also that $t(\lambda; \infty) = z(\lambda)$.

The data in this table are reprinted from E. T. Federighi [Sept. 1959], Extended Tables of the Percentage Points of Student's t-Distribution, *Journal of the American Statistical Association*, with the kind permission of the author.

Table B.3   Percentage Points $\chi^2[\lambda; \nu]$ of the χ^2 Distribution

ν	$\chi^2[\lambda; \nu]$					
	$\lambda = 0.005$	0.01	0.025	0.05	0.10	0.25
1	—	—	0.001	0.004	0.016	0.102
2	0.010	0.020	0.051	0.103	0.211	0.575
3	0.072	0.115	0.216	0.352	0.584	1.213
4	0.207	0.297	0.484	0.711	1.064	1.923
5	0.412	0.554	0.831	1.145	1.610	2.675
6	0.676	0.872	1.237	1.635	2.204	3.455
7	0.989	1.239	1.690	2.167	2.833	4.255
8	1.344	1.646	2.180	2.733	3.490	5.071
9	1.735	2.088	2.700	3.325	4.168	5.899
10	2.156	2.558	3.247	3.940	4.865	6.737
11	2.603	3.053	3.816	4.575	5.578	7.584
12	3.074	3.571	4.404	5.226	6.304	8.438
13	3.565	4.107	5.009	5.892	7.042	9.299
14	4.075	4.660	5.629	6.571	7.790	10.165
15	4.601	5.229	6.262	7.261	8.547	11.037
16	5.142	5.812	6.908	7.962	9.312	11.912
17	5.697	6.408	7.564	8.672	10.085	12.792
18	6.265	7.015	8.231	9.390	10.865	13.675
19	6.844	7.633	8.907	10.117	11.651	14.562
20	7.434	8.260	9.591	10.851	12.443	15.452
22	8.643	9.542	10.982	12.338	14.042	17.240
24	9.886	10.856	12.401	13.848	15.659	19.037
26	11.160	12.198	13.844	15.379	17.292	20.843
28	12.461	13.565	15.308	16.928	18.939	22.657
30	13.787	14.954	16.791	18.493	20.599	24.478
40	20.707	22.164	24.433	26.509	29.051	33.660
50	27.991	29.707	32.357	34.764	37.689	42.942
60	35.534	37.485	40.482	43.188	46.459	52.294
70	43.275	45.442	48.758	51.739	55.239	61.698
80	51.172	53.540	57.153	60.391	64.278	71.145
90	59.196	61.754	65.647	69.126	73.291	80.625
100	67.328	70.065	74.222	77.929	82.358	90.133
110	75.550	78.458	82.867	86.792	91.471	99.666
120	83.852	86.923	91.573	95.705	100.624	109.220
130	92.222	95.451	100.331	104.662	109.811	118.792
140	100.655	104.034	109.137	113.659	119.029	128.380
150	109.142	112.668	117.985	122.692	128.275	137.983
200	152.241	156.432	162.728	168.279	174.835	186.172
500	422.303	429.388	439.936	449.147	459.926	478.323

Table B.3   (*Continued*)

	$\chi^2[\lambda; \nu]$					
ν	$\lambda = 0.75$	0.90	0.95	0.975	0.99	0.995
1	1.323	2.706	3.841	5.024	6.635	7.879
2	2.773	4.605	5.991	7.378	9.210	10.597
3	4.108	6.251	7.815	9.348	11.345	12.838
4	5.385	7.779	9.488	11.143	13.277	14.860
5	6.626	9.236	11.071	12.833	15.086	16.750
6	7.841	10.645	12.592	14.449	16.812	18.548
7	9.037	12.017	14.067	16.013	18.475	20.278
8	10.219	13.362	15.507	17.535	20.090	21.955
9	11.389	14.684	16.919	19.023	21.666	23.589
10	12.549	15.987	18.307	20.483	23.209	25.188
11	13.701	17.275	19.675	21.920	24.725	26.757
12	14.845	18.549	21.026	23.337	26.217	28.299
13	15.984	19.812	22.362	24.736	27.688	29.819
14	17.117	21.064	23.685	26.119	29.141	31.319
15	18.245	22.307	24.996	27.488	30.578	32.801
16	19.369	23.542	26.296	28.845	32.000	34.267
17	20.489	24.769	27.587	30.191	33.409	35.718
18	21.605	25.989	28.869	31.526	34.805	37.156
19	22.718	27.204	30.144	32.852	36.191	38.582
20	23.828	28.412	31.410	34.170	37.566	39.997
22	26.039	30.813	33.924	36.781	40.289	42.796
24	28.241	33.196	36.415	39.364	42.980	45.559
26	30.435	35.563	38.885	41.923	45.642	48.290
28	32.620	37.916	41.337	44.461	48.278	50.993
30	34.800	40.256	43.773	46.979	50 892	53.672
40	45.616	51.805	55.758	59.342	63.691	66.766
50	56.334	63.167	67.505	71.420	76.154	79.490
60	66.981	74.397	79.082	83.298	88.379	91.952
70	77.577	85.527	90.531	95.023	100.425	104.215
80	88.130	96.578	101.879	106.629	112.329	116.321
90	98.650	107.565	113.145	118.136	124.116	128.299
100	109.141	118.498	124.342	129.561	135.807	140.169
110	119.608	129.385	135.480	140.917	147.414	151.948
120	130.055	140.233	146.567	152.211	158.950	163.648
130	140.482	151.045	157.610	163.453	170.423	175.278
140	150.894	161.827	168.613	174.648	181.840	186.847
150	161.291	172.581	179.581	185.800	193.208	198.360
200	213.102	226.021	233.994	241.058	249.445	255.264
500	520.950	540.930	553.127	563.852	576.493	585.207

* λ = area under curve from zero to $\chi^2[\lambda; \nu]$.

Data in the table are extracted from Owen, D. B. [1962], *Handbook of Statistical Tables*, Reading, MA: Addison-Wesley, and are reprinted with permission.

Table B.4 Percentage Points $F[\lambda; \nu_1, \nu_2]$ of the F Distribution*

ν_2	Cum. Prop.	$\nu_1 = 1$	2	3	4	5	6	7	8	9	10	11	12
1	.025	$.0^2 15$	.026	.057	.082	.100	.113	.124	.132	.139	.144	.149	.153
	.95	161	200	216	225	230	234	237	239	241	242	243	244
	.975	648	800	864	900	922	937	948	957	963	969	973	977
	.99	405^1	500^1	540^1	562^1	576^1	586^1	593^1	598^1	602^1	606^1	608^1	611^1
	.999	406^3	500^3	540^3	562^3	576^3	586^3	593^3	598^3	602^3	606^3	609^3	611^3
	.9995	162^4	200^4	216^4	225^4	231^4	234^4	237^4	239^4	241^4	242^4	243^4	244^4
2	.025	$.0^2 13$	.026	.062	.094	.119	.138	.153	.165	.175	.183	.190	.196
	.95	18.5	19.0	19.2	19.2	19.3	19.3	19.4	19.4	19.4	19.4	19.4	19.4
	.975	38.5	39.0	39.2	39.2	39.3	39.3	39.4	39.4	39.4	39.4	39.4	39.4
	.99	98.5	99.0	99.2	99.2	99.3	99.3	99.4	99.4	99.4	99.4	99.4	99.4
	.999	998	999	999	999	999	999	999	999	999	999	999	999
	.9995	200^1	200^1	200^1	200^1	200^1	200^1	200^1	200^1	200^1	200^1	200^1	200^1
3	.025	$.0^2 12$	.026	.065	.100	.129	.152	.170	.185	.197	.207	.216	.224
	.95	10.1	9.55	9.28	9.12	9.01	8.94	8.99	8.85	8.81	8.79	8.76	8.74
	.975	17.4	16.0	15.4	15.1	14.9	14.7	14.6	14.5	14.5	14.4	14.4	14.3
	.99	34.1	30.8	29.5	28.7	28.2	27.9	27.7	27.5	27.3	27.2	27.1	27.1
	.999	167	149	141	137	135	133	132	131	130	129	129	128
	.9995	266	237	225	218	214	211	209	208	207	206	204	204
4	.025	$.0^2 11$	.026	.066	.104	.135	.161	.181	.198	.212	.224	.234	.243
	.95	7.71	6.94	6.59	6.39	6.26	6.16	6.09	6.04	6.00	5.96	5.94	5.91
	.975	12.2	10.6	9.98	9.60	9.36	9.20	9.07	8.98	8.90	8.84	8.79	8.75
	.99	21.2	18.0	16.7	16.0	15.5	15.2	15.0	14.8	14.7	14.5	14.4	14.4
	.999	74.1	61.2	56.2	53.4	51.7	50.5	49.7	49.0	48.5	48.0	47.7	47.4
	.9995	106	87.4	80.1	76.1	73.6	71.9	70.6	69.7	68.9	68.3	67.8	67.4
5	.025	$.0^2 11$	.025	.067	.107	.140	.167	.189	.208	.223	.236	.248	.257
	.95	6.61	5.79	5.41	5.19	5.05	4.95	4.88	4.82	4.77	4.74	4.71	4.68
	.975	10.0	8.43	7.76	7.39	7.15	6.98	6.85	6.76	6.68	6.62	6.57	6.52
	.99	16.3	13.3	12.1	11.4	11.0	10.7	10.5	10.3	10.2	10.1	9.96	9.89
	.999	47.2	37.1	33.2	31.1	29.7	28.8	28.2	27.6	27.2	26.9	26.6	26.4
	.9995	63.6	49.8	44.4	41.5	39.7	38.5	37.6	36.9	36.4	35.9	35.6	35.2
6	.025	$.0^2 11$	.025	.068	.109	.143	.172	.195	.215	.231	.246	.258	.268
	.95	5.99	5.14	4.76	4.53	4.39	4.28	4.21	4.15	4.10	4.06	4.03	4.00
	.975	8.81	7.26	6.60	6.23	5.99	5.82	5.70	5.60	5.52	5.46	5.41	5.37
	.99	13.7	10.9	9.78	9.15	8.75	8.47	8.26	8.10	7.98	7.87	7.79	7.72
	.999	35.5	27.0	23.7	21.9	20.8	20.0	19.5	19.0	18.7	18.4	18.2	18.0
	.9995	46.1	34.8	30.4	28.1	26.6	25.6	24.9	24.3	23.9	23.5	23.2	23.0
7	.025	$.0^2 10$	.025	.068	.110	.146	.176	.200	.221	.238	.253	.266	.277
	.95	5.59	4.74	4.35	4.12	3.97	3.87	3.79	3.73	3.68	3.64	3.60	3.57
	.975	8.07	6.54	5.89	5.52	5.29	5.12	4.99	4.90	4.82	4.76	4.71	4.67
	.99	12.2	9.55	8.45	7.85	7.46	7.19	6.99	6.84	6.72	6.62	6.54	6.47
	.999	29.2	21.7	18.8	17.2	16.2	15.5	15.0	14.6	14.3	14.1	13.9	13.7
	.9995	37.0	27.2	23.5	21.4	20.2	19.3	18.7	18.2	17.8	17.5	17.2	17.0

Table B.4 (*Continued*)

ν_2	Cum. Prop.	$\nu_1 = 15$	20	24	30	40	50	60	100	120	200	500	∞
1	.025	.161	.170	.175	.180	.184	.187	.189	.193	.194	.196	.198	.199
	.95	246	248	249	250	251	252	252	253	253	253	254	254
	.975	985	993	997	100^1	101^1	101^1	101^1	101^1	101^1	102^1	102^1	102^1
	.99	616^1	621^1	623^1	626^1	629^1	630^1	631^1	633^1	634^1	635^1	636^1	637^1
	.999	616^3	621^3	623^3	626^3	629^3	630^3	631^3	633^3	634^3	635^3	636^3	637^3
	.9995	246^4	248^4	249^4	250^4	251^4	252^4	252^4	253^4	253^4	253^4	254^4	254^4
2	.025	.210	.224	.232	.239	.247	.251	.255	.261	.263	.266	.269	.271
	.95	19.4	19.4	19.5	19.5	19.5	19.5	19.5	19.5	19.5	19.5	19.5	19.5
	.975	39.4	39.4	39.5	39.5	39.5	39.5	39.5	39.5	39.5	39.5	39.5	39.5
	.99	99.4	99.4	99.5	99.5	99.5	99.5	99.5	99.5	99.5	99.5	99.5	99.5
	.999	999	999	999	999	999	999	999	999	999	999	999	999
	.9995	200^1	200^1	200^1	200^1	200^1	200^1	200^1	200^1	200^1	200^1	200^1	200^1
3	.025	.241	.259	.269	.279	.289	.295	.299	.308	.310	.314	.318	.321
	.95	8.70	8.66	8.63	8.62	8.59	8.58	8.57	8.55	8.55	8.54	8.53	8.53
	.975	14.3	14.2	14.1	14.1	14.0	14.0	14.0	14.0	13.9	13.9	13.9	13.9
	.99	26.9	26.7	26.6	26.5	26.4	26.4	26.3	26.2	26.2	26.2	26.1	26.1
	.999	127	126	126	125	125	125	124	124	124	124	124	123
	.9995	203	201	200	199	199	198	198	197	197	197	196	196
4	.025	.263	.284	.296	.308	.320	.327	.332	.342	.346	.351	.356	.359
	.95	5.86	5.80	5.77	5.75	5.72	5.70	5.69	5.66	5.66	5.65	5.64	5.63
	.975	8.66	8.56	8.51	8.46	8.41	8.38	8.36	8.32	8.31	8.29	8.27	8.26
	.99	14.2	14.0	13.9	13.8	13.7	13.7	13.7	13.6	13.6	13.5	13.5	13.5
	.999	46.8	46.1	45.8	45.4	45.1	44.9	44.7	44.5	44.4	44.3	44.1	44.0
	.9995	66.5	65.5	65.1	64.6	64.1	63.8	63.6	63.2	63.1	62.9	62.7	62.6
5	.025	.280	.304	.317	.330	.344	.353	.359	.370	.374	.380	.386	.390
	.95	4.62	4.56	4.53	4.50	4.46	4.44	4.43	4.41	4.40	4.39	4.37	4.36
	.975	6.43	6.33	6.28	6.23	6.18	6.14	6.12	6.08	6.07	6.05	6.03	6.02
	.99	9.72	9.55	9.47	9.38	9.29	9.24	9.20	9.13	9.11	9.08	9.04	9.02
	.999	25.9	25.4	25.1	24.9	24.6	24.4	24.3	24.1	24.1	23.9	23.8	23.8
	.9995	34.6	33.9	33.5	33.1	32.7	32.5	32.3	32.1	32.0	31.8	31.7	31.6
6	.025	.293	.320	.334	.349	.364	.375	.381	.394	.398	.405	.412	.415
	.95	3.94	3.87	3.84	3.81	3.77	3.75	3.74	3.71	3.70	3.69	3.68	3.67
	.975	5.27	5.17	5.12	5.07	5.01	4.98	4.96	4.92	4.90	4.88	4.86	4.85
	.99	7.56	7.40	7.31	7.23	7.14	7.09	7.06	6.99	6.97	6.93	6.90	6.88
	.999	17.6	17.1	16.9	16.7	16.4	16.3	16.2	16.0	16.0	15.9	15.8	15.7
	.9995	22.4	21.9	21.7	21.4	21.1	20.9	20.7	20.5	20.4	20.3	20.2	20.1
7	.025	.304	.333	.348	.364	.381	.392	.399	.413	.418	.426	.433	.437
	.95	3.51	3.44	3.41	3.38	3.34	3.32	3.30	3.27	3.27	3.25	3.24	3.23
	.975	4.57	4.47	4.42	4.36	4.31	4.28	4.25	4.21	4.20	4.18	4.16	4.14
	.99	6.31	6.16	6.07	5.99	5.91	5.86	5.82	5.75	5.74	5.70	5.67	5.65
	.999	13.3	12.9	12.7	12.5	12.3	12.2	12.1	11.9	11.9	11.8	11.7	11.7
	.9995	16.5	16.0	15.7	15.5	15.2	15.1	15.0	14.7	14.7	14.6	14.5	14.4

Table B.4   (*Continued*)

ν_2	Cum. Prop.	$F[\lambda; \nu_1, \nu_2]$											
		$\nu_1 = 1$	2	3	4	5	6	7	8	9	10	11	12
8	.025	$.0^2 10$	.025	.069	.111	.148	.179	.204	.226	.244	.259	.273	.285
	.95	5.32	4.46	4.07	3.84	3.69	3.58	3.50	3.44	3.39	3.36	3.31	3.28
	.975	7.57	6.06	5.42	5.05	4.82	4.65	4.53	4.43	4.36	4.30	4.24	4.20
	.99	11.3	8.65	7.59	7.01	6.63	6.37	6.18	6.03	5.91	5.81	5.73	5.67
	.999	25.4	18.5	15.8	14.4	13.5	12.9	12.4	12.0	11.8	11.5	11.4	11.2
	.9995	31.6	22.8	19.4	17.6	16.4	15.7	15.1	14.6	14.3	14.0	13.8	13.6
9	.025	$.0^2 10$	.025	.069	.112	.150	.181	.207	.230	.248	.265	.279	.291
	.95	5.12	4.26	3.86	3.63	3.48	3.37	3.29	3.23	3.18	3.14	3.10	3.07
	.975	7.21	5.71	5.08	4.72	4.48	4.32	4.20	4.10	4.03	3.96	3.91	3.87
	.99	10.6	8.02	6.99	6.42	6.06	5.80	5.61	5.47	5.35	5.26	5.18	5.11
	.999	22.9	16.4	13.9	12.6	11.7	11.1	10.7	10.4	10.1	9.89	9.71	9.57
	.9995	28.0	19.9	16.8	15.1	14.1	13.3	12.8	12.4	12.1	11.8	11.6	11.4
10	.025	$.0^2 10$	.025	0.69	.113	.151	.183	.210	.233	.252	.269	.283	.296
	.95	4.96	4.10	3.71	3.48	3.33	3.22	3.14	3.07	3.02	2.98	2.94	2.91
	.975	6.94	5.46	4.83	4.47	4.24	4.07	3.95	3.85	3.78	3.72	3.66	3.62
	.99	10.0	7.56	6.55	5.99	5.64	5.39	5.20	5.06	4.94	4.85	4.77	4.71
	.999	21.0	14.9	12.6	11.3	10.5	9.92	9.52	9.20	8.96	8.75	8.58	8.44
	.9995	25.5	17.9	15.0	13.4	12.4	11.8	11.3	10.9	10.6	10.3	10.1	9.93
11	.025	$.0^2 10$	.025	.069	.114	.152	.185	.212	.236	.256	.273	.288	.301
	.95	4.84	3.98	3.59	3.36	3.20	3.09	3.01	2.95	2.90	2.85	2.82	2.79
	.975	6.72	5.26	4.63	4.28	4.04	3.88	3.76	3.66	3.59	3.53	3.47	3.43
	.99	9.65	7.21	6.22	5.67	5.32	5.07	4.89	4.74	4.63	4.54	4.46	4.40
	.999	19.7	13.8	11.6	10.3	9.58	9.05	8.66	8.35	8.12	7.92	7.76	7.62
	.9995	23.6	16.4	13.6	12.2	11.2	10.6	10.1	9.76	9.48	9.24	9.04	8.88
12	.025	$.0^2 10$	.025	.070	.114	.153	.186	.214	.238	.259	.276	.292	.305
	.95	4.75	3.89	3.49	3.26	3.11	3.00	2.91	2.85	2.80	2.75	2.72	2.69
	.975	6.55	5.10	4.47	4.12	3.89	3.73	3.61	3.51	3.44	3.37	3.32	3.28
	.99	9.33	6.93	5.95	5.41	5.06	4.82	4.64	4.50	4.39	4.30	4.22	4.16
	.999	18.6	13.0	10.8	9.63	8.89	8.38	8.00	7.71	7.48	7.29	7.14	7.01
	.9995	22.2	15.3	12.7	11.2	10.4	9.74	9.28	8.94	8.66	8.43	8.24	8.08
15	.025	$.0^2 10$	.025	.070	.116	.156	.190	.219	.244	.265	.284	.300	.315
	.95	4.54	3.68	3.29	3.06	2.90	2.79	2.71	2.64	2.59	2.54	2.51	2.48
	.975	6.20	4.76	4.15	3.80	3.58	3.41	3.29	3.20	3.12	3.06	3.01	2.96
	.99	8.68	6.36	5.42	4.89	4.56	4.32	4.14	4.00	3.89	3.80	3.73	3.67
	.999	16.6	11.3	9.34	8.25	7.57	7.09	6.74	6.47	6.26	6.08	5.93	5.81
	.9995	19.5	13.2	10.8	9.48	8.66	8.10	7.68	7.36	7.11	6.91	6.75	6.60
20	.025	$.0^2 10$	.025	.071	.117	.158	.193	.224	.250	.273	.292	.310	.325
	.95	4.35	3.49	3.10	2.87	2.71	2.60	2.51	2.45	2.39	2.35	2.31	2.28
	.975	5.87	4.46	3.86	3.51	3.29	3.13	3.01	2.91	2.84	2.77	2.72	2.68
	.99	8.10	5.85	4.94	4.43	4.10	3.87	3.70	3.56	3.46	3.37	3.29	3.23
	.999	14.8	9.95	8.10	7.10	6.46	6.02	5.69	5.44	5.24	5.08	4.94	4.82
	.9995	17.2	11.4	9.20	8.02	7.28	6.76	6.38	6.08	5.85	5.66	5.51	5.38

Table B.4   (*Continued*)

ν_2	Cum. Prop.	$\nu_1 = 15$	20	24	30	40	50	60	100	120	200	500	∞
						$F[\lambda; \nu_1, \nu_2]$							
8	.025	.313	.343	.360	.377	.395	.407	.415	.431	.435	.442	.450	.456
	.95	3.22	3.15	3.12	3.08	3.04	3.02	3.01	2.97	2.97	2.95	2.94	2.93
	.975	4.10	4.00	3.95	3.89	3.84	3.81	3.78	3.74	3.73	3.70	3.68	3.67
	.99	5.52	5.36	5.28	5.20	5.12	5.07	5.03	4.96	4.95	4.91	4.88	4.86
	.999	10.8	10.5	10.3	10.1	9.92	9.80	9.73	9.57	9.54	9.46	9.39	9.34
	.9995	13.1	12.7	12.5	12.2	12.0	11.8	11.8	11.6	11.5	11.4	11.4	11.3
9	.025	.320	.352	.370	.388	.408	.420	.428	.446	.450	.459	.467	.473
	.95	3.01	2.94	2.90	2.86	2.83	2.80	2.79	2.76	2.75	2.73	2.72	2.71
	.975	3.77	3.67	3.61	3.56	3.51	3.47	3.45	3.40	3.39	3.37	3.35	3.33
	.99	4.96	4.81	4.73	4.65	4.57	4.52	4.48	4.42	4.40	4.36	4.33	4.31
	.999	9.24	8.90	8.72	8.55	8.37	8.26	8.19	8.04	8.00	7.93	7.86	7.81
	.9995	11.0	10.6	10.4	10.2	9.94	9.80	9.71	9.53	9.49	9.40	9.32	9.26
10	.025	.327	.360	.379	.398	.419	.431	.441	.459	.464	.474	.483	.488
	.95	2.85	2.77	2.74	2.70	2.66	2.64	2.62	2.59	2.58	2.56	2.55	2.54
	.975	3.52	3.42	3.37	3.31	3.26	3.22	3.20	3.15	3.14	3.12	3.09	3.08
	.99	4.56	4.41	4.33	4.25	4.17	4.12	4.08	4.01	4.00	3.96	3.93	3.91
	.999	8.13	7.80	7.64	7.47	7.30	7.19	7.12	6.98	6.94	6.87	6.81	6.76
	.9995	9.56	9.16	8.96	8.75	8.54	8.42	8.33	8.16	8.12	8.04	7.96	7.90
11	.025	.332	.368	.386	.407	.429	.442	.450	.472	.476	.485	.495	.503
	.95	2.72	2.65	2.61	2.57	2.53	2.51	2.49	2.46	2.45	2.43	2.42	2.40
	.975	3.33	3.23	3.17	3.12	3.06	3.03	3.00	2.96	2.94	2.92	2.90	2.88
	.99	4.25	4.10	4.02	3.94	3.86	3.81	3.78	3.71	3.69	3.66	3.62	3.60
	.999	7.32	7.01	6.85	6.68	6.52	6.41	6.35	6.21	6.17	6.10	6.04	6.00
	.9995	8.52	8.14	7.94	7.75	7.55	7.43	7.35	7.18	7.14	7.06	6.98	6.93
12	.025	.337	.374	.394	.416	.437	.450	.461	.481	.487	.498	.508	.514
	.95	2.62	2.54	2.51	2.47	2.43	2.40	2.38	2.35	2.34	2.32	2.31	2.30
	.975	3.18	3.07	3.02	2.96	2.91	2.87	2.85	2.80	2.79	2.76	2.74	2.72
	.99	4.01	3.86	3.78	3.70	3.62	3.57	3.54	3.47	3.45	3.41	3.38	3.36
	.999	6.71	6.40	6.25	6.09	5.93	5.83	5.76	5.63	5.59	5.52	5.46	5.42
	.9995	7.74	7.37	7.18	7.00	6.80	6.68	6.61	6.45	6.41	6.33	6.25	6.20
15	.025	.349	.389	.410	.433	.458	.474	.485	.508	.514	.526	.538	.546
	.95	2.40	2.33	2.39	2.25	2.20	2.18	2.16	2.12	2.11	2.10	2.08	2.07
	.975	2.86	2.76	2.70	2.64	2.59	2.55	2.52	2.47	2.46	2.44	2.41	2.40
	.99	3.52	3.37	3.29	3.21	3.13	3.08	3.05	2.98	2.96	2.92	2.89	2.87
	.999	5.54	5.25	5.10	4.95	4.80	4.70	4.64	4.51	4.47	4.41	4.35	4.31
	.9995	6.27	5.93	5.75	5.58	5.40	5.29	5.21	5.06	5.02	4.94	4.87	4.83
20	.025	.363	.406	.430	.456	.484	.503	.514	.541	.548	.562	.575	.585
	.95	2.20	2.12	2.08	2.04	1.99	1.97	1.95	1.91	1.90	1.88	1.86	1.84
	.975	2.57	2.46	2.41	2.35	2.29	2.25	2.22	2.17	2.16	2.13	2.10	2.09
	.99	3.09	2.94	2.86	2.78	2.69	2.64	2.61	2.54	2.52	2.48	2.44	2.42
	.999	4.56	4.29	4.15	4.01	3.86	3.77	3.70	3.58	3.54	3.48	3.42	3.38
	.9995	5.07	4.75	4.58	4.42	4.24	4.15	4.07	3.93	3.90	3.82	3.75	3.70

Table B.4   (*Continued*)

ν_2	Cum. Prop.	$F[\lambda; \nu_1, \nu_2]$											
		$\nu_1 = 1$	2	3	4	5	6	7	8	9	10	11	12
24	.025	$.0^210$	.025	.071	.117	.159	.195	.227	.253	.277	.297	.315	.331
	.95	4.26	3.40	3.01	2.78	2.62	2.51	2.42	2.36	2.30	2.25	2.21	2.18
	.975	5.72	4.32	3.72	3.38	3.15	2.99	2.87	2.78	2.70	2.64	2.59	2.54
	.99	7.82	5.61	4.72	4.22	3.90	3.67	3.50	3.36	3.26	3.17	3.09	3.03
	.999	14.0	9.34	7.55	6.59	5.98	5.55	5.23	4.99	4.80	4.64	4.50	4.39
	.9995	16.2	10.6	8.52	7.39	6.68	6.18	5.82	5.54	5.31	5.13	4.98	4.85
30	.025	$.0^210$	.025	.071	.118	.161	.197	.229	.257	.281	.302	.321	.337
	.95	4.17	3.32	2.92	2.69	2.53	2.42	2.33	2.27	2.21	2.16	2.13	2.09
	.975	5.57	4.18	3.59	3.25	3.03	2.87	2.75	2.65	2.57	2.51	2.46	2.41
	.99	7.56	5.39	4.51	4.02	3.70	3.47	3.30	3.17	3.07	2.98	2.91	2.84
	.999	13.3	8.77	7.05	6.12	5.53	5.12	4.82	4.58	4.39	4.24	4.11	4.00
	.9995	15.2	9.90	7.90	6.82	6.14	5.66	5.31	5.04	4.82	4.65	4.51	4.38
40	.025	$.0^399$	.025	0.71	.119	.162	.199	.232	.260	.285	.307	.327	.344
	.95	4.08	3.23	2.84	2.61	2.45	2.34	2.25	2.18	2.12	2.08	2.04	2.00
	.975	5.42	4.05	3.46	3.13	2.90	2.74	2.62	2.53	2.45	2.39	2.33	2.29
	.99	7.31	5.18	4.31	3.83	3.51	3.29	3.12	2.99	2.89	2.80	2.73	2.66
	.999	12.6	8.25	6.60	5.70	5.13	4.73	4.44	4.21	4.02	3.87	3.75	3.64
	.9995	14.4	9.25	7.33	6.30	5.64	5.19	4.85	4.59	4.38	4.21	4.07	3.95
60	.025	$.0^399$	.025	.071	.120	.163	.202	.235	.264	.290	.313	.333	.351
	.95	4.00	3.15	2.76	2.53	2.37	2.25	2.17	2.10	2.04	1.99	1.95	1.92
	.975	5.29	3.93	3.34	3.01	2.79	2.63	2.51	2.41	2.33	2.27	2.22	2.17
	.99	7.08	4.98	4.13	3.65	3.34	3.12	2.95	2.82	2.72	2.63	2.56	2.50
	.999	12.0	7.76	6.17	5.31	4.76	4.37	4.09	3.87	3.69	3.54	3.43	3.31
	.9995	13.6	8.65	6.81	5.82	5.20	4.76	4.44	4.18	3.98	3.82	3.69	3.57
120	.025	$.0^399$	.025	.072	.120	.165	.204	.238	.268	.295	.318	.340	.359
	.95	3.92	3.07	2.68	2.45	2.29	2.18	2.09	2.02	1.96	1.91	1.87	1.83
	.975	5.15	3.80	3.23	2.89	2.67	2.52	2.39	2.30	2.22	2.16	2.10	2.05
	.99	6.85	4.79	3.95	3.48	3.17	2.96	2.79	2.66	2.56	2.47	2.40	2.34
	.999	11.4	7.32	5.79	4.95	4.42	4.04	3.77	3.55	3.38	3.24	3.12	3.02
	.9995	12.8	8.10	6.34	5.39	4.79	4.37	4.07	3.82	3.63	3.47	3.34	3.22
∞	.025	$.0^398$	.025	.072	.121	.166	.206	.241	.272	.300	.325	.347	.367
	.95	3.84	3.00	2.60	2.37	2.21	2.10	2.01	1.94	1.88	1.83	1.79	1.75
	.975	5.02	3.69	3.12	2.79	2.57	2.41	2.29	2.19	2.11	2.05	1.99	1.94
	.99	6.63	4.61	3.78	3.32	3.02	2.80	2.64	2.51	2.41	2.32	2.25	2.18
	.999	10.8	6.91	5.42	4.62	4.10	3.74	3.47	3.27	3.10	2.96	2.84	2.74
	.9995	12.1	7.60	5.91	5.00	4.42	4.02	3.72	3.48	3.30	3.14	3.02	2.90

Table B.4   *(Continued)*

ν_2	Cum. Prop.	$\nu_1 = 15$	20	24	30	40	50	60	100	120	200	500	∞
24	.025	.370	.415	.441	.468	.498	.518	.531	.562	.568	.585	.599	.610
	.95	2.11	2.03	1.98	1.94	1.89	1.86	1.84	1.80	1.79	1.77	1.75	1.73
	.975	2.44	2.33	2.27	2.21	2.15	2.11	2.08	2.02	2.01	1.98	1.95	1.94
	.99	2.89	2.74	2.66	2.58	2.49	2.44	2.40	2.33	2.31	2.27	2.24	2.21
	.999	4.14	3.87	3.74	3.59	3.45	3.35	3.29	3.16	3.14	3.07	3.01	2.97
	.9995	4.55	4.25	4.09	3.93	3.76	3.66	3.59	3.44	3.41	3.33	3.27	3.22
30	.025	.378	.426	.453	.482	.515	.535	.551	.585	.592	.610	.625	.639
	.95	2.01	1.93	1.89	1.84	1.79	1.76	1.74	1.70	1.68	1.66	1.64	1.62
	.975	2.31	2.20	2.14	2.07	2.01	1.97	1.94	1.88	1.87	1.84	1.81	1.79
	.99	2.70	2.55	2.47	2.39	2.30	2.25	2.21	2.13	2.11	2.07	2.03	2.01
	.999	3.75	3.49	3.36	3.22	3.07	2.98	2.92	2.79	2.76	2.69	2.63	2.59
	.9995	4.10	3.80	3.65	3.48	3.32	3.22	3.15	3.00	2.97	2.89	2.82	2.78
40	.025	.387	.437	.466	.498	.533	.556	.573	.610	.620	.641	.662	.674
	.95	1.92	1.84	1.79	1.74	1.69	1.66	1.64	1.59	1.58	1.55	1.53	1.51
	.975	2.18	2.07	2.01	1.94	1.88	1.83	1.80	1.74	1.72	1.69	1.66	1.64
	.99	2.52	2.37	2.29	2.20	2.11	2.06	2.02	1.94	1.92	1.87	1.83	1.80
	.999	3.40	3.15	3.01	2.87	2.73	2.64	2.57	2.44	2.41	2.34	2.28	2.23
	.9995	3.68	3.39	3.24	3.08	2.92	2.82	2.74	2.60	2.57	2.49	2.41	2.37
60	.025	.396	.450	.481	.515	.555	.581	.600	.641	.654	.680	.704	.720
	.95	1.84	1.75	1.70	1.65	1.59	1.56	1.53	1.48	1.47	1.44	1.41	1.39
	.975	2.06	1.94	1.88	1.82	1.74	1.70	1.67	1.60	1.58	1.54	1.51	1.48
	.99	2.35	2.20	2.12	2.03	1.94	1.88	1.84	1.75	1.73	1.68	1.63	1.60
	.999	3.08	2.83	2.69	2.56	2.41	2.31	2.25	2.11	2.09	2.01	1.93	1.89
	.9995	3.30	3.02	2.87	2.71	2.55	2.45	2.38	2.23	2.19	2.11	2.03	1.98
120	.025	.406	.464	.498	.536	.580	.611	.633	.684	.698	.729	.762	.789
	.95	1.75	1.66	1.61	1.55	1.50	1.46	1.43	1.37	1.35	1.32	1.28	1.25
	.975	1.95	1.82	1.76	1.69	1.61	1.56	1.53	1.45	1.43	1.39	1.34	1.31
	.99	2.19	2.03	1.95	1.86	1.76	1.70	1.66	1.56	1.53	1.48	1.42	1.38
	.999	2.78	2.53	2.40	2.26	2.11	2.02	1.95	1.82	1.76	1.70	1.62	1.54
	.9995	2.96	2.67	2.53	2.38	2.21	2.11	2.01	1.88	1.84	1.75	1.67	1.60
∞	.025	.418	.480	.517	.560	.611	.645	.675	.741	.763	.813	.878	1.00
	.95	1.67	1.57	1.52	1.46	1.39	1.35	1.32	1.24	1.22	1.17	1.11	1.00
	.975	1.83	1.71	1.64	1.57	1.48	1.43	1.39	1.30	1.27	1.21	1.13	1.00
	.99	2.04	1.88	1.79	1.70	1.59	1.52	1.47	1.36	1.32	1.25	1.15	1.00
	.999	2.51	2.27	2.13	1.99	1.84	1.73	1.66	1.49	1.45	1.34	1.21	1.00
	.9995	2.65	2.37	2.22	2.07	1.91	1.79	1.71	1.53	1.48	1.36	1.22	1.00

$\ast \lambda$ = area under curve from zero to $F[\lambda; \nu_1, \nu_2]$. To obtain values of $F(0.05; \nu_1, \nu_2)$ and $F(0.01; \nu_1, \nu_2)$ one uses $F(\lambda; \nu_1, \nu_2) = 1/F(1 - \lambda; \nu_2, \nu_1)$.

Notation: $593^3 = 593 \times 10^3$, $.0^211 = 0.11 \times 10^{-2}$.

*From *Introduction to Statistical Analysis*, [1984], W. J. Dixon and F. J. Massey, McGraw-Hill Book Company. This material is reproduced with permission.

Table B.5   Values of $z = \frac{1}{2} \log_e[(1 + r)/(1 - r)]$*

r	0.00	0.01	0.02	0.03	0.04	0.05	0.06	0.07	0.08	0.09
.0	0.000	0.010	0.020	0.030	0.040	0.050	0.060	0.070	0.080	0.090
.1	0.100	0.110	0.121	0.131	0.141	0.151	0.161	0.172	0.182	0.192
.2	0.203	0.213	0.224	0.234	0.245	0.255	0.266	0.277	0.288	0.299
.3	0.310	0.321	0.332	0.343	0.354	0.365	0.377	0.388	0.400	0.412
.4	0.424	0.436	0.448	0.460	0.472	0.485	0.497	0.510	0.523	0.536
.5	0.549	0.563	0.576	0.590	0.604	0.618	0.633	0.648	0.662	0.678
.6	0.693	0.709	0.725	0.741	0.758	0.775	0.793	0.811	0.829	0.848
.7	0.867	0.887	0.908	0.929	0.950	0.973	0.996	1.020	1.045	1.071
.8	1.099	1.127	1.157	1.188	1.221	1.256	1.293	1.333	1.376	1.422

r	0.000	0.001	0.002	0.003	0.004	0.005	0.006	0.007	0.008	0.009
.90	1.472	1.478	1.483	1.488	1.494	1.499	1.505	1.510	1.516	1.522
.91	1.528	1.533	1.539	1.545	1.551	1.557	1.564	1.570	1.576	1.583
.92	1.589	1.596	1.602	1.609	1.616	1.623	1.630	1.637	1.644	1.651
.93	1.658	1.666	1.673	1.681	1.689	1.697	1.705	1.713	1.721	1.730
.94	1.738	1.747	1.756	1.764	1.774	1.783	1.792	1.802	1.812	1.822
.95	1.832	1.842	1.853	1.863	1.874	1.886	1.897	1.909	1.921	1.933
.96	1.946	1.959	1.972	1.986	2.000	2.014	2.029	2.044	2.060	2.076
.97	2.092	2.109	2.127	2.146	2.165	2.185	2.205	2.227	2.249	2.273
.98	2.298	2.323	2.351	2.380	2.410	2.443	2.477	2.515	2.555	2.599
.99	2.646	2.700	2.759	2.826	2.903	2.994	3.106	3.250	3.453	3.800

* Reprinted by permission from the Iowa State University Press, Ames, from *Statistical Methods*, 7th ed. [1980]: G. Snedecor and W. G. Cochran.

Table B.6 Percentiles of the Studentized Range*

ν	Cum. Prop.	k = 2	3	4	5	6	7	8	9	10	11	12	13	14	15	16	17	18	19	20
1	.95	18.0	27.0	32.8	37.1	40.4	43.1	45.4	47.4	49.1	50.6	52.0	53.2	54.3	55.4	56.3	57.2	58.0	58.8	59.6
	.99	90.0	135	164	186	202	216	227	237	246	253	260	266	272	277	282	286	290	294	298
2	.95	6.09	8.3	9.8	10.9	11.7	12.4	13.0	13.5	14.0	14.4	14.7	15.1	15.4	15.7	15.9	16.1	16.4	16.6	16.8
	.99	14.0	19.0	22.3	24.7	26.6	28.2	29.5	30.7	31.7	32.6	33.4	34.1	34.8	35.4	36.0	36.5	37.0	37.5	37.9
3	.95	4.50	5.91	6.82	7.50	8.04	8.48	8.85	9.18	9.46	9.72	9.95	10.2	10.4	10.5	10.7	10.8	11.0	11.1	11.2
	.99	8.26	10.6	12.2	13.3	14.2	15.0	15.6	16.2	16.7	17.1	17.5	17.9	18.2	18.5	18.8	19.1	19.3	19.5	19.8
4	.95	3.93	5.04	5.76	6.29	6.71	7.05	7.35	7.60	7.83	8.03	8.21	8.37	8.52	8.66	8.79	8.91	9.03	9.13	9.23
	.99	6.51	8.12	9.17	9.96	10.6	11.1	11.5	11.9	12.3	12.6	12.8	13.1	13.3	13.5	13.7	13.9	14.1	14.2	14.4
5	.95	3.64	4.60	5.22	5.67	6.03	6.33	6.58	6.80	6.99	7.17	7.32	7.47	7.60	7.72	7.83	7.93	8.03	8.12	8.21
	.99	5.70	6.97	7.80	8.42	8.91	9.32	9.67	9.97	10.2	10.5	10.7	10.9	11.1	11.2	11.4	11.6	11.7	11.8	11.9
6	.95	3.46	4.34	4.90	5.31	5.63	5.89	6.12	6.32	6.49	6.65	6.79	6.92	7.03	7.14	7.24	7.34	7.43	7.51	7.59
	.99	5.24	6.33	7.03	7.56	7.97	8.32	8.61	8.87	9.10	9.30	9.49	9.65	9.81	9.95	10.1	10.2	10.3	10.4	10.5
7	.95	3.34	4.16	4.68	5.06	5.36	5.61	5.82	6.00	6.16	6.30	6.43	6.55	6.66	6.76	6.85	6.94	7.02	7.09	7.17
	.99	4.95	5.92	6.54	7.01	7.37	7.68	7.94	8.17	8.37	8.55	8.71	8.86	9.00	9.12	9.24	9.35	9.46	9.55	9.65
8	.95	3.26	4.04	4.53	4.89	5.17	5.40	5.60	5.77	5.92	6.05	6.18	6.29	6.39	6.48	6.57	6.65	6.73	6.80	6.87
	.99	4.74	5.63	6.20	6.63	6.96	7.24	7.47	7.68	7.87	8.03	8.18	8.31	8.44	8.55	8.66	8.76	8.85	8.94	9.03
9	.95	3.20	3.95	4.42	4.76	5.02	5.24	5.43	5.60	5.74	5.87	5.98	6.09	6.19	6.28	6.36	6.44	6.51	6.58	6.64
	.99	4.60	5.43	5.96	6.35	6.66	6.91	7.13	7.32	7.49	7.65	7.78	7.91	8.03	8.13	8.23	8.32	8.41	8.49	8.57
10	.95	3.15	3.88	4.33	4.65	4.91	5.12	5.30	5.46	5.60	5.72	5.83	5.93	6.03	6.11	6.20	6.27	6.34	6.40	6.47
	.99	4.48	5.27	5.77	6.14	6.43	6.67	6.87	7.05	7.21	7.36	7.48	7.60	7.71	7.81	7.91	7.99	8.07	8.15	8.22
11	.95	3.11	3.82	4.26	4.57	4.82	5.03	5.20	5.35	5.49	5.61	5.71	5.81	5.90	5.99	6.06	6.14	6.20	6.26	6.33
	.99	4.39	5.14	5.62	5.97	6.25	6.48	6.67	6.84	6.99	7.13	7.25	7.36	7.46	7.56	7.65	7.73	7.81	7.88	7.95
12	.95	3.08	3.77	4.20	4.51	4.75	4.95	5.12	5.27	5.40	5.51	5.62	5.71	5.80	5.88	5.95	6.03	6.09	6.15	6.21
	.99	4.32	5.04	5.50	5.84	6.10	6.32	6.51	6.67	6.81	6.94	7.06	7.17	7.26	7.36	7.44	7.52	7.59	7.66	7.73
13	.95	3.06	3.73	4.15	4.45	4.69	4.88	5.05	5.19	5.32	5.43	5.53	5.63	5.71	5.79	5.86	5.93	6.00	6.05	6.11
	.99	4.25	4.96	5.40	5.73	5.98	6.19	6.37	6.53	6.67	6.79	6.90	7.01	7.10	7.19	7.27	7.34	7.42	7.48	7.55
14	.95	3.03	3.70	4.11	4.41	4.64	4.83	4.99	5.13	5.25	5.36	5.46	5.55	5.64	5.72	5.79	5.85	5.92	5.97	6.03
	.99	4.21	4.89	5.32	5.63	5.88	6.08	6.26	6.41	6.54	6.66	6.77	6.87	6.96	7.05	7.12	7.20	7.27	7.33	7.39

*Data extracted from Table 18 of W. J. Dixon and F. J. Massey, *Introduction to Statistical Analysis*, 2nd Ed., McGraw-Hill, 1957. Used with permission of McGraw-Hill Book Company.

Index

WILEY SERIES IN PROBABILITY AND STATISTICS

The *Wiley Series in Probability and Statistics* is well established and authoritative. It covers many topics of current research interest in both pure and applied statistics and probability theory. Written by leading statisticians and institutions, the titles span both state-of-the-art developments in the field and classical methods.

Reflecting the wide range of current research in statistics, the series encompasses applied, methodological and theoretical statistics, ranging from applications and new techniques made possible by advances in computerized practice to rigorous treatment of theoretical approaches.

This series provides essential and invaluable reading for all statisticians, whether in academia, industry, government, or research.

ABRAHAM and LEDOLTER · Statistical Methods for Forecasting
AGRESTI · Analysis of Ordinal Categorical Data
AGRESTI · An Introduction to Categorical Data Analysis
AGRESTI · Categorical Data Analysis, *Second Edition*
ALTMAN, GILL, and McDONALD · Numerical Issues in Statistical Computing for the
    Social Scientist
AMARATUNGA and CABRERA · Exploration and Analysis of DNA Microarray and
    Protein Array Data
ANDĚL · Mathematics of Chance
ANDERSON · An Introduction to Multivariate Statistical Analysis, *Third Edition*
*ANDERSON · The Statistical Analysis of Time Series
ANDERSON, AUQUIER, HAUCK, OAKES, VANDAELE, and WEISBERG ·
    Statistical Methods for Comparative Studies
ANDERSON and LOYNES · The Teaching of Practical Statistics
ARMITAGE and DAVID (editors) · Advances in Biometry
ARNOLD, BALAKRISHNAN, and NAGARAJA · Records
*ARTHANARI and DODGE · Mathematical Programming in Statistics
*BAILEY · The Elements of Stochastic Processes with Applications to the Natural
    Sciences
BALAKRISHNAN and KOUTRAS · Runs and Scans with Applications
BARNETT · Comparative Statistical Inference, *Third Edition*
BARNETT and LEWIS · Outliers in Statistical Data, *Third Edition*
BARTOSZYNSKI and NIEWIADOMSKA-BUGAJ · Probability and Statistical Inference
BASILEVSKY · Statistical Factor Analysis and Related Methods: Theory and
    Applications
BASU and RIGDON · Statistical Methods for the Reliability of Repairable Systems
BATES and WATTS · Nonlinear Regression Analysis and Its Applications
BECHHOFER, SANTNER, and GOLDSMAN · Design and Analysis of Experiments for
    Statistical Selection, Screening, and Multiple Comparisons
BELSLEY · Conditioning Diagnostics: Collinearity and Weak Data in Regression

*Now available in a lower priced paperback edition in the Wiley Classics Library.

BELSLEY, KUH, and WELSCH · Regression Diagnostics: Identifying Influential Data and Sources of Collinearity

BENDAT and PIERSOL · Random Data: Analysis and Measurement Procedures, *Third Edition*

BERRY, CHALONER, and GEWEKE · Bayesian Analysis in Statistics and Econometrics: Essays in Honor of Arnold Zellner

BERNARDO and SMITH · Bayesian Theory

BHAT and MILLER · Elements of Applied Stochastic Processes, *Third Edition*

BHATTACHARYA and JOHNSON · Statistical Concepts and Methods

BHATTACHARYA and WAYMIRE · Stochastic Processes with Applications

BILLINGSLEY · Convergence of Probability Measures, *Second Edition*

BILLINGSLEY · Probability and Measure, *Third Edition*

BIRKES and DODGE · Alternative Methods of Regression

BLISCHKE AND MURTHY (editors) · Case Studies in Reliability and Maintenance

BLISCHKE AND MURTHY · Reliability: Modeling, Prediction, and Optimization

BLOOMFIELD · Fourier Analysis of Time Series: An Introduction, *Second Edition*

BOLLEN · Structural Equations with Latent Variables

BOROVKOV · Ergodicity and Stability of Stochastic Processes

BOULEAU · Numerical Methods for Stochastic Processes

BOX · Bayesian Inference in Statistical Analysis

BOX · R. A. Fisher, the Life of a Scientist

BOX and DRAPER · Empirical Model-Building and Response Surfaces

*BOX and DRAPER · Evolutionary Operation: A Statistical Method for Process Improvement

BOX, HUNTER, and HUNTER · Statistics for Experimenters: An Introduction to Design, Data Analysis, and Model Building

BOX and LUCEÑO · Statistical Control by Monitoring and Feedback Adjustment

BRANDIMARTE · Numerical Methods in Finance: A MATLAB-Based Introduction

BROWN and HOLLANDER · Statistics: A Biomedical Introduction

BRUNNER, DOMHOF, and LANGER · Nonparametric Analysis of Longitudinal Data in Factorial Experiments

BUCKLEW · Large Deviation Techniques in Decision, Simulation, and Estimation

CAIROLI and DALANG · Sequential Stochastic Optimization

CHAN · Time Series: Applications to Finance

CHATTERJEE and HADI · Sensitivity Analysis in Linear Regression

CHATTERJEE and PRICE · Regression Analysis by Example, *Third Edition*

CHERNICK · Bootstrap Methods: A Practitioner's Guide

CHERNICK and FRIIS · Introductory Biostatistics for the Health Sciences

CHILÈS and DELFINER · Geostatistics: Modeling Spatial Uncertainty

CHOW and LIU · Design and Analysis of Clinical Trials: Concepts and Methodologies, *Second Edition*

CLARKE and DISNEY · Probability and Random Processes: A First Course with Applications, *Second Edition*

*COCHRAN and COX · Experimental Designs, *Second Edition*

CONGDON · Applied Bayesian Modelling

CONGDON · Bayesian Statistical Modelling

CONOVER · Practical Nonparametric Statistics, *Second Edition*

COOK · Regression Graphics

COOK and WEISBERG · Applied Regression Including Computing and Graphics

COOK and WEISBERG · An Introduction to Regression Graphics

CORNELL · Experiments with Mixtures, Designs, Models, and the Analysis of Mixture Data, *Third Edition*

COVER and THOMAS · Elements of Information Theory

*Now available in a lower priced paperback edition in the Wiley Classics Library.

COX · A Handbook of Introductory Statistical Methods
*COX · Planning of Experiments
CRESSIE · Statistics for Spatial Data, *Revised Edition*
CSÖRGŐ and HORVÁTH · Limit Theorems in Change Point Analysis
DANIEL · Applications of Statistics to Industrial Experimentation
DANIEL · Biostatistics: A Foundation for Analysis in the Health Sciences, *Sixth Edition*
*DANIEL · Fitting Equations to Data: Computer Analysis of Multifactor Data,
    Second Edition
DASU and JOHNSON · Exploratory Data Mining and Data Cleaning
DAVID and NAGARAJA · Order Statistics, *Third Edition*
*DEGROOT, FIENBERG, and KADANE · Statistics and the Law
DEL CASTILLO · Statistical Process Adjustment for Quality Control
DENISON, HOLMES, MALLICK and SMITH · Bayesian Methods for Nonlinear
    Classification and Regression
DETTE and STUDDEN · The Theory of Canonical Moments with Applications in
    Statistics, Probability, and Analysis
DEY and MUKERJEE · Fractional Factorial Plans
DILLON and GOLDSTEIN · Multivariate Analysis: Methods and Applications
DODGE · Alternative Methods of Regression
*DODGE and ROMIG · Sampling Inspection Tables, *Second Edition*
*DOOB · Stochastic Processes
DOWDY, WEARDEN, and CHILKO · Statistics for Research, *Third Edition*
DRAPER and SMITH · Applied Regression Analysis, *Third Edition*
DRYDEN and MARDIA · Statistical Shape Analysis
DUDEWICZ and MISHRA · Modern Mathematical Statistics
DUNN and CLARK · Basic Statistics: A Primer for the Biomedical Sciences,
    Third Edition
DUPUIS and ELLIS · A Weak Convergence Approach to the Theory of Large Deviations
*ELANDT-JOHNSON and JOHNSON · Survival Models and Data Analysis
ENDERS · Applied Econometric Time Series
ETHIER and KURTZ · Markov Processes: Characterization and Convergence
EVANS, HASTINGS, and PEACOCK · Statistical Distributions, *Third Edition*
FELLER · An Introduction to Probability Theory and Its Applications, Volume I,
    Third Edition, Revised; Volume II, *Second Edition*
FISHER and VAN BELLE · Biostatistics: A Methodology for the Health Sciences
*FLEISS · The Design and Analysis of Clinical Experiments
FLEISS · Statistical Methods for Rates and Proportions, *Third Edition*
FLEMING and HARRINGTON · Counting Processes and Survival Analysis
FULLER · Introduction to Statistical Time Series, *Second Edition*
FULLER · Measurement Error Models
GALLANT · Nonlinear Statistical Models
GIESBRECHT and GUMPERTZ · Planning, Construction, and Statistical Analysis of
    Comparative Experiments
GIFI · Nonlinear Multivariate Analysis
GHOSH, MUKHOPADHYAY, and SEN · Sequential Estimation
GIFI · Nonlinear Multivariate Analysis
GLASSERMAN and YAO · Monotone Structure in Discrete-Event Systems
GNANADESIKAN · Methods for Statistical Data Analysis of Multivariate Observations,
    Second Edition
GOLDSTEIN and LEWIS · Assessment: Problems, Development, and Statistical Issues
GREENWOOD and NIKULIN · A Guide to Chi-Squared Testing
GROSS and HARRIS · Fundamentals of Queueing Theory, *Third Edition*
*HAHN and SHAPIRO · Statistical Models in Engineering

*Now available in a lower priced paperback edition in the Wiley Classics Library.

*Now available in a lower priced paperback edition in the Wiley Classics Library.

KAUFMAN and ROUSSEEUW · Finding Groups in Data: An Introduction to Cluster Analysis

KEDEM and FOKIANOS · Regression Models for Time Series Analysis

KENDALL, BARDEN, CARNE, and LE · Shape and Shape Theory

KHURI · Advanced Calculus with Applications in Statistics, *Second Edition*

KHURI, MATHEW, and SINHA · Statistical Tests for Mixed Linear Models

KLEIBER and KOTZ · Statistical Size Distributions in Economics and Actuarial Sciences

KLUGMAN, PANJER, and WILLMOT · Loss Models: From Data to Decisions

KLUGMAN, PANJER, and WILLMOT · Solutions Manual to Accompany Loss Models: From Data to Decisions

KOTZ, BALAKRISHNAN, and JOHNSON · Continuous Multivariate Distributions, Volume 1, *Second Edition*

KOTZ and JOHNSON (editors) · Encyclopedia of Statistical Sciences: Volumes 1 to 9 with Index

KOTZ and JOHNSON (editors) · Encyclopedia of Statistical Sciences: Supplement Volume

KOTZ, READ, and BANKS (editors) · Encyclopedia of Statistical Sciences: Update Volume 1

KOTZ, READ, and BANKS (editors) · Encyclopedia of Statistical Sciences: Update Volume 2

KOVALENKO, KUZNETZOV, and PEGG · Mathematical Theory of Reliability of Time-Dependent Systems with Practical Applications

LACHIN · Biostatistical Methods: The Assessment of Relative Risks

LAD · Operational Subjective Statistical Methods: A Mathematical, Philosophical, and Historical Introduction

LAMPERTI · Probability: A Survey of the Mathematical Theory, *Second Edition*

LANGE, RYAN, BILLARD, BRILLINGER, CONQUEST, and GREENHOUSE · Case Studies in Biometry

LARSON · Introduction to Probability Theory and Statistical Inference, *Third Edition*

LAWLESS · Statistical Models and Methods for Lifetime Data, *Second Edition*

LAWSON · Statistical Methods in Spatial Epidemiology

LE · Applied Categorical Data Analysis

LE · Applied Survival Analysis

LEE and WANG · Statistical Methods for Survival Data Analysis, *Third Edition*

LePAGE and BILLARD · Exploring the Limits of Bootstrap

LEYLAND and GOLDSTEIN (editors) · Multilevel Modelling of Health Statistics

LIAO · Statistical Group Comparison

LINDVALL · Lectures on the Coupling Method

LINHART and ZUCCHINI · Model Selection

LITTLE and RUBIN · Statistical Analysis with Missing Data, *Second Edition*

LLOYD · The Statistical Analysis of Categorical Data

MAGNUS and NEUDECKER · Matrix Differential Calculus with Applications in Statistics and Econometrics, *Revised Edition*

MALLER and ZHOU · Survival Analysis with Long Term Survivors

MALLOWS · Design, Data, and Analysis by Some Friends of Cuthbert Daniel

MANN, SCHAFER, and SINGPURWALLA · Methods for Statistical Analysis of Reliability and Life Data

MANTON, WOODBURY, and TOLLEY · Statistical Applications Using Fuzzy Sets

MARCHETTE · Random Graphs for Statistical Pattern Recognition

MARDIA and JUPP · Directional Statistics

MASON, GUNST, and HESS · Statistical Design and Analysis of Experiments with Applications to Engineering and Science, *Second Edition*

McCULLOCH and SEARLE · Generalized, Linear, and Mixed Models

McFADDEN · Management of Data in Clinical Trials

*Now available in a lower priced paperback edition in the Wiley Classics Library.

McLACHLAN · Discriminant Analysis and Statistical Pattern Recognition
McLACHLAN and KRISHNAN · The EM Algorithm and Extensions
McLACHLAN and PEEL · Finite Mixture Models
McNEIL · Epidemiological Research Methods
MEEKER and ESCOBAR · Statistical Methods for Reliability Data
MEERSCHAERT and SCHEFFLER · Limit Distributions for Sums of Independent Random Vectors: Heavy Tails in Theory and Practice
MICKEY, DUNN, and CLARK · Applied Statistics: Analysis of Variance and Regression, *Third Edition*
*MILLER · Survival Analysis, *Second Edition*
MONTGOMERY, PECK, and VINING · Introduction to Linear Regression Analysis, *Third Edition*
MORGENTHALER and TUKEY · Configural Polysampling: A Route to Practical Robustness
MUIRHEAD · Aspects of Multivariate Statistical Theory
MULLER and STOYAN · Comparison Methods for Stochastic Models and Risks
MURRAY · X-STAT 2.0 Statistical Experimentation, Design Data Analysis, and Nonlinear Optimization
MURTHY, XIE, and JIANG · Weibull Models
MYERS and MONTGOMERY · Response Surface Methodology: Process and Product Optimization Using Designed Experiments, *Second Edition*
MYERS, MONTGOMERY, and VINING · Generalized Linear Models. With Applications in Engineering and the Sciences
NELSON · Accelerated Testing, Statistical Models, Test Plans, and Data Analyses
NELSON · Applied Life Data Analysis
NEWMAN · Biostatistical Methods in Epidemiology
OCHI · Applied Probability and Stochastic Processes in Engineering and Physical Sciences
OKABE, BOOTS, SUGIHARA, and CHIU · Spatial Tesselations: Concepts and Applications of Voronoi Diagrams, *Second Edition*
OLIVER and SMITH · Influence Diagrams, Belief Nets and Decision Analysis
PALTA · Quantitative Methods in Population Health: Extensions of Ordinary Regressions
PANKRATZ · Forecasting with Dynamic Regression Models
PANKRATZ · Forecasting with Univariate Box-Jenkins Models: Concepts and Cases
*PARZEN · Modern Probability Theory and Its Applications
PEÑA, TIAO, and TSAY · A Course in Time Series Analysis
PIANTADOSI · Clinical Trials: A Methodologic Perspective
PORT · Theoretical Probability for Applications
POURAHMADI · Foundations of Time Series Analysis and Prediction Theory
PRESS · Bayesian Statistics: Principles, Models, and Applications
PRESS · Subjective and Objective Bayesian Statistics, *Second Edition*
PRESS and TANUR · The Subjectivity of Scientists and the Bayesian Approach
PUKELSHEIM · Optimal Experimental Design
PURI, VILAPLANA, and WERTZ · New Perspectives in Theoretical and Applied Statistics
PUTERMAN · Markov Decision Processes: Discrete Stochastic Dynamic Programming
*RAO · Linear Statistical Inference and Its Applications, *Second Edition*
RAUSAND and HØYLAND · System Reliability Theory: Models, Statistical Methods, and Applications, *Second Edition*
RENCHER · Linear Models in Statistics
RENCHER · Methods of Multivariate Analysis, *Second Edition*
RENCHER · Multivariate Statistical Inference with Applications
RIPLEY · Spatial Statistics
RIPLEY · Stochastic Simulation

*Now available in a lower priced paperback edition in the Wiley Classics Library.

ROBINSON · Practical Strategies for Experimenting

ROHATGI and SALEH · An Introduction to Probability and Statistics, *Second Edition*

ROLSKI, SCHMIDLI, SCHMIDT, and TEUGELS · Stochastic Processes for Insurance and Finance

ROSENBERGER and LACHIN · Randomization in Clinical Trials: Theory and Practice

ROSS · Introduction to Probability and Statistics for Engineers and Scientists

ROUSSEEUW and LEROY · Robust Regression and Outlier Detection

RUBIN · Multiple Imputation for Nonresponse in Surveys

RUBINSTEIN · Simulation and the Monte Carlo Method

RUBINSTEIN and MELAMED · Modern Simulation and Modeling

RYAN · Modern Regression Methods

RYAN · Statistical Methods for Quality Improvement, *Second Edition*

SALTELLI, CHAN, and SCOTT (editors) · Sensitivity Analysis

*SCHEFFE · The Analysis of Variance

SCHIMEK · Smoothing and Regression: Approaches, Computation, and Application

SCHOTT · Matrix Analysis for Statistics

SCHOUTENS · Levy Processes in Finance: Pricing Financial Derivatives

SCHUSS · Theory and Applications of Stochastic Differential Equations

SCOTT · Multivariate Density Estimation: Theory, Practice, and Visualization

*SEARLE · Linear Models

SEARLE · Linear Models for Unbalanced Data

SEARLE · Matrix Algebra Useful for Statistics

SEARLE, CASELLA, and McCULLOCH · Variance Components

SEARLE and WILLETT · Matrix Algebra for Applied Economics

SEBER and LEE · Linear Regression Analysis, *Second Edition*

SEBER · Multivariate Observations

SEBER and WILD · Nonlinear Regression

SENNOTT · Stochastic Dynamic Programming and the Control of Queueing Systems

*SERFLING · Approximation Theorems of Mathematical Statistics

SHAFER and VOVK · Probability and Finance: It's Only a Game!

SMALL and McLEISH · Hilbert Space Methods in Probability and Statistical Inference

SRIVASTAVA · Methods of Multivariate Statistics

STAPLETON · Linear Statistical Models

STAUDTE and SHEATHER · Robust Estimation and Testing

STOYAN, KENDALL, and MECKE · Stochastic Geometry and Its Applications, *Second Edition*

STOYAN and STOYAN · Fractals, Random Shapes and Point Fields: Methods of Geometrical Statistics

STYAN · The Collected Papers of T. W. Anderson: 1943–1985

SUTTON, ABRAMS, JONES, SHELDON, and SONG · Methods for Meta-Analysis in Medical Research

TANAKA · Time Series Analysis: Nonstationary and Noninvertible Distribution Theory

THOMPSON · Empirical Model Building

THOMPSON · Sampling, *Second Edition*

THOMPSON · Simulation: A Modeler's Approach

THOMPSON and SEBER · Adaptive Sampling

THOMPSON, WILLIAMS, and FINDLAY · Models for Investors in Real World Markets

TIAO, BISGAARD, HILL, PEÑA, and STIGLER (editors) · Box on Quality and Discovery: with Design, Control, and Robustness

TIERNEY · LISP-STAT: An Object-Oriented Environment for Statistical Computing and Dynamic Graphics

TSAY · Analysis of Financial Time Series

UPTON and FINGLETON · Spatial Data Analysis by Example, Volume II: Categorical and Directional Data

VAN BELLE · Statistical Rules of Thumb

*Now available in a lower priced paperback edition in the Wiley Classics Library.

VESTRUP · The Theory of Measures and Integration

VIDAKOVIC · Statistical Modeling by Wavelets

WEISBERG · Applied Linear Regression, *Second Edition*

WELSH · Aspects of Statistical Inference

WESTFALL and YOUNG · Resampling-Based Multiple Testing: Examples and Methods for *p*-Value Adjustment

WHITTAKER · Graphical Models in Applied Multivariate Statistics

WINKER · Optimization Heuristics in Economics: Applications of Threshold Accepting

WONNACOTT and WONNACOTT · Econometrics, *Second Edition*

WOODING · Planning Pharmaceutical Clinical Trials: Basic Statistical Principles

WOOLSON and CLARKE · Statistical Methods for the Analysis of Biomedical Data, *Second Edition*

WU and HAMADA · Experiments: Planning, Analysis, and Parameter Design Optimization

YANG · The Construction Theory of Denumerable Markov Processes

*ZELLNER · An Introduction to Bayesian Inference in Econometrics

ZHOU, OBUCHOWSKI, and McCLISH · Statistical Methods in Diagnostic Medicine

*Now available in a lower priced paperback edition in the Wiley Classics Library.

CPSIA information can be obtained at www.ICGtesting.com
Printed in the USA
BVOW031428011212

306984BV00002B/19/P

9 780470 571255